OBESITY AND DL ~~~~~~IUN
IN THE ENLIGHTENMENT

Oklahoma Project for Discourse and Theory
Series for Science and Culture

OBESITY AND DEPRESSION
IN THE ENLIGHTENMENT

Anita Guerrini

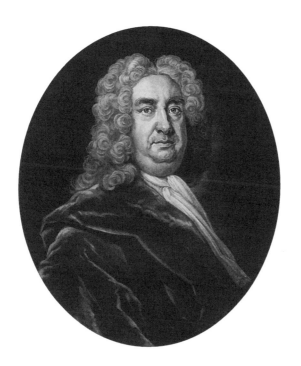

THE LIFE AND TIMES
OF GEORGE CHEYNE

University of Oklahoma Press : Norman

Also by Anita Guerrini
Natural History and the New World, 1524–1770 (Philadelphia, 1986)

Published with the assistance of the National Endowment for the Humanities, a federal agency which supports the study of such fields as history,
philosophy, literature, and language.

Library of Congress Cataloging-in-Publication Data

Guerrini, Anita, 1953–
     Obesity and depression in the enlightenment : the life and times
of George Cheyne / Anita Guerrini.
          p.   cm. — (Oklahoma project for discourse and theory. Series
for science and culture ; v. 3)
     Includes bibliographical references and index.
     ISBN 0-8061-3159-4 (cloth - alk. paper)
     ISBN 0-8061-3201-9 (pbk - alk. paper)
     1. Cheyne, George, 1673–1743.   2. Physicians—Great Britain
Biography.   3. Medicine—Great Britain—History—18th century.
I. Title.   II. Series.
R489.C45G84   2000
610'.92—dc21
     [B]   99-35909
                                                                          CIP

On the Title Page: George Cheyne. Mezzotint by J. Farber, Jr., 1732, after J. van Diest.
Courtesy Wellcome Institute Library, London.

Text design by Gail Carter.

Obesity and Depression in the Enlightenment: The Life and Times of George Cheyne is Volume 3 of the
Oklahoma Project for Discourse and Theory, Series for Science and Culture.

1   2   3   4   5   6   7   8   9   10

To
Michael, Paul, and Henry
with love

CONTENTS

EDITORS' FOREWORD

Since its inception in 1987, the Oklahoma Project for Discourse and Theory has challenged and helped to redefine the boundaries of traditional disciplinary structures of knowledge. Employing various approaches, ranging from feminism and deconstruction to sociology and nuclear studies, books in this series have offered their readers opportunities to explore our postmodern condition. In the Series on Science and Culture, the Oklahoma Project extends its inquiries into the postdisciplinary areas of the complex relations among the humanities, social sciences, and sciences. The term *postdisciplinary* is meant to suggest that we have entered an era of rapid sociocultural and technological change in which "common sense" divisions between, say, physics and literature no longer seem as sensible as they once did. The values and assumptions, methods and technologies, that we had been taught were "natural" and "universal" are being challenged, reworked, and demystified to demonstrate the ways in which they are culturally constructed. All coherence may not be gone, but what counts as coherence is being redefined in provocative ways.

In recent years, the study of science, both within and outside of the academy, has undergone a sea change. Traditional approaches to the history and philosophy of science treated science as an insular set of procedures concerned to reveal fundamental truths or laws of the physical universe. In contrast, the postdisciplinary study of science emphasizes its cultural embeddedness, the ways in which particular laboratories, experiments, instruments, scientists, and procedures are historically and socially situated. Science is no longer a closed system that generates carefully plotted paths proceeding asymptotically toward the truth, but an open system that is everywhere penetrated by contingent and even competing accounts of what constitutes our world. These include—but are by no means limited to—the discourses of race, gender, social class, politics, theology, anthropology, sociology, and literature. In the phrase of the Nobel laureate Ilya Prigogine, we have moved from a science of being to a science of becoming. This becoming is the ongoing concern of the volumes in the Series on Science and Culture. Their purpose is to open up possibilities for further inquiries rather than to close off debate.

The members of the editorial board of the series reflect our commitment to reconceiving the structures of knowledge. All are prominent in their fields, although in every case what their "field" is has been redefined, in large measure by their own work. The departmental or program affiliations of these distinguished scholars—Sander Gilman, Donna Haraway, N. Katherine Hayles, Bruno Latour, Richard Lewontin, Michael Morrison, Mark Poster, G. S. Rousseau, and Donald Worster—seem to tell us less about what they do than where, institutionally, they have been. Taken together as a set of strategies for rethinking the relationships between science and culture, their work exemplifies the kind of careful, self-critical scrutiny within fields such as medicine, biology, anthropology, history, physics, and literary criticism that leads us to a recognition of the limits of what and how we have been taught to think. The postdisciplinary aspects of our board members' work stem from their professional expertise within their home disciplines and their willingness to expand their studies to other, seemingly alien fields. In differing ways, their work challenges the basic divisions within Western thought between metaphysics and physics, mind and body, form and matter.

Robert Markley

University of West Virginia

Robert Con Davis
Ronald Schleifer

University of Oklahoma

ACKNOWLEDGMENTS

Although writing is a solitary enterprise, writing history is certainly a collective one. I could not have written this book without the assistance of many people: friends, colleagues, librarians, archivists, and the unsung employees of granting agencies. I would not be a historian at all if not for the inspiration of my teachers, especially David Bennett, Helen Mulvey, Jenifer Hart, and the late Richard S. Westfall. I began this project with the assistance of a grant from the National Science Foundation (SES-87-04646), and along the way received assistance in the form of a Fletcher Jones Fellowship at the Huntington Library and a Bernadotte Schmitt grant from the American Historical Association.

I am grateful to the staffs of many libraries and archives in the United States and Great Britain. At the University of California, Santa Barbara, I especially thank the staff of Interlibrary Loans. I also used the University Research Library and the Biomedical Library at the University of California, Los Angeles; the History of Medicine Division, National Library of Medicine; the Firestone Library at Princeton University; the Historical Library of the College of Physicians, Philadelphia; and the Wangensteen Library at the University of Minnesota. The Huntington Library, San Marino, California, confirmed for me its reputation as scholar's heaven. I am particularly grateful to Mary Robertson and Mary-of-the-chocolates.

In Britain, I wish especially to thank Colin McLaren of the Aberdeen University Library; Mrs. J. Currie of the Edinburgh University Library; Colin Johnston, Bath City Archivist; Clive Quinnell of the Royal National Hospital for Rheumatic Diseases, Bath; and David Brown and Tristram Clarke of the Scottish Record Office, Register House. Kathleen Cann of

Cambridge University Library and J. S. Williams, Bristol City Archivist, were also very helpful, as was the staff at the library of the Wellcome Institute for the History of Medicine. I also used the British Library, the Public Record Office (Chancery Lane), the library of the College of Surgeons, Edinburgh, the National Library of Scotland, the library of Christ Church, Oxford, and the Bodleian Library at Oxford.

I am grateful to the Huntington Library for permission to quote from the Hastings and Stowe manuscripts, and to Francis G. A. Ogilvy for permission to quote from the Ogilvy of Inverquharity papers on deposit at the Scottish Record Office.

Several people read this book in draft; I wish especially to acknowledge Roger Emerson, Francine Graves, J. Sears McGee, Roy Porter, and Jeffrey Burton Russell. Mirjam deBaar shared her research on Antoinette Bourignon with me. Thanks too to Natalie Zemon Davis, who introduced me to Mirjam. Henry Sefton and Paul Wood shared their knowledge of Aberdeen, while Robert Erickson, Linda Veronika Troost, and Frederic V. Bogel helped with literary matters. James Lattis, Jole Shackelford, and especially Peter Sobol assisted with Latin translations, though I must emphasize that they are in no way responsible for any mangled translations herein. Special thanks are owed to Jill Meekins for heroic editorial work. Marilyn Post and Linda Hulten gave me their friendship. I am especially in debt to Robert Markley, who persuaded me to send my manuscript to Oklahoma, and for his editorial skills. Kimberly Wiar at OU Press has been a model editor.

Portions of this book were delivered at various conferences; I thank in particular David Cressy for inviting me to present an early version of chapter 5 at the Huntington Library British History seminar.

I am especially grateful to my family for enduring Cheyne for so long. My husband, Michael Osborne, read every word I wrote, often several times, and invariably gave me his love and support. Our son Paul Osborne has put up with Mommy's and Daddy's books with grace, and with his new brother, Henry, reminds me that there is more to life than academe.

INTRODUCTION

I first began to examine the theme of Newtonianism, religion, and the body in my Ph.D. dissertation on Newtonian medicine. As I examined the Newtonian virtuosi in my dissertation and in subsequent articles, George Cheyne increasingly emerged as the critical figure on that topic.[1] Among the cluster of young natural philosophers jostling for position in the London of 1700, George Cheyne was not the most prepossessing. Overweight and overbearing, he seemed more fit for derision than celebrity.

Yet this 450-pound physician who advocated temperance among the neurotic upper classes in Bath is both a mirror and a window to his era. Scientist and mystic, patient and healer, libertine and scholar, Cheyne is a mirror to the obsessions and passions of his patients. His obsessions, reflected in such writings as his *Essay on Gout* (1720) and *Essay of Health and Long Life* (1724), were food and religion: recognizably modern, yet also age-old. Conspicuously missing from his work is any mention of sex, although an author more Freudian than I might be able to find it. Cheyne is a window to the age of Anne and the early Hanoverians through his own experiences with religion, politics, society, and intellectual life. The vexed relationship between science, religion, and the body, between matter, spirit, and flesh, is most fully expressed in his *English Malady* (1733).

Remarkably little has been written on so pivotal a figure in British cultural history. Today Cheyne is remembered—if he is known at all—as a physician, one of that bewigged bedside regiment so beloved by the caricaturists Hogarth and Cruickshank. A recent work referred to Cheyne "promulgating his diet at Bath, creating a fad like the Beverly Hills diet."[2]

Yet such a description makes Cheyne seem both too modern and too simple. In his life and work, Cheyne uniquely epitomizes the transition between premodern and modern culture. He crosses back and forth over the boundaries between the view of a world governed by God and one governed by the laws of Newtonian physics; between a medicine that intervened and one that merely observed; between the distant God of deism and the immanent deity of the mystics; between animistic and mechanistic views of the human body; between old and new ideas of female character and physiology.

In the first half of the eighteenth century George Cheyne was much admired. His obituary in the *Gentleman's Magazine* in 1743 described him as "that learned Physician, sound Christian, deep Scholar, and warm Friend."[3] Cheyne enjoyed wide fame as a physician. In the cutthroat atmosphere of the eighteenth-century medical marketplace, his writings on self-care and preventive medicine, particularly the immensely popular *Essay of Health and Long Life* (1724), gained him a vast audience and a medical practice that made him a wealthy man.[4]

But Cheyne's importance in his time lay equally in those other aspects of his career—Christianity, scholarship, friendship—which his obituarist linked in a characteristically premodern fashion. On none of these scores, including medicine, could Cheyne be called conventional. Self-help was not a new medical approach, but few elite physicians (of which Cheyne was one) preached it with his fervor. His Christian beliefs ranged over the course of his life from the broad and loosely defined Anglicanism of the latitudinarians to an eclectic mysticism that borrowed from medieval saints as well as contemporary philosophers, although he remained nominally attached to the Anglican confession. As the historian Jonathan Clark has recently reminded us, religion did not suddenly disappear in the eighteenth century, and the dialectic, or perhaps dialogue, between science and religion is a recurring cultural theme in that era.[5]

As a scholar, Cheyne was among the first to apply Newtonian ideas to explain human physiology in such contentious works as his *New Theory of Fevers* (1701). While he retained the hydraulic imagery of tubes and fluids in later works, he subtly modified his ideas to reflect both his own renewed interest in the spirit and Newton's alterations to his physics in

the second editions of the *Principia* (1713) and the *Opticks* (1718), which led
to an emphasis on an immaterial ether. By the time Cheyne published the
Essay on Regimen in 1740, his views had become overtly Platonic or
Neoplatonic, describing an infinite chain between matter and spirit.

Cheyne's friends ranged from the Scots mystics James and George
Garden to the bookseller and novelist Samuel Richardson, from Isaac
Newton to Robert Walpole, the prime minister. He discussed religion
with the Countess of Huntingdon, a leading Methodist, and philosophy
with the Scottish politician the Duke of Roxburghe. In an age of violent
and contentious dispute in politics, religion, and society, Cheyne was as
contentious as anyone. But he managed to retain the respect of most of
his contemporaries and the affection of many. Above all, he presented
himself to his patients, both male and female, as a sympathetic and empa-
thetic friend, and in this age of sociability he offered conversation, either
written or face to face, as the most effective therapy.

In an autobiography attached to his book on melancholy, *The English
Malady* (1733), Cheyne laid his life open to his readers and patients in
endearing (if at times excruciating) detail, revealing himself as a fellow
sufferer and sinner in his *Pilgrim's Progress* of the body. Cheyne's lifelong
battle with obesity and depression and their cure revealed his vision of
melancholy and "the spleen" as a complex amalgam of physical, mental,
and spiritual influences at a time when most believed it to be largely
physical in origin.[6]

Those who have written on Cheyne are both few and heterogeneous,
approaching his life from various disciplinary orientations. A nineteenth-
century biographer included him in a series on "Christian lives" as a particular example of piety.[7] The British *Dictionary of National Biography* emphasized his medical practice, scorning his theories, "the barren speculation
of an obsolete school of medical thought."[8] These theories were already
out of fashion when *Biographia Britannica* included Cheyne in the 1780s.[9]
More recently, the historian of science Theodore Brown has exhumed
these theories and placed them under the historical gaze in his valuable
dissertation *The Mechanical Philosophy and the "Animal Oeconomy"*.[10] In their
articles, historians of medicine including Henry Viets and Lester King
have situated Cheyne among the throng of eighteenth-century medical

men."¹¹ In his brilliant survey of eighteenth-century madness, *Mind-forg'd Manacles*, the historian of medicine Roy Porter has focused on Cheyne as psychiatrist, lighting up along the way new avenues to be explored.¹² Following the pioneering work of the Scottish religious historian G. D. Henderson in the 1930s, the literary historian G. S. Rousseau has attempted to disentangle the thread of Cheyne's religion from the thick web of his life in his 1988 article "Mysticism and Millenarianism."¹³ Another literary scholar, David Shuttleton, continued this program in his Ph.D. thesis, completed in 1992.¹⁴ Another recent dissertation and a thesis assess Cheyne's writing in the context of eighteenth-century literature.¹⁵

My goal in this book is to construct a coherent account of Cheyne's life and work. The first three chapters, which deal with Cheyne's life up to the age of thirty-four, begin with his religious crisis in 1705 and go back to his Scottish origins, the natural philosophy of his time, and his attempts to build a scientific and medical career. Chapter 4 analyzes Cheyne's major early work, the *Philosophical Principles of Natural Religion* (1705) and its heavily revised second edition, the *Philosophical Principles of Religion, Natural and Revealed* (1715), tracing the changes in Cheyne's and Newton's Newtonianism in relation to religion. Chapter 5 reconstructs his medical practice in Bath, particularly analyzing his method of practice as illustrated by the case of Catherine Walpole, daughter of Robert Walpole. A rich series of letters from Cheyne to the London physician Hans Sloane allows this case to be analyzed in detail, highlighting Cheyne's particular appeal to women patients. Chapter 6 looks at Cheyne's two most important works of popular medicine, the *Essay of Health and Long Life* (1724) and his work on madness, *The English Malady* (1733), discussing the central role of the passions in both these works. The final chapter follows Cheyne through the last decade of his life. The conclusion assesses his significance and influence.

I write narrative history, which I see as more than a mere recounting of events. Almost twenty years ago, Lawrence Stone announced "the revival of narrative" in history as a counterweight to "the analytical and structural approach." Stone's assertion of the increased importance of *mentalité* and "the narration of a very detailed story of a single incident or personality" seems prophetic.¹⁶ But he did not predict the equally important growth of

the so-called linguistic turn, with its emphasis on the text not as a representation of reality but simply as a collection of symbols whose meaning
is highly unstable.[17] The challenge of the "linguistic turn" is especially relevant to the history of science, which relies heavily on the scientific text as
a historical source. Between Stone's definition of narrative history as
merely descriptive and the minute but ultimately self-referential textual
analysis of deconstruction, I seek a middle ground that analyzes the text
or the event in itself but also places it in a broader context.[18] In this I
emulate Cheyne himself, who constantly sought a via media among the
political, intellectual, and religious extremes of his time.

The primary texts for this work are Cheyne's own writings, supplemented by his surviving correspondence, which includes about 150 letters.
I employ the tools of several disciplines in my analysis of these texts. I
subject the texts themselves to a close reading, but supplement that
reading with attention to the social, political, and intellectual contexts
found in other primary sources and interpreted over a wide range of
historiography. Such a "mixed" reading seems essential to gaining a sensitive historical understanding of a topic that crosses several disciplines.[19]

For example, I look at Cheyne's natural philosophy both in terms of
the content of his theories as well as their social construction within the
tensions of politics and patronage.[20] In discussing Cheyne's medical
practice I use anthropological concepts of illness narratives developed by
the medical anthropologist Arthur Kleinman.[21] My analysis of the interaction of Cheyne's religion and his therapeutics is informed by feminist
perspectives of mysticism and the body, particularly the medieval
historian Caroline Walker Bynum's *Holy Feast and Holy Fast*.[22] Thus this
work moves toward a cross-disciplinary history of aspects of eighteenth-
century culture that have been too long ignored.

Born near Aberdeen in about the year 1671, Cheyne grew to maturity in
Restoration Scotland. It was an era of burgeoning intellectual activity,
when many of the ideas and institutions of the Scottish enlightenment
began to take root. Yet this time was marked by deep social and political
turmoil between Presbyterians and Episcopalians, Whigs and Tories, a
turmoil exacerbated by the Glorious Revolution of 1688–89, which added

the Jacobites, the followers of the deposed King James II, to this tumult. The major influence on Cheyne's intellectual and social development was the Jacobite physician Archibald Pitcairne of Edinburgh, who is discussed in chapter 2. Pitcairne was the first, though not the last, to attempt to graft Newtonian physics onto medicine and physiology, disciplines dominated at the time by mechanistic theories derived from the French philosopher René Descartes. Pitcairne's work not only initiated a research program but also catapulted his students and followers, among them Cheyne, into Newton's orbit in London. Yet Pitcairne's deeply conservative political and social philosophy strongly colored his natural philosophy, and his "Newtonianism" differed both from that of Newton and from that of many other "Newtonians," particularly in his discussion of scientific method.

Cheyne followed a horde of Scots to London at the turn of the eighteenth century and joined the nascent Newtonian circle at the Royal Society, which elected him a fellow in 1702. Continuing his natural philosophical inquiries, he struggled to establish a medical practice amid the chaotic marketplace of London medicine. Cheyne also inherited Pitcairne's contentious nature, and he became embroiled in a number of professional disputes.

My story opens in medias res, when Cheyne began his life anew following a physical and emotional crisis in 1705–6, described in his autobiography, which led him to abandon London. He returned to his native Aberdeen, where he encountered the second major influence on his life, the Scottish theologians George and James Garden.

The Gardens, like Pitcairne, supported the deposed King James II after 1689. But unlike him, they responded to the turbulence of the 1690s by retreating to a Quaker-like religious "Quietism" that emphasized inner faith and individual piety. In this they drew inspiration from native Scottish traditions dating back to the turn of the seventeenth century as well as from medieval mystics and the more recent works of the Fleming Antoinette Bourignon (1616–80) and the Frenchwoman Jeanne Guyon (1648–1717), both notorious in their day for their unconventional lives and ideas.[21] Under their influence, Cheyne experienced a religious conversion, in the course of which he abandoned the quasi-deism of his youth for a more deeply felt mysticism. Cheyne joined a circle of mystical correspondents focused on the Gardens. Like them, he remained within the Episcopalian faith but occupied what increasingly became its outer fringes.

Having healed his soul, Cheyne then traveled to Bath both to heal his body and to build a medical practice. He married and began a family. At Bath, at the beginning of its fame as a health spa, Cheyne at last established a successful practice, dealing mainly with gout and nervous afflictions. Women especially suffered from the latter, under the general rubric of "the vapours." Cheyne's popularity as doctor stems from his combination of two modes of experience: mysticism and a mechanical concept of physiology. Cheyne based his therapeutic and theoretical stance on his personal spiritual resolution of the mind-body problem, which included healing the soul as well as the body. This idea had particular resonance with the changing concepts of femininity and the female body. The spiritual capacity of women had been the subject of much debate. Women had often been viewed as primarily matter or flesh, closer to beasts; now women were increasingly seen as the more spiritual gender. On the other hand, behaviors previously viewed as particularly feminine, including sensitivity and the expression of emotion, now became desirable aspects of male character.[24]

Cheyne became a household word in the 1720s, when he published such popular medical works as the *Essay on Gout* (1720) and the *Essay of Health and Long Life* (1724). With his intimate writing style and his urgings to self-maintenance, he appealed to the consuming classes who frequented Bath. Cheyne argued that much illness was a result of overindulgence and exhorted his patients to abstinence. His continued problems with weight and depression only made his arguments more convincing, as the result of direct experience. Certainly many found the notion of a thirty-two-stone diet doctor to be ridiculous; but Cheyne's evident sincerity and his sympathetic stance as a fellow sufferer won over many others. His popular appeal reflected both the growth of middle-class culture and the changes taking place in the practice of medicine, as the physician was no longer an unquestioned authority, but one among many therapeutic options.

In 1733 appeared Cheyne's most original work, *The English Malady*, a treatise on that popular complex of diseases which included hysteria, hypochondria, and "the spleen." The book includes the author's lengthy autobiographical account of his own bouts with melancholy. Cheyne's mingling of somatic and spiritual explanations for the cause and cure of this illness places him in the center of debates, both contemporary and historiographical, about eighteenth-century madness and its cultural place. Against the gloomy views of the historians Andrew Scull and Michael MacDonald, the latter of whom found the eighteenth century to be "a disaster for the insane,"[25] my reading of Cheyne's work tends to support the more optimistic assessments of Roy Porter, who points to the eclectic nature of eighteenth-century theories and therapies as a sign of the emergence of practical psychiatry.[26] Unlike Porter, however, who emphasizes the process of secularization in his discussions of eighteenth-century therapeutics, I give more weight to the continued influence of religion in this period.[27]

During the 1730s Cheyne's influence grew. He advised Alexander Pope on his health and Samuel Richardson on *Pamela*. His circle of mystical friends included the philanthropist Lady Elizabeth Hastings and the spiritual writer William Law. Through his patient the Countess of Huntingdon (Lady Betty's sister-in-law), Cheyne made the acquaintance of John Wesley, the founder of Methodism, whose ideas in many ways complemented his own. Wesley and Cheyne drew their theologies of the "inner light" and the "religion of the heart" from many of the same sources, including medieval mystics, Bourignon, and Guyon; and Wesley borrowed aspects of the Methodist emphasis on personal regimen from Cheyne's works. When he died at Bath in 1743 at the age of seventy-two, Cheyne was planning an edition of mystical works with Samuel Richardson. He was at the height of his fame.

Yeats wrote, "The intellect of man is forced to choose/Perfection of the life, or of the work." Cheyne tried to do both: his life was his work. This book tells the story of a single intellectual life. But this life encompasses many lives of the early eighteenth century in Britain. It is a world on the edge of becoming our own. Together, the stories of these lives tell us something about both the world we have lost and the world we have made.

OBESITY AND DEPRESSION
IN THE ENLIGHTENMENT

1

A SOUL IN CRISIS

In the early years of the eighteenth century, Britain was rife with prophets and millennial predictions. The English clergyman John Mason had claimed that Jesus would appear in 1694. Francis Mercury van Helmont, an alchemist and friend of Henry More, Robert Boyle, and Anne Conway, predicted that the reign of the saints would commence in 1702. In the 1690s the millenarian prophet Jane Lead (or Leade) gained many followers for her mystical sect known as the Philadelphians, which followed the teachings of the German mystic Jacob Boehme (1575–1624). This sect labeled itself a "Religious Society for the Reformation of Manners, for the Advancement of an Heroical Christian Piety, and Universal Love towards All." Two years later, the millenarian Camisards or French Prophets first visited London.[1] The Newtonian William Whiston calculated that the world would end in 1736.

The Glorious Revolution may temporarily have removed the threat of popery, but the Anglican Church was far from secure. Rent from within by squabbles between high and low church, Tory and Whig, on issues ranging from toleration to the succession, the church also struggled against the external threats of dissenters, deists, and atheists. Voluntary groups such as the religious societies and the Society for Promoting Christian Knowledge were formed to combat what seemed to be an increasing tide of doctrinal indifference.[2] The suspension of licensing in 1695 opened the door to every kind of pamphlet debate, not the least of which concerned religious matters.

And all around, said observers, society was in decay: morals declined, drunkenness and disorder abounded. Ned Ward's popular *London Spy*, written at the turn of the century from the vantage point of his King's

Head Tavern, described a world of drunkards and gamblers, whore-mongers and strumpets, in which the old order of society stood in disarray: a 'prentice metamorphosed into a young buck who washed his hands only in orange juice and Hungary water, and the young gentle-woman was in fact a seasoned jade. The physician Bernard Mandeville complained in *The Fable of the Bees* of the predominance of "Sharpers, Parasites, Pimps, Players, Pick-Pockets, Coiners, Quacks, Sooth-Sayers." "All Trades and Places knew some Cheat," he bemoaned; "No Calling was without Deceit."[3] On the one hand, this perception of decay led to the formation in the 1690s of the Societies for the Reformation of Manners, which attempted to enforce legal restrictions on behavior; on the other, radicals such as the Philadelphians saw signs of imminent millennium, when the old order would collapse and the thousand-year rule of the saints commence.[4]

In 1705 a large, bumptious, and talkative young Scottish physician named George Cheyne attempted, like many others of his generation, to resolve the social and religious tensions of his age by means of natural philosophy. He published in that year what he hoped was his magnum opus, *The Philosophical Principles of Natural Religion*. It was largely ignored, but its failure proved to be the turning point in Cheyne's life.

The failure of the *Philosophical Principles* led to a physical, spiritual, and intellectual crisis from which Cheyne emerged reborn. It defined the triangle of food, flesh, and spirit that dictated his subsequent life and career. Cheyne described his crisis in an autobiographical study, "The Case of the Author," appended to his 1733 work on nervous disorders, *The English Malady*. By this account, despite being "dispos'd to *Corpulence*" with the rest of his family, Cheyne had led a remarkably healthy existence up to the time of his crisis. He had noted in his youth, he said, that "the slightest *Excesses*" led him to "slippery Bowels, or a Spitting," signs that "my *Glands* were naturally *lax*, and my *Solids feeble*"—signs, in other words, of a sensitive, nervous nature, despite his beefy appearance. Nonetheless, his youth and a robust constitution had allowed him to retain his health through the excesses of his earlier years in Scotland, when he had followed the hard-drinking and high-living example of his mentor, the Edinburgh physician Archibald Pitcairne.[5]

He continued to follow this lifestyle in London, embracing the culture of the coffeehouse and tavern, "nothing being necessary for that Purpose, but being able to *Eat* lustily, and swallow down much *Liquor*." "I was tempted to continue *this Course*," he added, "no doubt, from a *Liking*, as well as to force a *Trade*, which Method I had observ'd to succeed with some others." Mandeville observed, "if you can Chat, and be a good Companion, you may drink yourself into Practice . . . [or] you must . . . keep a set of Coffee-Houses, observe your certain Hours, and take care you are often sent for where you are, and ask'd for where you are not."[6]

With such a regimen, Cheyne's physical collapse in 1705 was probably inevitable. By "constantly Dineing and Supping in *Taverns*, and in the Houses of my Acquaintances of *Taste* and *Delicacy*," Cheyne exacerbated his tendency toward obesity, becoming, as he said, "excessively *fat, short-breath'd, Lethargic* and *Listless*." The first warning signs of disaster soon appeared in the guise of an "*autumnal intermittent Fever*." The date of its appearance is not clear but perhaps may be placed in the autumn of 1703, following another professional failure, the disastrous appearance of Cheyne's book on Newtonian calculus, which was roundly criticized and disowned by Newton himself. This was the first time, but not the last, that Cheyne's health paralleled his professional fortunes.[7] Although he recovered from this bout, he spent the next year feeling "*jumbled* and *turbid*." The following autumn the mathematician Abraham de Moivre offered a devastating refutation of Cheyne's book, to which he responded by falling victim to a "*vertiginous Paroxysm*." His vertigo was so severe that "I was forced . . . to lay hold on the Posts of my Bed, for fear of tumbling out."[8]

The attacks of vertigo resolved themselves into "a constant violent *Head-Ach, Giddiness, Lowness, Anxiety* and *Terror*, so that I went about like a *Malefactor* condemn'd, or one who expected every Moment to be crushed by a *ponderous* Instrument of Death, hanging over his Head." Plainly this was no ordinary illness. Cheyne well knew in 1733 that he had suffered from the disease in which he came to specialize, that vague cluster of nervous ailments referred to as "the vapours."[9]

"The vapours," often known as "hypochondria" in men or "hysteria" in women, was preeminently an eighteenth-century disease. As Stanley

Jackson explains, in the seventeenth century both Thomas Willis and Thomas Sydenham had decoupled hypochondria from melancholia and instead linked it with hysteria; Sydenham asserted the virtual equivalence of the two.[10] On a continuum of nervous illness, "the vapours" constituted a minor disturbance, while melancholia itself could lead to madness and the loss of all reason. Hypochondria and hysteria came to refer, in fact, to a broad complex of symptoms, both physical and mental. Cheyne later referred to "the Hyp" as "a true *Proteus*."[11] Traditionally, hypochondria was a somatic dysfunction centering on the "hypochondria," the region just below the rib cage, where the liver, gallbladder, and spleen are located. In humoral terms, hypochondria was associated with black bile, produced by the spleen, and "spleen" came to be a shorthand for this disorder. Black bile contributed both to digestive upset and to melancholy; indeed, the imperfect digestion that led to an excess of black bile often could cause melancholy, because its disturbing fumes rose to the head.[12] Humoral explanations had been redefined in mechanical terms by 1700, and Sydenham referred to the "irregular motions of the animal spirits."[13] Yet the symptoms, and the connection with digestion, remained, and "the vapours" continued to be viewed as a somatic disorder, even when evidence existed to the contrary. In 1707 Dr. John Purcell vividly described a complex of symptoms resembling Cheyne's:

Those who are troubled with Vapours, generally perceive them approach in the following manner: first, they feel a Heaviness upon their Breast, a Grumbling in their Belly; they belch up, and sometimes vomit sower, sharp, or bitter Humours: They sometimes have a Difficulty in Breathing; and think they feel something that comes up into their Throat, which is ready to choak them. . . . They perceive a Swimming in their Heads: a Dimness comes over their Eyes, they turn pale; are scarce able to stand: their Pulse is weak; they shut their Eyes; fall down; and remain senseless for some time.[14]

In his *Treatise of the Hypchondriack and Hysterick Passion* (1711), Bernard Mandeville noted "an extraordinary *Consensus* between the Brain and the Stomach."[15]

The psychiatrist and anthropologist Arthur Kleinman has identified in the symptoms of depression a modern counterpart of "the vapours," as the "somatized" product of cultural and social stress.[16] Cheyne recognized an interrelationship between his mental and physical states that was something more than merely somatic. In *The English Malady* and other works, he helped to relocate these symptoms as nervous and to connect them to the nascent culture of sensibility.[17]

Like hypochondria in men, hysteria in women referred to a complex of nervous ailments with physical symptoms. By 1700 hypochondria and hysteria were virtually indistinguishable in their symptoms, but the gendered cause of each ailment remained problematic. Sydenham pointed out that both women and men suffered from these symptoms, although the weaker female constitution was more susceptible. Mandeville commented, "I never dare speak of Vapours, the very Name is become a Joke; and the general Notion the Men have of them, is, that they are nothing but a malicious Mood, and contriv'd Sullenness of willful extravagant and imperious Women, when they are denied, or thwarted in their unreasonable Desires."[18] Yet Mandeville did not deny the reality of its symptoms. As its name indicates, hysteria had been thought to originate in the womb, which in Hippocratic physiology was believed to wander through the trunk. A hysteric fit, with its feeling of choking or suffocation, was an effect of this wandering womb.[19] By Cheyne's time the notion of a wandering womb had long been discarded, although Friedrich Hoffmann believed the uterus was nonetheless implicated, and the French physician Jean Astruc, writing in 1740, attributed hysteria to "Impressions made on the *Uterus*, whereby certain sensations are raised in the Brain."[20] However, most physicians agreed with Sydenham that what "in men we call Hypochondricall, in women Hystericall" proceeded "from an Ataxy or Shatteredness of the Animall Spirits."[21]

At the first sign of illness, Cheyne's "*Bouncing, protesting, undertaking* Companions forsook me," he wrote, "and dropt off like *autumnal Leaves*," leaving him "to pass the melancholy Moments with my own *Apprehensions* and *Remorse*." Cheyne was "forc'd to retire into the Country quite alone," forced, no doubt, by financial as well as medical reasons. Cheyne had planned to return to Scotland in the summer of 1705 to write, with his mentor Pitcairne, the *Principia* of medicine. But as at so many times in Cheyne's life, his expectations far exceeded reality. He returned to Scotland in the summer of 1705 not in triumph but in despair.[22]

Cheyne's narrative of events can be seen as a spiritual autobiography, ending with the experience of conversion.[23] Unlike Calvinist autobiographies such as John Bunyan's *Grace Abounding*, Cheyne's conversion did not commence in a feeling of predestinarian guilt but originated in the body. The sixteenth-century Italian Luigi Cornaro, as well as Galen himself, had written similar personal histories that ended not in religious conversion but in a kind of secular conversion to a moderate regimen. Cheyne's conversion contained elements of both approaches. He reconstructed himself both in the older religious sense of the imitation of Christ and in terms of his relationship with contemporary secular culture, including medical theory.[24]

Following Pitcairne's mechanistic medical theories, Cheyne attributed his initial symptoms to "an *anomalous* Fit of my relapsing *Intermittent* [fever]." His headache and giddiness had, he believed, somatic causes.[25] Yet, at thirty-two stone (448 pounds), Cheyne's body also displayed his moral decay, for the cause of his illness was his profligate lifestyle. The moral shallowness of his life became evident when his friends abandoned him at the first sign of illness. Even those whom he had assisted in their extremities "did now entirely relinquish and abandon me." When friendship is based merely on "*sensual Pleasures* and mere *Jollity*," he concluded morosely, such were the consequences.[26] Like all converts, Cheyne entered the dark night of the spirit alone.

In his account, Cheyne's journey back toward God progressed in Platonic steps from body, to mind, to spirit. The mystical writers he read during this period described such a course: "The order of spiritual regeneration is divided by the mystic doctors, and that very justly, into the *purgative*, the *illuminative*, and the *unitive* states; but, as such must be the actual course of experience of all the truly and fully regenerate."[27] As Cheyne unencumbered himself from the flesh, the spirit emerged. Carol Flynn has argued that in the eighteenth century, "A sense of frustration informs many of the attempts to rationalize, utilize, and eventually get rid of the bodies that bind";[28] Cheyne here seems to be an exception to this generalization, although, as we shall see, the body continually returned to haunt him. Because his obesity was a major cause of his illness, in his case the shedding of the flesh was quite literal. While his body diminished, his mind became more and more detached from it, entering a state of "undisturbed *Meditation* and *Reflection*," which he had not been able to reach amid the bustle of London.

Cheyne's meditation very shortly led him into an *"Unknown State of Things."* In this receptive state Cheyne sought out spiritual guidance from a trusted mentor, a friend of his youth, who led him toward appropriate texts. Cheyne's spirit was calmed, and he resolved always *"To neglect nothing to secure my eternal Peace."*[29] This seems a mild act of religious conversion. Yet these texts led Cheyne to a Quaker-like recognition of an "inner light," the notion of God working in the soul.

Cheyne downplayed his mysticism in his 1733 account, undoubtedly with a view toward his intended audience of potential patients. Cheyne presented his autobiography as a medical case study in a book on melancholy, and his own case was an example not only of hypochondria but also of another recognized illness, religious melancholy. As such, he emphasized the somatic causes of his ailment and minimized aspects that might be interpreted as religious enthusiasm.[30] His subsequent postconversion narrative continued a tale of repeated failings and successes but focused on Cheyne's body, not his soul. He is a turning point in the process described by Flynn when "Christian contempt for the body was giving way to a secular concern for the bodily container."[31]

His account nonetheless made clear the parallel between spiritual and bodily healing. The body could not be healed, said Cheyne, without healing the soul; nor could the soul reach perfection without attention to the suffering body. By 1733 Cheyne's therapeutic persona was priest as much as healer.[32] Thus Cheyne stands at the intersection of spiritual, mental, and physical explanations of mental disorder.

In London, where street preachers demanded repentance, Cheyne's conversion may have been less surprising. But in the serene granite surroundings of his native Aberdeen, the final retribution seemed less near. In contrast to the millenarian aspirations of the English capital, Cheyne's friend and fellow Scot John Craig had placed the apocalypse far in the future, setting 3150 as the earliest year in which it could occur.[33] Craig's conservative estimate illustrated a Scottish rejection of fanaticism and sectarianism that Cheyne shared, extending a particular theme in Scottish Episcopalian theology. Cheyne's conversion took place within a specific local context, and he would connect his experience to the wider world only later.

In Aberdeen, Cheyne "liv'd very low."[34] He put in his neck a seton—a thread or cord drawn through a fold of skin, often in the neck, to maintain a constant discharge of fluid—a symbol, perhaps, that his body remained tied to the world. To relieve his physical symptoms—caused, he knew, by his excessive weight—he took the standard purging therapy to great lengths, consciously attempting to get rid of the body that so plagued him. His contemporary Defoe raged against "The unmortified pampered Carkass" as the source of "all these raging, tyrannizing Inclinations."[35] Defoe referred to sexual passion, but Cheyne recognized that the body could be tyrannized by other passions as well, such as a craving for food. His rejection of the body and its demands was the first step of the *imitatio Christi* as outlined by his religious mentors. He dosed himself with increasingly strong medicines. Since the usual purges and mineral waters availed little, he tried various mercurial compounds, including "Prince's Powder," Turbith mineral, and calomel, all violent cathartics and emetics. "Lightsomer indeed" from this course, Cheyne's stomach rebelled, and the vomits he used to quell it pumped up "*Oceans of Choler,*" an apt metaphor for the dregs of his former life, which he now ritually shed.[36] Cheyne shed not only weight but also his old personality, which was strongly "choleric" in the traditional humoral description of angry, aggressive, and argumentative.

With his body "melting away like a *Snow-ball* in Summer," Cheyne turned to the more compelling problem of his spiritual state. His retirement to the country afforded him the opportunity for undisturbed introspection, an activity in which he had not indulged during his hectic years in London. To his surprise, Cheyne found himself "infallibly entering into an *Unknown State of Things.*" What was there not to know? He had had the benefit of a "*liberal* and *regular Education,*" and "the Instruction and example of pious Parents." From them he had gained knowledge of the basis of "all *Virtue* and *Morality*: viz. the *Existence* of a *supreme and infinitely perfect Being*, the *Freedom* of the *Will*, the *Immortality* of the Spirits of all intelligent Beings, and the Certainty of *future Rewards* or *Punishments*." Such reasonable tenets formed the basis of the latitudinarian "natural religion" Cheyne had defended in his *Philosophical Principles of Natural Religion*. He had confirmed these doctrines "from *abstracted* Reasonings, as well as from the best *natural Philosophy*," and the contrivance of the world described in his *Philosophical Principles* had proven their "Truth and Necessity."[37]

His country reflections led Cheyne to realize that his proof of a deity by natural philosophy came dangerously close to deism's denial of revelation. Had not the well-known clergyman Samuel Clarke recently argued that deists claimed to gain all their knowledge "by the light of Nature alone"? The warm security of natural religion abandoned him, and he wondered whether "there might not be more required" of him. Had God revealed "higher, more noble, and more enlightening Principles" than he knew? Were there not more "encouraging and enlivening *Motives* proposed, to form a more extensive and *Heroic* virtue upon, than those arising from *natural* Religion only"?[38]

Cheyne groped for guidance. He displayed symptoms of religious melancholy, that "dark lanthorn of the Spirit," in which the sufferer's guilty conscience led, according to Robert Burton, to "great pain and horror of mind, distraction of soul, restless, full of continual fears . . . they can neither eat, drink, nor sleep." Burton had distinguished two varieties of religious melancholy, caused either by "deficit" of belief or its "excess."[39] In his autobiography, Cheyne described his case as one of deficit. He had previously discussed "that kind of *Melancholy*, which is called *Religious*, because 'tis conversant about matters of *Religion*; although, often the Persons so distempered have little *solid Piety*." Such an ailment arose from "a *Disgust* or *Disrelish* of worldly *Amusements* and *Creature-comforts*." He recommended for this malady first physical regimen and then spiritual meditation.[40] In his own case, Cheyne sought "some clear Accounts discoverable of that State I was then apparently going into [i.e., religious melancholy], than could be obtained from the mere Light of

Nature and *Philosophy*."[41] He turned to the friend of his youth, George Garden, whom he had met as an undergraduate in Aberdeen. In "The Case of the Author" Cheyne identified him only as "a worthy and learned *Clergyman* of the *Church of England*, sufficiently known and distinguished in the *Philosophical* and *Theological* World (whom I dare not name, because he is still living, tho' now extreamly old)."[42] When Cheyne wrote in 1732, Garden was over eighty, and near death. He had published several papers in the *Philosophical Transactions*, corresponded with Scottish virtuosi, and was sufficiently distinguished in natural philosophy to have been proposed for fellowship in the Royal Society in 1695, although his political leanings probably derailed his election.[43] Cheyne had relied on Garden's account of generation (published in the *Philosophical Transactions* in 1691) for his own discussion of that topic in the *Philosophical Principles*.[44]

While his natural philosophy followed the mainstream, Garden had placed himself well beyond the pale in theology and politics by the time Cheyne encountered him again in 1705. Both he and his brother James had followed a well-worn Scottish theological path toward personal religion, but events during Cheyne's absence from Aberdeen in the 1690s led them farther and farther from the religious mainstream. The aftermath of the Glorious Revolution in Scotland was the reestablishment of the Presbyterian religion in 1689. As Episcopalians, the Gardens did not accept the Presbyterian settlement and refused the required oaths. Aberdeen itself was slow to accept the new form of worship, and Presbyterian services were not held there until 1704.[45]

Cheyne undoubtedly had heard George Garden preach from his usual pulpit at the city church of St. Nicholas. In 1692 the Scottish Privy Council removed him from St. Nicholas for his refusal both to pray for William and Mary and to read proclamations that referred to them. He was also barred from serving as a minister elsewhere in Scotland. But he continued to minister to his followers, even after the General Assembly of the Church of Scotland deposed him from the ministry in 1701. Meanwhile, James Garden had been deprived of his post as professor of divinity at King's College, Aberdeen, in 1696 for refusing to sign the Westminster Confession, the doctrinal basis of Scottish Presbyterianism.[46]

Critical for both brothers was their discovery in the mid-1690s of the works of the Flemish mystic Antoinette Bourignon (1616–80). To those as steeped in local mystical traditions as the Gardens, Bourignon represented but a small leap; but to others, she was a rank heretic. James Garden's *Comparative Theology*, published as a Latin dissertation in 1699 and in English in 1700, clearly shows the influence of Bourignon but did not name her. George Garden's 1699 *Apology for Mme. Bourignon* directly defended her doctrines and led to his defrocking.[47]

The roots of the Gardens' apostasy lay deep in Scots religious culture.[48] The seventeenth-century Scottish Kirk was continually subject to political tides. James VI and I imposed Episcopal authority on the Calvinist Presbyterian Church established by John Knox in the sixteenth century, but Scottish Episcopalianism fell to the Presbyterian Covenanters in 1638, only to be reimposed in 1660. In 1689 the Calvinist William III welcomed the disestablishment of the bishops, most of them Jacobites, in favor of renewed Presbyterianism.

Each of these shifts instigated new rounds of persecution and reprisals, creating successive sets of martyrs. Such turmoil, or its threat, also led to the construction among Scots Episcopalians of a unique body of theological writings that aimed at a middle way between the extremes of sectarianism. Calvinist in conviction, the doctrines of Scottish Episcopalianism fell somewhere between the more extreme Calvinism of Presbyterianism and the more moderate Anglican Church.[49]

The revolt of the Covenanters decisively split Episcopalians from Presbyterians. Thereafter, Scottish Episcopalians felt continually threatened. Many leading Episcopalians began to look inward rather than outward for religious affirmation and faith. The succession of mystics leading to James and George Garden began with Patrick Forbes of Corse (1564–1635), consecrated bishop of Aberdeen in 1618.[50] The works of these mystics and others they recommended, including Bourignon, constituted Cheyne's theological education in the summer and autumn of 1705.

Patrick Forbes's son John (1593–1648), professor of divinity at King's College, Aberdeen, was one of the "Aberdeen Doctors" who objected to the Covenant in 1638. They were deposed from their positions and went

into exile.[51] John Forbes expressed his mystical side most fully in the diary
he kept from 1624 until 1647. Known as the *Spiritual Exercises*, this work
was published (in a Latin translation) by George Garden in his edition of
Forbes's collected works only in 1702–3. This text helped establish a
legitimate ancestry for the Gardens' claim to a uniquely Scots strain of
mysticism.[52]

Even more important was Henry Scougal's *Life of God in the Soul of Man*,
first published in 1677, a year before Scougal's early death at the age of
twenty-eight. George Garden had been a friend of Scougal since their
undergraduate days at King's, and both were regents there in the early
1670s. Garden's sermon at Scougal's funeral became another text in the
mystical tradition.[53]

Like John Forbes, Scougal held the king's divinity chair; and Scougal's
father, Patrick (?1607–82), like Patrick Forbes also bishop of Aberdeen,
had ordained Garden into the ministry.[54] His friend was Bishop Robert
Leighton (1611–84), whose Presbyterian father had been horribly tortured
by Laud's men in the 1630s.[55] Leighton helped establish the strong
connection between Scottish Episcopalianism and certain French mystics.
While in France, he was linked to the Jansenists, and he gained knowledge
too of the mystics François de Sales and the Baron de Renty.[56] In his
writings, Leighton added to Calvinism a diverse range of mystical influences stretching back to the Middle Ages, including these as well as
Bernard of Clairvaux, Thomas à Kempis, and Theresa of Avila. Like them,
he emphasized the value of the individual experience of God over
theological divisiveness or empty debate over ceremony. Leighton's works,
published posthumously in 1692, provided another link in the Gardens'
chain.[57]

Like Leighton and John Forbes, Henry Scougal turned toward personal religion as an antidote to sectarianism. In his introduction to *The
Life of God in the Soul of Man*, Gilbert Burnet pointed to Scougal's emphasis
on the value of the imitation of Christ as a counterweight to factional
strife.[58] Scougal's *imitatio Christi* marked out a typically Scots middle way.
In *The Life of God in the Soul of Man*, he listed several "mistakes about
religion." Some Christians, he said, believed it to inhere in "Orthodox
Notions and Opinions"; others, in "a constant course of external duties";

yet others "put all Religion in the affections, in rapturous heats, and
extatick [*sic*] devotion." But true religion, he wrote, was simply "an Union
of the Soul with God." If the seeker of truth will listen to his heart, he
will naturally incline to the good and lead a life of moderation in all
things.[59] G. D. Henderson has emphasized the influence of the Cambridge Platonists, particularly John Smith, on these views, also noting the
influence of Henry More on Scougal's ethics course at Aberdeen. His
lectures continued to be repeated by others long after his death, and
Cheyne undoubtedly heard them as an undergraduate.[60]

Forbes, Scougal, and Leighton emphasized attaining purity of spirit
through the conduct of daily life. Like all mystics, they argued that one
fully conscious of God's presence within cannot lead a normal life. Such
a person must give up the things of the world. Leighton commented:
"This, then, should be our main study, first to search out our iniquities,
the particular defilements of our nature; not only gross filthiness, drunkenness, lasciviousness, &c., but our love of this earth, or of air or vanity
of mind, our self-will and self-seeking."[61] His message of rejection, even
mortification, of the body in order to redeem the spirit spoke directly to
the sick and obese Cheyne. A subtext in Scougal and Leighton, this
notion took center stage in the work of Antoinette Bourignon, to which
George Garden was introduced around 1695 by her disciple Pierre Poiret
(1646–1719).[62] By the time Cheyne reencountered Garden in 1705–6, he
had translated several of Bourignon's works and published his *Apology for
Mme Bourignon*, whose title page bore a motto from Leighton.

Much of Antoinette Bourignon's early life is known only through her
autobiography, written in 1663 and later supplemented by Poiret.[63]
According to this account Bourignon exhibited signs of sanctity from
early childhood. She was the daughter of a wealthy merchant of Lille. At
twenty she ran away from home to avoid an arranged marriage. Unable to
join a convent because her father refused to provide her a dowry, she
spent much of her life wandering, persecuted at various times for heresy
and sorcery. She arrived in the tolerant United Provinces in 1667, and
soon thereafter a stream of writings began to appear. In Amsterdam she
was exposed to the full spectrum of seventeenth-century religious believers,
ranging from Calvinists to Quakers, from Catholics to Mennonites.

Although she absorbed many ideas, what Garden referred to as this "*Babel*" of opinions, "where the Language is confounded, and the Builders do not understand one another" also convinced her that the true Church was fatally corrupted, shattered beyond repair into sects.[64]

Earlier she had been influenced by the Jansenist movement within French Catholicism and its emphasis on individual conversion and reform of personal life.[65] In Amsterdam she developed a more expansive view of Christianity and rejected the Jansenist (and Calvinist) notions of election and predestination, both of which seemed to prevent the exercise of free will. At the same time, her experience of sectarianism led her to reject all established doctrine, relying solely on the "inner light" of the spirit as her guide. Rather than embracing a particular church or doctrine, Bourignon simply abandoned herself to the action of the Holy Spirit.[66]

Bourignon advocated a personal mystical union with God devoid of theological hairsplitting or empty organized devotion. But salvation required an ongoing effort, and spiritual passivity was insufficient without physical involvement. Like the Scottish mystics, Bourignon emphasized the imitation of Christ as a model for personal life; Jesus had shown the path to salvation, which the individual could choose to follow. She compared Christ to a physician, who gave "medicines for the various maladies of their souls." As illness is a "privation of health," so the only evil or moral illness is the privation of God.[67] This was a theme to which Cheyne would return in his popular medical writings.

Bourignon argued that the corruption of the world in general, and the body in particular, formed the barrier between the human soul and the spirit of God. Her writings gave specific instructions on the conduct of life. Her personal regimen revolved around material asceticism, especially in matters of food and drink. Attention to the body—"this miserable lump of flesh"—was a distraction from attending to God.

For when [Man] suffereth himself to be governed by his own Passions, he stumbleth, and falleth into all manner of Mischief every Step . . . if any one eats and drinks according to his Passions, he runneth into many Excesses which will bring upon him divers Diseases and other Inconveniences: and if he is carried out to Luxury and carnal Pleasures, he cannot hope for long Life, but must expect the Gout and other shameful Maladies.[68]

"They who are Christ's," preached Bourignon, "have crucified the Flesh, with its Affections and Lusts."[69] Mortification of the body, along with complete spiritual passivity, were both intended particularly to tame the bestial nature of women. The sins of gluttony, sloth, and lust, she declared, were specifically feminine.[70] In this she took her cues, consciously or unconsciously, from medieval female mystics, who had established the close relationship between bodily activities, particularly eating, and spirituality. Such figures as Catherine of Siena and Angela da Foligno figured prominently in the "Catalogue" of mystical works published by Bourignon's disciple Poiret in 1708 and have been discussed more recently in Caroline Walker Bynum's *Holy Feast and Holy Fast*.[71] Like the medieval saints, in her youth Bourignon had secretly fasted and mixed what little food she ate with ashes to disguise its taste. As Garden noted, however, Bourignon later in life moderated this ascetic program, greatly aiding her appeal to Garden and later to Cheyne.[72]

The personal religion Bourignon described would lead, she said, not only to a moral regeneration of humanity but also to a physical transformation. As with the great medieval female mystics, this transformation involved a literal replacement of flesh with spirit. In addition, Bourignon argued, this ideal spiritual state was androgynous; but she altered the Quaker definition of the genderless soul to emphasize its female nature.[73] "All Mens souls are the spouses of Jesus Christ," she wrote, and the apostle's epithet of "captive silly women," enslaved by the flesh, applied to both sexes. As Bynum has pointed out, Jesus himself had often been depicted in the Middle Ages as a lactating mother.[74] At the second coming, which Bourignon believed to be near at hand, male and female would be transformed into a more perfect being that partook of both sexes, like Adam before the birth of Eve. At the level of the pre-millennium present, this also meant that men and women were spiritually equal. In her own life, Bourignon had demonstrated this essential equality; when she left her family to embark on a spiritual life, it was in the guise of a male pilgrim.[75] Elizabeth Castelli has noted that among early female saints, "gender ambiguity [became] a sign of special holiness," and that their piety, based on sexual renunciation and virginity, amounted to a rejection of traditional gender roles. Yet some theologians viewed this blurring of gender lines as dangerous.[76] Cheyne later acknowledged the balance between male and female natures in himself, and this recognition was an important element of the culture of sensibility.

Between 1696 and 1708, George Garden translated several of Bourignon's works, to which he added lengthy prefaces that summarized Bourignon's dense and repetitive prose and, in later works, responded to his critics. At least ten works critical of Bourignon appeared in England and Scotland between 1696 and 1710, an indication both of the popularity of her doctrines and the threat they posed to the established order, whether Episcopalian or Presbyterian.[77]

John Cockburn, a Scottish Episcopalian clergyman resident in Amsterdam and the Gardens' brother-in-law, delivered a particularly pointed critique in two 1698 pamphlets, *Bourignianism Detected*. He lumped Bourignon together with "all other Enthusiastical Impostures and Delusions. Our *Quakers* and *Philadelphians*, as well as the *Quietists* and *Pietists* abroad, are of the same kidney."[78] Cockburn dismissed Garden's claims for Bourignon's sanctity, based on her early practices of austerity and mortification, claiming that mortifications are only performed by "Hypocrites and Fools," and that such modern saints as Teresa of Avila and Catherine of Siena were inferior to the biblical prophets in holiness.[79] George White, an Episcopalian clergyman in Aberdeenshire, wrote an *Advertisement annent the Reading of the Books of Antonia Bourignon* in 1700. He claimed that her ideas had spread "like a devouring fire, leading sundry well-meaning persons to vent many errors, and causing young men of good expectations to have their melancholly heightened to an excessive degree."[80] He could have described Cheyne.

George Garden's *Apology for M. Antonia Bourignon* and James Garden's *Comparative Theology* responded to these critics. Both found in Bourignon's doctrines a resolution of the sectarianism that plagued the Scottish church as well as a return to the doctrines of primitive Christianity, a true Reformation. These learned men now rejected learning as the basis of their faith, and even placed knowledge of Scripture far below faith, repentance, and the mortification of the body as the means of attaining salvation. George Garden listed the "Three Means, which have caused Men to abandon God: Their Want of True Love to one another, their Love of this present Life, and their being addicted to their sensual Appetites; the Pleasures of the Mouth and Belly." The imitation of Christ meant "humility and self-denial." Similarly, James Garden argued that "the inward Manifestations of the Holy Ghost do require a calm and composed Mind; and the soft Whispers cannot be heard and observed by unregenerate Men, because of the obstreperous Noise, and din of blustring and tumultuating Passions and Lusts."[81]

These were the "Spiritual and Dogmatic *Authors*" recommended by Cheyne's unnamed mentor. Their words reverberated through his being, so much so that decades later the cadences of their prose and even phrases from their works echo through Cheyne's autobiography. With James Garden, Cheyne sought "higher, more noble, and more enlightening principles."[82] Scougal discussed those whose religion was based on "natural reason." These individuals

will many times disdain the grosser sort of vices, and spring up into fair imitations of Virtue and Goodness: if a man have but so much reason as to consider the prejudice which intemperance and inordinate lust doth bring unto his health, his fortune and his reputation, self-love may suffice to restrain him. . . . this natural principle [i.e., self-love] by the help of reason may take a higher flight, and come nigher the instances of Piety and Religion; it may incline a man to the diligent study of Divine Truths.

Yet however pleasant this intellectualized faith seemed, it was not sufficient for salvation: the reasonable man may "all the while continue a stranger to the holy temper and spirit of the Blessed Jesus, and so instead of a Deity he may embrace a cloud."[83]

Cheyne wrote of this period that he had always had "a firm Perswasion of the great and fundamental Principles of all *Virtue* and *Morality*." Even in his "loosest Days," he reflected, he had never "*pimp'd* to the *Vices* or *Infidelity* of any." Although he had carefully examined the doctrines of Christianity, confirming them "from abstracted Reasonings, as well as from the best *natural Philosophy*," at the depth of his crisis he began to realize, as Scougal had instructed, that reasonable religion alone was inadequate.[84] Mainstream Anglicanism had emphasized the ease of conversion and the imitation of Christ.[85] The more Calvinistic Scottish Episcopalians, like the Puritans, thought this was more difficult; but unlike the Puritans or the Scots Presbyterians, they did not feel that their attempt was predestined to fail.

The Gardens' heresy found a ready response among those Scots who, like Cheyne, sought deeper spiritual meaning than could be found in the established church, particularly the Presbyterian Church of Scotland, and who moreover sought to escape the bitterly divisive political scene. For a time, George Garden led a group of followers of Bourignon who lived communally in the village of Rosehearty near Aberdeen, on the estate of Alexander, Lord Forbes of Pitsligo, a follower and later Cheyne's patient. Garden also became the center of a circle of correspondence on mystical matters.[86] It focused not merely on Bourignon but also on the eclectic collection of mystical authors Poiret catalogued in 1708. As Shuttleton has pointed out, most of the members of this circle were also Jacobites, but the relationship between the politics and the religion of this group remains unclear.[87]

Cheyne was joined in this circle by another Scottish physician, James Keith (?–1726), who migrated to London in 1704.[88] Keith acted as the London emissary for the Aberdeen circle, and his letters to another member of the group, Lord Deskford, heir to the Earl of Seafield, are filled with news and gossip of Scottish affairs in London.[89] Keith's London acquaintances included several physicians as well as the Philadelphian Francis Lee and the orientalist and suspected Arian Simon Ockley.[90] Keith served as Cheyne's London contact, for after the crisis of 1705 Cheyne never again resided permanently in London. Cheyne described Keith as "a wise & good man, who knows spiritual matters more distinctly & without the animal heat & ferment." At about this time Cheyne also met Andrew Michael Ramsay (?1686–1743), another member of Garden's circle, with whom he shared his spiritual crises. They remained friends even after Ramsay moved to France in 1710.[91]

In the spring of 1706 Cheyne traveled to Bath to continue his cure with a course of the waters. The waters worked only too well, for he found himself again slipping into his old bad habits of excess. Exchanging Bath water for Bristol water helped, but on his next return to Bath in the spring of 1707 he heard of a "wonderful Cure" administered by another self-medicating doctor, a Dr. Taylor of Croydon, who had cured himself in "an *Epileptick Case*" by a milk diet. In the winter of 1707–8 he visited Taylor in Croydon and became a convert to his dietary therapy. He ate abstemiously and exercised regularly, usually by riding. Cheyne's resolutions, however, were characteristically short-lived, and his health and weight for the next decade seesawed back and forth with depressing regularity.[92]

Cheyne nonetheless found in Bath a place where he could remake himself and, at last, build a medical practice. He followed the increasingly popular migration to Bath in the summer and back to London in the winter for the next dozen years, finally settling in Bath in 1718. Keith wrote of him in that year, "Dr. Ch. is indeed extreamly fat but yet has pretty good health. He writes that he has for ever bid an adieu to London." During this period, Cheyne wrote, "I followed the Business of my *Profession*, with great Diligence and Attention," and he began to specialize in the "low and nervous *Cases*" with which he had gained close familiarity from his own sufferings.[93]

Cheyne the failed Newtonian, the tortured soul, the obese buffoon, the successful physician, rang the changes of many lives over the course of his single life. His crisis of 1705, and the nexus of food, flesh, and spirit that it delineated, determined the man he became and played a critical role in the development of the successful medical works he published in the 1720s and 1730s. When he described this crisis in 1733, he intended to demonstrate to his patients that redemption, both physical and spiritual, was possible. As we shall see in the next chapters, he himself took a long time to learn this lesson.

2

THE EDUCATION
OF A NEWTONIAN

Tall, florid, and heavily built, Cheyne alighted from the Edinburgh coach onto the London pavement on a November day in 1701. The city rumbled with rumors of war. The deposed king James II had died in Paris in September, and Louis XIV had declared his young son to be James III and VIII, king of England and Scotland—a deliberate provocation to all patriotic Britons. King William returned home from Holland in November and dissolved Parliament, and pamphlets flew between Whig and Tory.

Cheyne's family tendency to corpulence had begun to manifest itself in the thirty-year-old physician.[1] He might have reflected during his two weeks on the London coach at his good fortune in being alive and healthy in an era when as many as half of his generation had not lived to see the age of ten.[2] As a physician, he knew that surviving childhood did not lead to any greater security; fevers, poxes, and plagues awaited the unwary, and the great Scottish famine of 1695–99 had exacted its toll.[3] The young man's soon-to-be-employer, the earl of Roxburghe, owed his title to the untimely death of his brother from a fever at the age of nineteen.

Socially, too, young Cheyne was better off than most of his compatriots. He rode a coach over the rutted and stony roads of pre-turnpike England and no doubt stayed at inns along the way, rather than riding horseback or walking and sleeping rough. He had attended a university, and if his medical degree had been purchased rather than earned, it was no less valuable. Far from wealthy, he had scratched out a living as a mathematics tutor and would do so again. His life revolved around books and learned discourse, drink and tavern gossip; a masculine life, in which few women appeared.

Cheyne carried with him a letter of introduction to Hans Sloane, secretary of the Royal Society and editor of the *Philosophical Transactions*. Sloane was also preeminent among the London physicians whose patronage could make or break a budding medical career.[4] Cheyne's recommendation bore the signature of Archibald Pitcairne, a well-known—some would say notorious—Edinburgh physician. Pitcairne described Cheyne as "a knowing man & good mathematicien," adding, "he is very desirous to be knowne to yow a patron of learn'd men."[5]

Cheyne was born, probably in 1671 or 1672, in the parish of Methlick, north of Aberdeen.[6] He later claimed descent from the Cheynes of Esslemont, a prominent family in the area, going so far as to matriculate arms under this rubric. But his own branch had experienced a reversal of fortune during the seventeenth century. Cheyne's father, James, was a tenant of his kinsman Patrick Maitland of Auchencruive. Their kinship stemmed from the powerful Burnet family. James Cheyne's mother was Isobel Burnet, sister of Robert Burnet, Lord Crimond. Her sister Katherine married Patrick Maitland. When the Cheynes lost their own land, they moved to Auchencruive. Among Isobel and Katherine Burnet's brothers were Gilbert, later bishop of Salisbury, and Thomas, a prominent Edinburgh physician.[7]

Twenty-five years after George Cheyne's birth, his father, James, was listed in the 1696 Aberdeenshire poll tax list. As a tenant, he paid a hundredth part of the laird's valuation; this came to £2 13s, more than most tenants in the parish paid. "Classing himself as ane gentleman," Cheyne paid an additional assessment of £3 6s. Along with the seven servants listed, these assessments mark James Cheyne as a substantial citizen. By 1696 he was married to his second wife and raising a second family. George Cheyne eventually assumed responsibility for the education of his half-brother William, born in 1704.[8]

Even though in economic terms he was the equal of most of his medical contemporaries, in terms of status the Cheynes occupied a lower rung. They were the sons of professionals or magistrates, minor lairds or younger sons of the nobility. George Cheyne's continued consciousness of his humble origins is evidenced by the pains he took in 1720 to establish his descent from the Cheynes of Esslemont.[9]

He left behind little evidence of his earlier life. He had, he later wrote, "a *liberal* and *regular Education*, with the Instruction and Example of pious Parents." Following in the footsteps of his great-uncle Gilbert Burnet, he entered Marischal College, Aberdeen, around 1686, since he is listed as a "tertian" or third-year student in 1688–89. His parents intended him to study divinity; the ministry had long been a means of social mobility for clever boys of lower status, and unlike in other fields, bursaries existed to fund such study.[10] Cheyne did not, however, take a degree at Marischal. Even if he had completed the four-year course, he may not, like many, have been able to afford the fees for graduation.

In Aberdeen, as at the other Scots universities, the new philosophy became part of the curriculum long before it did at Oxford or Cambridge. Judging by student notebooks from the era, teaching focused on Cartesian physics and included discussion of recent experiments, including those of Boyle.[11] The ethics course in the third year included Henry Scougal's moral philosophy lectures, which continued to be read long after his death. Scougal's main source was Henry More's *Enchiridion ethicum* and the work of other Cambridge Platonists, but he also referred to Descartes.[12]

Under the Scots system of regents, Cheyne would have spent his four-year course under the tutelage of a single regent. His regent, James Moir, was described as a "student of divinitie."[13] During his years in Aberdeen he also made the acquaintance of James and George Garden. Archibald Pitcairne later referred to his protégé Thomas Bower as Cheyne's "master" in mathematics, but Bower's formal association with the Aberdeen universities began long after Cheyne's student days.[14] Bower was hired in 1703 "to teach mathematicks both publickly and privately" at King's College, and was named professor of mathematics in 1707.[15] Bower's instruction of Cheyne, if it occurred, must have been informal and private.

When Cheyne stepped off the London coach, both friends and enemies awaited him. Most of them were somehow connected with Archibald Pitcairne, his mentor, father figure, and alter ego. Pitcairne not only taught Cheyne what he knew about medicine but also launched Cheyne's career as a pugnacious defender of his own "modern" medical theories, which appropriated the ideas of Isaac Newton. But Pitcairne's

importance both to Cheyne and to the wider cultural scene owed at least
as much to his personality and politics as it did to the content of his
theories. Pitcairne's Edinburgh was the political, religious, and social
milieu that shaped Cheyne in his twenties.

When Archibald Pitcairne returned to Edinburgh from Paris in 1680, he
found a city astir with intellectual activity. Scotland in the 1680s verged
on a cultural explosion. An era of peace and even prosperity had succeeded the strife of midcentury. Religious turmoil, after the uprisings of
1679–80, was in abeyance under the hegemony of the Scottish
Episcopalian bishops. Under the patronage of James, Duke of York, sent
to Scotland by his brother between 1679 and 1682 as royal commissioner,
learning flourished in the Scottish towns and their colleges.[16] Natural
philosophy, the new science of Bacon, Descartes, Galileo, and Harvey,
was, as across Europe, central to this cultural crisis.[17] The town of
Edinburgh and its college, soon to become a university under its new
charter, fostered the progressive, improving Scottish physicians who
began to meet in 1679 at the home of Dr. Robert Sibbald, the most
active of the local virtuosi. Sibbald's circle, like other provincial scientific
groups of the period, modeled itself on the Royal Society.[18] In 1681 he
founded an Edinburgh College of Physicians, modeled on the London
College.

A young member of Sibbald's circle and the new college, Archibald
Pitcairne was born in Edinburgh in 1652. His father was a merchant and
magistrate, and also a minor landholder. Pitcairne studied in the Town
College of Edinburgh and later in Paris, where he decided to enter medicine.[19] Around 1680 he met a young mathematician, David Gregorie
(1659–1708), the eldest son of the laird of Kinnairdie near Aberdeen. His
uncle, James Gregorie (1638–75), a fellow of the Royal Society, was
named the first professor in the new mathematics chair at Edinburgh in
1674. Following his death in 1675 his mathematical papers, which
included correspondence with Newton, passed to his nephew.[20] David
Gregory studied, like Cheyne, at Marischal College in Aberdeen. At the
age of twenty-four he was appointed to his uncle's chair in mathematics
in Edinburgh.[21]

Pitcairne and Gregory taught each other medicine and mathematics and vied with each other in their admiration for the work of Isaac Newton. Gregory sent a copy of his first book to Newton in 1684, setting the tone for their future relationship: "S[i]r yee will exceedingly oblidge mee, if yee will spare so much time from your Philosophical and Geometrical studies, as to allow me your free thoughts and character of this exercitation, which I assure you I will justly value more than that of all the rest of ye world."[22] Gregory's recognition of Newton's potential as a patron would pay off handsomely.

The social life of Pitcairne and Gregory revolved around the tavern; Pitcairne even consulted patients there.[23] Both were accused of drunkenness. Upon hearing of Pitcairne's death in 1713, the Calvinist clergyman Robert Wodrow commented, "He gote a vast income, but spent it upon drinking, and was twice drunk every day."[24] Wodrow was hardly a sympathetic witness, but Pitcairne's and Gregory's correspondence reveal a deep devotion to the bottle. When Pitcairne was arrested in 1699 for writing a seditious letter to his London friend Robert Gray, he pleaded that he wrote "through the Influence of a small Excess," that he had been, in other words, "in Cups"; and this plea was accepted.[25] Both Pitcairne and Gregory frequently mention the latest shipment of claret from Bordeaux. Since England was at war with France for much of this period, such shipments not only were an act of political defiance but also demonstrate how much these Augustans drank.[26] Such was the lifestyle in which the young Cheyne immersed himself, and against which he later rebelled.

Contemporaries also accused Gregory and Pitcairne of atheism. Wodrow claimed that Pitcairne profaned the sabbath with mock services ridiculing Scripture, and that he believed in ghosts and even claimed to have seen one. A Scot once sought out Edmond Halley to "see the man that has less religion than Dr. Gregory." Atheism was among the charges leveled against Gregory by the 1690 university visitors.[27] Yet these charges are evidence of deeper differences within Scottish society. A Covenanting regent of the University of Glasgow had referred to Descartes as a "very ignorant atheist," a "fatuous heretic."[28] Pitcairne and Gregory were at least nominally Episcopalians.

The Glorious Revolution of 1688–89 shattered their comfortable existence. The revolutionary settlement in Scotland favored neither Episcopalians nor the supporters of the departed King James, the Jacobites. The Restoration of 1660 had dismantled the Presbyterian ascendancy of the Commonwealth years in favor of episcopacy,[29] but the settlement of 1689 abolished episcopacy in Scotland, leading to the restoration of Presbyterianism as the Church of Scotland.[30] In a reversal of the situation at the Restoration, Episcopalian ministers were now ejected for refusing the new oaths of allegiance to the Presbyterian church or to William and Mary.

The Convention Parliament in Edinburgh passed the Act for Visitation, requiring a visitation of the universities by a commission that was, like the university visitors of the late 1640s in England, instructed to enforce allegiance to the new regime. All university professors were required to swear an oath of allegiance to William and Mary and to "submitt to the government of the Church now settled by Law"—the Presbyterian Church. The "Presbyterian inquisition"—so labeled by Alexander Monro, the Jacobite principal of the University of Edinburgh—ejected him and several others. At Cheyne's Aberdeen, James Garden was the only one in that hotbed of Jacobitism to refuse the oaths.[31]

Pitcairne and Gregory both left Edinburgh in the early 1690s: Gregory for Oxford in 1691, Pitcairne for Leiden shortly thereafter. While Gregory had been under considerable suspicion from the university visitors, he did not lose his Edinburgh chair. Pitcairne had no official positions from which he could threaten the new order, but his Jacobitism was no secret.[32] He described the continued unrest in the university in his satirical play *The Assembly*, written in 1692, blaming the visitors, who "scurvily thrust out the old masters."[33] *The Assembly* reveals not only Pitcairne's Jacobite politics but the role he felt "mathematick learning" could play in the struggle against sectarian enthusiasts, a lesson Cheyne learned and applied in his *Philosophical Principles of Natural Religion*. Pitcairne valued Episcopalianism less on doctrinal grounds than for its lack of fanaticism; if Gilbert Rule, the university's new principal, could question the teaching of Cartesian logic, then Edinburgh was on its way back to the bad old covenanting days, when the mad mob ruled.[34] The fear of fanaticism expressed in this work proved to be a governing principle for Cheyne.

In Pitcairne's play, Gilbert Rule became "Salathiel Little Sense," who claimed that God ordered the universities purged because "they were all over-grow [*sic*] with *Cartle's* [i.e., Descartes's] Mathematicks and humane Reasoning; yea some of them were so blasphemous, as to maintain that the King was supream and unaccountable."[35] To Pitcairne, the latter point was critical: like other Jacobites, he believed that if hereditary right was violated, the nation would be subverted and the order of society over-turned.[36] Against enthusiasts' railing against "mathematical *Atheists*," Pitcairne replied that "all are *Atheists* except Mathematicians." His Presbyterian answered with Pitcairne's nightmare of the ignorant fanatic mob: "I am told that the *First Prob[lem]* in Euclid does prove, That the World is eternal; and the *Second*, That there is not a God: Besides, one must have a compact with the *Devil* ere he can understand them."[37]

Throughout this turbulent period, Cheyne has disappeared from historical view. The only reference to the decade between his appearance as a student in Aberdeen in 1689 and his reappearance in Edinburgh in 1699 as Pitcairne's protégé is in the introduction and dedication to his *Philosophical Principles of Natural Religion*, published in 1705. There Cheyne stated that at some time in the past—he did not say when—he had acted as a tutor to the young John Ker, who in 1696 succeeded his brother as earl of Roxburghe. By 1705 Roxburghe, still only in his midtwenties, was a leader of the "squadrone" group of Scots politicians, one of the secretaries of state for Scotland, and would soon be elevated to a dukedom.[38]

Subsequent accounts of Cheyne's life have woven a substantial cloth from this small thread, dating Cheyne's tutoring as early as 1690. In 1690 Roxburghe would have been about ten years old, a precocious age for engaging in learned exchange on philosophical topics. Historians have further hypothesized the influence of Gilbert Burnet and George Garden on this appointment and waxed eloquent about the pious atmosphere of "Roxburgh House," where Cheyne imbibed "millenarian talk" that turned his mind toward mysticism, or alternately about the "salubrious hunting country" around Floors Castle, a Roxburghe residence.[39] This weave vanishes like a cobweb, however, on closer examination. There was a Roxburghe residence at Floors, but Floors Castle was not built until 1718, and there was no "great country estate" known as Roxburgh House. There is no evidence that Cheyne had any connection with the Roxburghe family until after he moved to London in 1701.[40]

The correspondence of the widowed countess of Roxburghe with her father, the earl of Tweeddale, gives a rather different picture.[41] The beleaguered countess, widowed at the age of twenty-four, devoted herself to her three young sons—the young earl Robert, John, and Will—their estate, and their education, frequently consulting her father for advice. In the early 1690s, as the Ker brothers reached adolescence, their education became an increasingly pressing problem. The name of Cheyne, however, does not figure in her ruminations, nor does anyone else seem to be in residence as a tutor until 1694, when James Gray entered the Roxburghe household.[42] While this is not conclusive proof of Cheyne's absence, it is highly suggestive. He did act as a tutor during the 1690s, but he was dismissed, as we shall see, under circumstances that were best left unsaid.

Cheyne has also been identified as one "Georgius Heill" who enrolled as a medical student at the University of Leiden in December 1691.[43] Since Pitcairne began teaching at Leiden in April 1692, this could have been their meeting place. However, this identification can only be regarded as tentative. Neither Cheyne nor Pitcairne ever mentioned being at Leiden together, and Cheyne would surely have noted his attendance at Leiden's prestigious medical school when he was later criticized for his lack of medical training.

Pitcairne's career as a medical professor at the University of Leiden was, in any case, short. In the summer of 1693, little more than a year after his arrival, he left for Scotland and did not return. In his letter of resignation he spoke only of "unexpected obstacles" that prevented his return to Leiden.[44] Upon his return to Scotland, he immediately plunged into controversy, and this controversy eventually involved Cheyne. In September 1694 Pitcairne wrote to his friend Robert Gray, "I send yow by Mr Kinkead a copie of a discourse De curatione febrium &c. It is writ only to lay the pride of some pratlers here."[45] The "pratlers" were some Edinburgh physicians who had been involved since 1691 in a pamphlet dispute concerning the proper treatment for fevers.[46]

Pitcairne delivered his contribution to the debate, the *Dissertatione de curatione febrium, quae per evacuationes instituitur* (Dissertation on the cure of fevers, initiated by evacuations), as one of the monthly lectures to the Royal College of Physicians of Edinburgh in November 1694 and published it soon after. *De curatione febrium* closely resembled the public dissertations Pitcairne had delivered at Leiden.[47]

In his Leiden dissertations Pitcairne had emphasized theory over practice, declaring that only mathematics could provide a basis of authority and certainty for medicine. In *The Assembly* Pitcairne had argued in addition that mathematical learning provided the basis of authority to uphold traditional values, including hereditary right, against religious sectarianism and rule by parliament. In terms of theory, each side in the debate claimed expertise in the new mechanical philosophy. The real issue was therapy: not so much in specifics, which varied only slightly, but in how it was derived. Andrew Brown, who initiated the debate, claimed to follow the empirical method of the English physician Thomas Sydenham, while Pitcairne claimed that his therapy came not from experience but from his superior learning. Pitcairne believed that the empirical medicine espoused by his opponents had potentially subversive implications: under dispute were not merely conflicting medical theories but conflicting visions of society. Empirical medicine implied a lack of respect for traditional authority, both intellectual (as the College of Physicians upheld) and political.[48]

As Theodore Brown has shown, the London College of Physicians had adopted iatromechanism over Galenism as its governing theory by the 1690s, although therapies remained largely unchanged. The Royal Society had declared their allegiance to the mechanical philosophy in the 1670s, yet the experimental program that might have provided this theory with some empirical proofs had peaked in the late 1660s and then rapidly declined.[49] Brown traces the College's acceptance of iatromechanism to Thomas Willis (1621–75), whose *Diatribae duae* (1659) had developed a mechanical explanation for fevers that also justified standard therapeutics. Fever was a model for all disease, and Willis's explanation, which involved chemical fermentations in the blood, placed it within the context of Harvey's theory of the circulation.[50]

At the same time as iatromechanism became the favored theory, however, another physician, Thomas Sydenham (1642–89), challenged the validity of any theory in the clinical context. Sydenham urged a return to the Hippocratic ideal of bedside observation and case histories. He employed a Baconian methodology of collecting clinical observations in order to build a picture of disease. Declaring himself independent of any theory, he actively urged against a reliance on physiology as a basis for medical knowledge. But he retained the Galenic doctrine of the humors as the model for disease and therapy.[51] Sydenham was an extremely successful practitioner, and his many writings detailed his ideas. The tension between theory and practice, between iatromechanism and neo-Hippocratism, was evident by the 1690s; although knowledge of theory was the mark of the learned physician, the success of Sydenham and other atheoretical practitioners such as John Radcliffe could not be ignored.

The Edinburgh fevers debate was one example of this continuing tension. The so-called empirics self-consciously identified with Sydenham. While Pitcairne wished to replace both traditional Galenic authority and Willis-style iatromechanism with the new authority of mathematics, he fervently believed in authority, and believed that knowledge of theory must be the distinguishing mark of a physician over a quack. Pitcairne's dissertation on the cure of fevers, delivered with his usual brashness, provoked an uproar in the Edinburgh College of Physicians. Since he defended learning and traditional therapies against the empirics, he assumed the college would agree with him. But he justified his therapeutics with an unconventional theory based on mathematics and attractions and invoking Newton's natural philosophy. The college, already torn over political issues, split in two over Pitcairne's paper.[52]

Despite a favorable summary of *De curatione febrium* in the *Philosophical Transactions* of the Royal Society, two anti-Pitcairne works quickly appeared from within the college and continued the pamphlet war. The satirical *Apollo Mathematicus; or, The Art of Curing Diseases by the Mathematics* was written by Robert Sibbald's protégé Edward Eizat. He probably also penned a hostile translation of *De curatione febrium* entitled *Apollo Staticus*. The latter work concluded, "By what here is said, any Body may see the vast difference that is between one that takes his Observations from Nature, and one that takes his Marks from the Moon, that is, between a Rational and Mathematical Physician."[53] Pitcairne, in other words, was not to be allowed to assume the mantle of the learned, rational physician with his newfangled theories. Pitcairne's Leiden student George Hepburn countered with a pamphlet, *Tarrugo Unmasked*, and other pamphlets followed. The Edinburgh College closed ranks and expelled Pitcairne and his faction from the college late in 1695.[54] Pitcairne's arrogance had not endeared him to his Edinburgh colleagues, and his scientific pretensions, as Eizat's satires made clear, seemed like so much grandstanding.

Cheyne's name does not appear in the course of the fevers dispute in the college. If he had indeed been a student of Pitcairne in Leiden it seems likely that in Edinburgh he would have been, with George Hepburn, a prominent supporter of Pitcairne in the dispute. Since Cheyne later assumed this role, he was probably unacquainted with Pitcairne before his expulsion from the college.

By 1699 Cheyne knew Pitcairne and his theories sufficiently to enter the fevers dispute. A new chapter in that struggle had recently been initiated by Charles Oliphant (?1666–1720), author of *A Short Discourse to Prove the Usefulness of Vomiting in Fevers*. Oliphant, a brother-in-law of David Gregory, had been one of Pitcairne's allies and had been ousted from the Edinburgh College with Pitcairne's party.[55] Oliphant claimed in his *Short Discourse* to defend the "Useful Ingenious and Demonstrative Discoveries of a most Learned *Physician*," whose identity remained hidden. Apparently "*Apollo* the *Mathematician*" (or possibly the author of that work, Edward Eizat) had publicly criticized Oliphant's treatment of a fever patient. Oliphant did not mention that the patient subsequently died.[56] Yet such was the confusion engendered by the fever dispute, with the "modern" Pitcairne defending traditional therapeutics against the college, that both sides in the dispute assumed Oliphant attacked them.

The pamphlet debate raged first between Eizat and Oliphant. A further anonymous pamphlet, *An Answer to the Pretended Refutation of Dr Olyphant's Defence*, replied to both of them. It was written by a supporter of Pitcairne, probably either James Johnston, a former Leiden student who wrote several more pamphlets in 1701–2, or George Cheyne.[57] Oliphant did not reply to the *Answer to the Pretended Refutation*, but he was enraged by the next contribution, Cheyne's *New Theory of Fevers*, published anonymously in 1701. For the next two years the controversy raged at its fiercest level, and ad hominem arguments became the rule.

At the end of 1702 Oliphant wrote a long letter to a friend, detailing "that scurvy affair I am engaged in," with particular reference to "this Cheyne." Although he had not met Cheyne, he described him as having "all the Impudence of the North centred in him, he is a big lubbardly fellow, I believe understands the Mathematicks pretty well but knows as little of Medecine as he does of Magick." Cheyne, he said, had been "in Ingliston's family for some years but was dismist for those reasons told in the Answer."[58] This was Oliphant's *Short Answer to Two Lybels Lately Published against D.O. by Drs. Cheyne and Pitcairn*, published in 1702, and the evidence he provided was damning.

During the late 1690s Cheyne was employed as a tutor. Oliphant's reference to "Ingliston" points to Ingliston House outside Edinburgh, the home of Hugh Wallace, writer to the signet and formerly cash keeper to Charles II and James II. The cash keeper was responsible for disbursing government funds, and Wallace received this appointment around 1681–82, a period coinciding with the residence of James Duke of York in Scotland. Wallace's fortunes were tied to those of James. His seat in the Scottish Parliament, held since 1689, was declared vacant in 1693 because he had not signed the oath to William and Mary. Wallace's seat was from a district in the northeast, possibly Aberdeen, and family connections may have been responsible for Cheyne's employment as a tutor in Wallace's household. Wallace had married for a second time in 1678 and could have had an adolescent son to be tutored.[59] He owned land near Ingliston, but did not possess vast estates.[60] Ingliston's proximity to Edinburgh meant that Cheyne could easily participate in the life of the city.

According to Oliphant's account, Cheyne's social life with the hard-drinking Pitcairne resulted in his dismissal from Wallace's employ. Oliphant surmised that Cheyne's otherwise inexplicable hostility to himself must have stemmed from his loss of employment, for which Cheyne held him responsible. Did Oliphant squeal to Wallace about Cheyne's carousing with Pitcairne? According to Oliphant, Pitcairne sent

Cheyne "nightly home Reeling with these nauseous Loads he had burthened himself with to comply with his Patron, and to animat his unwieldy Carcass, which he often, to the scandal of the whole Family, disgorged in his Pupil's Bosom, and gave him of his Cheer what he wanted of his Conversation."[61]

Neither Cheyne nor Pitcairne ever denied this unedifying account. With reference to his works against Oliphant, Cheyne later wrote, "I heartily condemn and detest all personal Reflexions, all malicious and unmannerly Turns, and all false and unjust Representations, as unbecoming Gentlemen, Scholars, and Christians," an acknowledgment of how close to the truth Oliphant trod.[62] In his 1733 autobiography, Cheyne disingenuously wrote, "I passed my *Youth* in close Study, and almost constant application to the *abstracted Sciences* (wherein my chief Pleasure consisted) and consequently in great *Temperence* and a *sedentary Life*; yet not so much but that I sometimes kept *Holiday*, diverted myself with the Works of *Imagination*, and roused *Nature* by agreeable Company and *good Cheer*." He added, "I was near *thirty years* old before I drank scarce any thing strong, at least, for a Continuance."[63]

Yet his life could not have been merely an alcoholic debauch, for during this period—probably while still in Wallace's household—Cheyne wrote his first substantial work, *A New Theory of Fevers*. A mathematically sophisticated defense of Pitcairne's ideas, the *New Theory* was published in London early in 1701. Pitcairne wrote Robert Gray in November 1700, "Yee shall have a new theory of continow'd fevers from this place. When it comes owt I shall write about it. the author—he must not be knowne. I'l answer for its sufficiencie. it will be owt in a month, 5 sheets. Speak not of it, especially to the Oliphant-men."[64] Pitcairne arranged for the book to be printed in Edinburgh, but sent to London for sale. He told Gregory and Gray in February 1701 that three hundred copies had been sent to George Strachan or Strahan, a Scots émigré bookseller who would remain Cheyne's publisher for life.[65] Pitcairne thus brought the debate before the Royal Society, a new and potentially more favorable audience than could be found in Edinburgh.

Cheyne soon followed his book to London. With his disgrace publicly trumpeted by Oliphant, another tutoring position was probably not in

the offing. Controversy, while amusing, was not lucrative, and Cheyne
had no independent source of income. London and medical practice
seemed the next step. Pitcairne arranged for Cheyne to receive a medical
degree from King's College, Aberdeen. King's and Marischal, as well as
the University of St. Andrews, granted medical degrees on the basis of
recommendations from established physicians. As Oliphant commented,
such a degree was "no great tryal of skill," yet it sufficed to enter many
Scots into medical careers, including Cheyne's friend John Arbuthnot.[66]
Undoubtedly on Pitcairne's recommendation, Cheyne was awarded his
degree in September 1701, and the customary fee of sixty pounds Scots
(about five pounds sterling) was waived, according to the degree
proclamation,

because he's not onely our owne countreyman and at present not rich, but is
recommended by the ablest and most learned Physitians in Edinburgh, as one of
the best Mathematicians in Europe and for his skill in Medecine he hath given a
sufficient indication of that by his learned tractat *De Febribus*, which hath made
him famous abroad as well as at home, and he being just now goeing to England
upon invitation from some members of the Royal Society, in all probability he
may prove ane ornament to our Nation as well as to our Society.[67]

With these high hopes on his broad shoulders, and Pitcairne's letter to
Hans Sloane in his baggage, Cheyne boarded the London coach to seek
his fortune.

Cheyne carried with him Pitcairne's hopes and desires as well as his
intellectual legacy. In his writings, he first imitated and then built upon
the natural philosophy of Pitcairne, with its particular social, political,
and religious biases. Cheyne never entirely abandoned this worldview.

Michel Foucault urged that historians distinguish between mechan-
ization, mathematization, and what he called *mathesis* in seventeenth-
century culture. If we take seriously Foucault's contention that the
"fundamental element" of late Baroque culture was *mathesis*, defined as the
use of mathematics as a model for political, social, and physical order,
then the activities of Pitcairne and others during the 1690s can be viewed

as attempts at the realization of this ideal, which encompasses natural history, natural philosophy, and such activities as Newton's work (unpublished in his lifetime) on biblical chronology and the interpretation of the books of Daniel and Revelation.[68] Pitcairne's contribution to this program (aided by Gregory) was his theory of "iatromathematics," which would unify medicine, mathematics, and mechanics into a single system explaining all activities of the human body.[69] Mathematics also carried an important political dimension for Pitcairne.

Gregory, Pitcairne, and Cheyne had especially good reason to be attracted to a mathematical, demonstrative style of natural philosophy rather than an experimental, empirical one.[70] Scots culture was influenced as much by continental, especially French, developments as by English. By the last quarter of the seventeenth century, Cartesian natural philosophy, with its emphasis on mathematical proof and deductive rationalism, formed a prominent part of the curricula of the Scottish universities.[71] To this Cartesian tradition (reinforced by his French medical training) Pitcairne, followed by Cheyne, added his version of Newton's natural philosophy. The resulting "Newtonianism" was one of many such in the disputed territory of London natural philosophy in 1700.

Pitcairne developed his ideas in the late 1680s, while Cheyne was still a student in Aberdeen. In 1687, that critical year for natural philosophy, Pitcairne took rooms with Gregory, beginning a period of intense intellectual activity. While Pitcairne studied the Italian iatromechanists, particularly Giovanni Alfonso Borelli (1608–79) and Lorenzo Bellini (1643–1707), Gregory devoted himself to Newton's *Principia*. He had received a copy soon after its publication in July 1687 and immediately began to write a commentary, the massive *Notae in Isaaci Newtoni Principia*, which he continued to add to for several years. Gregory and Pitcairne drained more than one bottle of red Bordeaux wine in their ensuing discussions.[72]

From both Borelli and Newton, Pitcairne gained the central methodological dictum that the only certain knowledge—certain in the sense of being guaranteed by God—was that obtained by mathematical demonstration. In his *De motu animalium* (1680–81), Borelli followed Descartes's assertion of the "conceptual equivalence" of geometry and physics and argued that his mechanical theory of animal motion was true on the grounds of method. Following "mechanical necessity" was methodologically and epistemologically equivalent to a mathematical demonstration.[73]

Borelli's pupil Bellini published a book of essays in 1683 that included works on secretion and fevers. Bellini's implied precision and his reference to physical laws convinced Pitcairne that this was the sought-after path to mathematized medicine. Gregory brought a further dimension to his "iatromathematics" with his study of Newton, leading Pitcairne to an ideal of a Newtonian medicine along the lines set up by Borelli and Bellini. Borelli's emphasis on mathematics as the foundation of certainty resonated strongly with Pitcairne's bent toward authoritarian politics; the absolute certainty of mathematics paralleled the absolute authority of the divinely anointed monarch. While both Pitcairne and Newton believed that mathematics was true because God-given, Newton did not connect mathematical with political authority. A Whig M.P. in the 1689 Parliament, Newton was no absolutist. His message could be read in many ways, and as Cheyne found, Pitcairne's version soon entered a highly contested battleground for the "true" Newtonianism.[74]

In the fevers dispute, Pitcairne in addition attempted to redefine medical learning in Newtonian terms. In his first published work in 1688, the pamphlet "Solutio problematis de historicis; seu, De inventoribus dissertatio" (Solution of historical problems; or, A dissertation on inventors), Pitcairne already raised those issues of the status and learning of medical men that would be debated in the fevers dispute. He called for replacing the learning of the ancients with his new Newtonian mathematical medicine as the basis for learned, elite practice.[75] Empiricism, he said, was not a viable alternative to Galen. He aimed to show "those who are willing to cultivate Truth and Honour a Way to vindicate themselves from so base a Slavery" as empiricism. Only those gentlemanly practitioners "of better Skill, and who are enflamed with a Desire of attaining higher Arts" need pay him attention; "For the endeavour to bring the Vulgar to the Right, were an Undertaking of a Mad Man."[76]

He had published nothing since the appearance of the *Principia*, but by the early 1690s Isaac Newton was pursuing mathematics, optics, and alchemy with feverish intensity.[77] A small but significant fruit of this labor was the short essay "De natura acidorum." On his way to Leiden in the spring of 1692, Pitcairne visited Newton in Cambridge. Although they had not directly corresponded, Pitcairne was well acquainted with Newton's works through Gregory. During the course of this short visit Newton gave Pitcairne a copy of "De natura acidorum." Pitcairne sent a copy of the essay, with notes of his conversations with Newton, to Gregory.[78] As the first self-proclaimed "Newtonians" to reach prominence, Gregory and Pitcairne marked the beginning of a new intellectual era and the first of many "Newtonianisms."

By the early 1690s, "Newtonianism" had already moved beyond a determination of Newton's own intentions to become a contested territory, a complex and conflicted discourse in which Newton and many others participated. The stakes were high, for those who would be able to impose their definitions of "Newtonianism" and "mathematics" on the language and practice of natural philosophy or medicine would also be able to appropriate the considerable capacity for patronage that, by the early eighteenth century, had accrued to Newton himself and the image of Newtonianism. Thus "Newtonianism" designated no single set of concepts, no single ideology, but a constantly shifting dialogue among many, often conflicting, views of natural philosophy, medicine, religion, and politics.[79]

"De natura acidorum" was for over a decade at the center of the debate about Newton's theories and their contribution to an understanding of the body.[80] Newton's Latin *Opticks*, published in 1706, effectively superseded "De natura acidorum" with its more detailed account of matter theory in query 24 (later renumbered as 31). Pitcairne's and Gregory's acquisition and dissemination of "De natura acidorum" in the 1690s initiated a research program in which they and many of their students participated. R. S. Westfall and B. J. T. Dobbs have each detailed Newton's activities leading up to the composition of "De natura acidorum," and both emphasize the central role played by alchemical studies in the formation of Newton's theory of matter.[81] Pitcairne did not know about this activity, but he seized upon Newton's ideas with alacrity. Cheyne's *Philosophical Principles*, published in 1705, relied heavily on "De natura acidorum" and Pitcairne's interpretation of it.

A short and abrupt document, "De natura acidorum" established several tenets of Newton's theory of matter. He combined the corpuscularian chemistry of Boyle, which incorporated a hierarchical arrangement of matter, with the older "chymistry" of specific substances or principles. To this amalgam he added the crucial concept of a short-range attractive force analogous but not identical to gravity. Acids, assuming the role played by the alchemical sulfur, acted as the bearers of this force and the origin of chemical activity. All substances were composed of acid and earthy parts—the alchemical sulfur and mercury—in a hierarchical arrangement of increasing complexity. By this argument, transmutation was indeed possible, but it would not be a simple task.[82]

Pitcairne's conversations with Newton in March 1692, notes of which he appended to the manuscript, elicited further details on the hierarchical arrangement of matter and on some points in physiology such as the secretion of urine.[83] A few days after this meeting, Gregory delivered his theses at Oxford for his M.D. degree, preparatory to assuming the Savilian chair of astronomy. Perhaps referring to these theses, Gregory wrote in his memoranda,

if it be necessary that I emitt Theses at Act. I am resolved to have them de secretione Animali. and for that Cause to look over Wharton de glandulis, Coles de secretione Animali, Bayle, and Willis if they have written any thing or any thing thats newer, to destroy the parts indifferently figured as naively geometrical and either to establish the mutual attraction of homogeneous Bodys, or the meer different bigness of pores and for the ancient termes to read Senerti institutiones medicinae.[84]

In the event, Gregory perhaps decided that such a task was too arduous. He drew the theses he submitted from his Edinburgh lectures on optics and only mentioned secretion in their opening sentences, as a topic amenable to geometrical analysis.[85]

Gregory's memorandum succinctly outlined Pitcairne's ideas about the body, upon which Cheyne later relied. Glandular secretion was a prototypical mechanical theme. A month after Gregory's theses, secretion figured prominently in Pitcairne's inaugural lecture at Leiden. He called the interpretation of secretion the predominant error of current medical thinking, an error based on faulty scientific method. He also rejected the search for ultimate causes pursued by "philosophical sects": "our Knowledge of Things is confined to the Relations they bear to one another, and the Laws and Properties of Powers, which enable them to produce Changes in some things, and to become altered by other things." Were these "Powers" (*vires*) forces such as Newton's gravity and the interparticulate force described in "De natura acidorum"? Like Newton, Pitcairne's concern was the effects of the "Powers," not their causes.[86] He continued,

> it [is not] unreasonable to suppose, that lesser Bodies, which are the Objects of Medical Enquiries, are subject to the same Laws that Astronomers have discovered in the Greater. The Nature of all Bodies is certainly the same, and every Body is capable of being changed into the Body of another of any Kind whatsoever; and by consequence all Bodies, of whatsoever Magnitude or Minuteness, are liable to the common Effects of Motion, or Change.[87]

He here cited three principal elements of Newton's theory of matter: the analogy of the microcosm to the macrocosm, the possibility of limitless transmutation, and the inertness of matter, which was independent of force and activity.[88] In this lecture he did not mention Newton by name or the concept of attraction, perhaps because to physicians, this name did not yet hold much significance.

On the basis of the method he outlined, Pitcairne went on to reject every current physiological concept. The "infamous Mark of *Uncertainty*," he promised, was about to be removed from medicine for good; nor would "the Honour of our Profession" lay anymore at "the Mercy of the Vulgar." The exact science of mathematics, rather than vague iatromechanism or empiricism, would form the basis of medicine.[89]

Pitcairne's inflammatory lecture was received with great applause at Leiden; on the same day, the university governors voted to increase his salary.[90] He wasted no time in fulfilling his promise to place medicine on the track of scientific respectability. In a series of "dissertations" presented and published in Leiden in 1693, he presented his new "iatromathematics," defined as a Newtonian, fully mathematized physiology of forces. These dissertations were "exercitii gratia," staged performances at which selected students responded to the master's exposition. They supplemented the lectures Pitcairne read as professor, and unlike those lectures, the dissertations were immediately rushed into print.[91]

In his dissertations Pitcairne presented mathematics as the only certain method for dealing with submicroscopic entities, such as the unobserved and, in contemporary conditions, unobservable particles of the blood. He asserted, "And this Simplicity, and those few *Postulata's* which distinguish our Hypothesis, is a genuine Evidence of that Truth, which the Greatest and Best Geometrician has been pleased to affix to it." The greatest and best geometrician was God, but he also mentioned Newton a few lines later. He attributed to Newton the "geometrical method" of the first "Hypothesis" of the *Principia*: to admit no more causes than such as are both true and sufficient. Even attractive forces could be an unnecessary multiplication of entities.[92]

In this essay, Pitcairne demonstrated his mechanical theory of secretion with numerical proportions but not actual quantities.[93] Had he adhered strictly to his own dictum—that only mathematical statements are possible about invisible entities—he could not have said anything about actual animal structure or function. He did not have, nor could he acquire, enough concrete, quantifiable data to fill in his new system of "iatromathematics." While both Pitcairne and Newton assumed an analogy between the macrocosm and the microcosm, atoms could not be observed as could planets. In "De natura acidorum" Newton's very general statements about the submicroscopic world could not be pressed beyond the most elementary level without flying off into speculation.

Pitcairne believed that his description of the human body in the Leiden dissertations was not merely probable but true, since, following Borelli, he demonstrated a "mechanical necessity" by a "mathematical method." He believed that he followed Newton in describing a world that reified the ideal world of mathematics and was therefore not merely a hypothesis. Cheyne later drew out the consequences of the Platonism implicit in this belief.[94]

The truth of Pitcairne's conclusions was moreover guaranteed by God, who had created a world of geometrical proportion and symmetry. The same God who sanctioned the divine right of kings gave the mathematician the priestly role of interpreting his creation to those without learning; the ignorant Presbyterians Pitcairne had satirized in *The Assembly* could not serve in this capacity. Mathematics, as Plato had visualized, served as the intermediary between God and nature. Pitcairne's and Cheyne's friend John Craig, influenced by Locke, similarly valued Newtonian method for its power of "deductive demonstration." His *Mathematical Principles of Christian Theology* (1699) conceptually linked Newton's natural philosophy to theology in a manner Cheyne would imitate in his *Philosophical Principles.*[95]

Pitcairne's statutory lectures as professor at Leiden reiterated the themes of his dissertations. Although these lectures were copied by more than one generation of students, they were published only in 1717 as *Elementa medicinae.*[96] Unlike other mechanists, and like Newton, Pitcairne rejected the existence of an ether, although Newton later revived this idea in the "General Scholium" to the second edition of the *Principia*, which appeared in 1713, the year of Pitcairne's death. Pitcairne urged his students to study mathematics and dismissed Cartesian mechanism.[97]

But Pitcairne did not fully endorse Newton in Descartes's place. Attractions had no role in his mechanistic scheme. In his self-appointed role as Harvey's heir, Pitcairne turned to the heartbeat—the cause of circulation—as his central mechanism. The body was composed of "*Canals* and *Fluids*," and the hydraulics of this arrangement provided the proper realm of physic.[98] While Pitcairne drew his underlying metaphor from astronomy, he drew an analogy between gravity and the heartbeat, not, as Newton had in "De natura acidorum," between gravity and local, short-range attractions. Andrew Cunningham has suggested that Pitcairne's politics formed another facet of this analogy. The absolute monarch upon whom the life of the state depended in Jacobite political theory had long been compared to the sun. In his dedicatory letter to Charles I prefaced to *De motu cordis*, Harvey—a royal physician and a royalist in the English civil war—had compared the king to both the sun and the heart. Moreover, the heartbeat, gravity, and the power of the hereditary monarch all came directly from God.[99]

Pitcairne derived function from structure, and from function he derived design. In the circulation of the blood and the motion of the heart he found evidence of divine intervention much as had Newton in his account of gravity.[100] Newton explained planetary motion in a 1693 letter to Richard Bentley: "So then gravity may put ye planets into motion but without ye divine power it could never put them into such a Circulating motion as they have about ye Sun, & therefore for this as well as other reasons I am compelled to ascribe ye frame of this Systeme to an intelligent agent."[101]

Although Pitcairne could not have seen this letter, he may have read Bentley's last Boyle lecture, published in May 1693, which expounded the same theme. A year later Pitcairne wrote to his friend Robert Gray, "I have desired Gregorie to procure me a scheme of Mr Neuton's divine thoughts (I hope yee'll not laugh) that I may write a demonstration for our religion: but this will be a tale of two drinks. I am confident tho that better things may be said to that purpose than hitherto has been said." He added in a postscript, "I am serious in seeking an account of Mr Neuton's thoughts anent differences in religion, for I am truly resolved to doe something that way."[102]

Pitcairne knew of Newton's notions of the original religion and how this had disintegrated into sects. In May 1694 Gregory followed Pitcairne's footsteps to Newton's rooms and took notes of their conversations on the origins of religions. According to Newton, the beginning of religion and the beginning of natural philosophy were one and the same. The most ancient natural philosophy was heliocentrist and "observed the gravitation of all bodies towards all," and the original religion was based on the worship of a single God represented by a central fire. The original temples were modeled on the structure of the heavens. Newton argued therefore that his natural philosophy was simply a rediscovery of the true natural philosophy. In his many manuscripts on theology, he attempted to perform the same feat of rediscovery for the true religion.[103]

In both natural philosophy and religion he sought historical sanction for his modern practice. In natural philosophy he sought to show that gravitation and the Copernican system had in fact been known by the ancients, the *prisci theologi*, but that this knowledge had been obscured by subsequent commentators. He sought the historical origins of Christianity to demonstrate that the doctrine of the Trinity was a theological aberration, and that the true church, as Protestants had been arguing for nearly two centuries, had been corrupted.[104]

In his inaugural lecture at Leiden, Pitcairne had argued that mathematical method was valid because it was the most ancient method. Like Newton, Pitcairne claimed that astronomy was the first science, and ancient physicians and philosophers both employed its "Method of Reasoning." Medicine, indeed, was prior to all philosophy, and the practice of physic became corrupted when it was exposed to philosophical "sects" and neglected proper mathematical reasoning. Pitcairne drew forcefully the parallel to the religious sectarianism of his own day: philosophical sectarianism could lead only to a "Tyranny" over reason and "the most insolent internal Slavery."[105]

In this way Pitcairne justified his claim that only from mathematical method could a physician derive true statements about the body and its functions. In Newton's theogony, natural philosophy and true religion were the same thing, and its truth was guaranteed by God. To Pitcairne, true government, true religion, and true learning all depended upon the single God-given authority of mathematics. *Mathesis* was the governing principle of the universe. However widely they diverged in practice, Pitcairne and Newton thus agreed strongly in principle.

Most historians of science have presented physics and astronomy as the model sciences of the Scientific Revolution. Thomas Kuhn has argued further that physical sciences may be divided into "classical" and "Baconian" traditions, the former highly mathematical and the latter more qualitative and experimental.[106] While this distinction may be valid for the end of the eighteenth century, it is not as useful a description for the early years of the century as Foucault's term *mathesis*, which includes activities that we now do not consider "scientific." Under this definition, Pitcairne's use of mathematical method in medicine, Newtonian physics, and the impulse to collect, name, and classify the productions of man and nature can be viewed as facets of the same cultural imperative. As Simon Schaffer has urged, natural philosophy was a "prescientific" activity.[107]

Like Newton, Pitcairne saw theology as the indispensable anchor of natural philosophy and religious practice as the essential glue of society.[108] In the face of the dual threats of atheism and enthusiasm, the search led by Newton for the origins of the true church was not mere antiquarianism but a search for the vital underpinnings of a society in peril. If knowledge was to remain entire and not fragment into "atomies" as John Donne had feared a century earlier, theology, natural history, and natural philosophy had all to take their rightful places within it. Nothing less than the coherence and stability of society were at stake.[109]

Their program crossed political boundaries and doctrinal lines to confront the common enemy of fanaticism, whether atheistic or enthusiastic. At the turn of the century, the Tory apprehension of a church in danger found assent across a wide swath of society. If Newton's cry was "no popery," then the ignorant mob feared by Pitcairne was Presbyterian, and the Gardens in Aberdeen similarly feared the Covenanting zealots.[110] In *The Assembly* Pitcairne had declared mathematics to be the key to certain knowledge and therefore to social stability. Newton went another step: mathematics could provide the key to God's plan for the world, as it could provide the key to alchemy. John Craig followed this idea to one logical conclusion. In his *Theologia christianae principia mathematica* (1699) he produced a *Principia* of theology, calculating the time of the Second Coming—a calculation in which Newton also engaged himself. As we have seen, against the millenarian tide, Craig placed that time far in the future.[111] Two years later, Cheyne entered a London scene that included individuals with considerably less moderate expectations.

3

THE PURSUIT OF FAME

In its sprawling dimensions, from the broad new streets and squares of its West End to the docks of Rotherhithe, London offered a distinct contrast to the austere gray granite of Aberdeen, and to medieval Edinburgh with its cramped and winding streets, where, reported Defoe, "in no [other] city in the world [do] so many people live in so little room."[1] The largest city in Europe and by far the largest city in Britain, London was the center of political, economic, and cultural life, a magnet for the poor, the ambitious, the gentry, the dispossessed. "London," wrote the chronicler Thomas Brown, "is a World by it self."[2]

Its importance increased dramatically around 1700. The founding of the Bank of England in 1694, the financing of King William's War, and the continued growth of foreign, domestic, and colonial trade made London the indisputable locus of wealth and power.[3] The web of finance and politics, of parliament, court, and church, grew ever more tangled as the century turned, and kept politicians as well as financiers close to London's newspapers and its centers of gossip, the coffeehouses.[4]

Even before the union of the Scottish and English Parliaments in 1707, London lured Scottish politicians with its scent of power. Lady Roxburghe complained in the 1690s that her father, Lord Tweeddale, having spent three consecutive years in London, was neglecting his family and estates. Her son, the earl of Roxburghe, followed his grandfather's example and left his mother to manage the family holdings.[5]

Above all, London consumed. Into its great maw poured the fruits of English agriculture, manufacture, and trade. According to the contemporary observer Ned Ward, its inhabitants consumed entertainments, from prizefighting to the theater, with the same intensity they devoted to politics or commerce.[6] Defoe likened London to England's heart, drawing in nourishment and then pumping it out again for the benefit of the nation.[7] The post-Restoration growth of national wealth centered on London; its shopkeepers and innkeepers, and even its servants and laborers, were much better off than their provincial counterparts. London inspired a new upper class whose wealth derived from trade and not land, whose focus fixed on the city and not the country. At the same time, the "middling sort" of merchants and traders, those "petty capitalists" once defined by the guild, were growing enormously in numbers, wealth, and influence.[8]

London society appeared far more open to a newcomer than the provinces. Gregory King's multiple steps of rank seemed easily scaled when merchant and gentry, poet and preacher jostled one another in the coffeehouses. The entrepreneurial and the energetic might succeed on their own, but patronage still greased the wheels, and London in 1700 was hardly a meritocracy. As the center of wealth and power, the city was preeminently the center of patronage.[9]

London loomed large on the mental horizon of the aspiring natural philosopher in 1700. There he could seek patrons for one of the scarce fellowships at Oxford or Cambridge or for an ill-paying curacy in a remote village. Increasingly, London became an end in itself. The peculiar mix of learned scholars and wealthy dilettantes at the Royal Society pointed to potential sources of employment outside both university and church. Both the improving middle ranks and the leisured gentry of London supported natural philosophy, whether as names on a subscription list or as students of such enterprising men as John Harris, who conducted a lecture and demonstration course at a coffeehouse.[10]

Many natural philosophers were, like Cheyne, also physicians, and sought in London both a medical practice and intellectual recognition. The court, the London season, and the commercial exchanges kept the wealthiest patients in the capital for at least part of the year. Only in London could one attain the fabulous success of Dr. John Radcliffe, whose wealth at his death in 1714 exceeded eighty thousand pounds, in an era when one hundred pounds per year was an adequate middle-class income.[11] Radcliffe and his colleagues such as Hans Sloane acted as patrons of younger physicians, to whom they provided introductions and referred patients.

George Cheyne's move to London was practically inevitable, and he followed a long line of Scots in this migration. Scotland's economy could not support its intellectuals. In the 1690s economic depression descended, exacerbated by the collapse of the ill-fated Darien colony in 1700.[12] The continuing stream of Scots medical graduates of French and Dutch universities showed no sign of abating, and the large numbers of surgeons who emerged from apprenticeship could not be absorbed by a country whose population barely topped one million.[13]

The political and religious consequences of 1689 in Scotland accelerated the long-standing brain drain to the south. David Gregory had moved to Oxford in 1692, and a number of Episcopalian physicians and natural philosophers, many of them connected with him or Pitcairne, followed in his wake. Gregory's student John Keill, a mathematician, accompanied him to Oxford. Keill's brother James and Pitcairne's brother David, both physicians, soon joined them. Gregory's friend John Arbuthnot, son of an ejected Episcopalian minister, moved to London in 1692, and Pitcairne's Leiden student William Cockburn followed. George Hepburn, one of Pitcairne's bulldogs in the fevers dispute, made the journey south at the turn of the century, as did Cheyne. Charles Oliphant succumbed to the blandishments of London and his patron, the duke of Argyll, arriving in London in 1708.[14]

London medical practice reflected the new pressures on traditional society. The development of capitalism and of market behaviors, the growth of an affluent middle rank, the "urban renaissance" all influenced the organization of medical practice. The traditional hierarchies epitomized by the Royal College of Physicians of London gave way to a more open system as the distinctions, never clear-cut, between physicians, surgeons, and apothecaries faded. The historic functions of the College of Physicians as a regulatory body for medicine as a whole and as a privileged professional organization of physicians were disappearing. After the Restoration, the College's influence waned against the intellectual competition of the Royal Society and an onslaught of competing practitioners. The expiration in 1695 of the Licensing Act effectively ended the College's censorship of medical books, while the Rose decision in 1703, which legitimized the de facto medical practice of the apothecaries in London, dealt a fatal blow to the College's regulatory function.[15]

The increasing numbers of the populace who could pay for medical attention could choose from a broad range of healers at the turn of the eighteenth century, from collegiate physicians to illiterate herb sellers. Far from dictating the bounds of medical practice, members of the College competed with a welter of healers. The entry of Scots physicians onto the scene only exacerbated this competition, for they could claim similar social status and—with their continental educations—perhaps superior knowledge to the English physicians.

Learning, in the classics or more lately in the new philosophy, had long been part of the university-educated physician's bag of tools, differentiating him from other practitioners. The London College of Physicians enforced these distinctions by restricting its fellowships to men with degrees from Oxford or Cambridge who could moreover afford its hefty entrance fees. This policy was relaxed somewhat by the end of the seventeenth century to accommodate royal physicians and other celebrated practitioners. The College's licensing of licentiates was somewhat less restrictive but confined to those whom the College deemed worthy in learning.[16] As we have seen, in the second half of the century Galenist physicians debated the followers of the new mechanical philosophy over matters of medical theory. Since the College's standing as an intellectual body was being challenged by the Royal Society, while at the same time its regulatory function was being put to the test, the outcome of this debate was central to the College's very survival. By 1700 the mechanical ideas of the new philosophy were firmly ensconced as the College's official dogma.[17] But "iatromechanism" covered a wide range of opinion, and the Edinburgh fevers dispute, in which both sides claimed mechanical knowledge, demonstrated instead the tension between different methodological models for deriving therapy: "Baconian" empiricism and induction versus Pitcairne's deductive, "mathematical" approach.

In their practice, most British physicians, with the notable exception of Pitcairne, paid at least lip service to Thomas Sydenham, the "English Hippocrates," who had declared himself the least theoretical of physicians.

Although Sydenham claimed simply to describe symptoms, he in fact often assumed the guise of a learned physician and attributed causes as well.[18] Sydenham's successors stretched his mantle very far, to cover such self-consciously "Baconian" practitioners as Andrew Brown. In the highly competitive atmosphere of London medicine, however, mere empiricism was not enough. While John Radcliffe owed his success to his effective bedside manner, he bequeathed his lucrative London practice to Richard Mead, who had made his name as a natural philosopher, with several treatises applying Newtonian theory to medical problems.[19]

One model of the successful Scots medical migrant was David Hamilton (1663–1721). The youngest son of a landowner, Hamilton graduated M.D. from Rheims. Migrating to London, he took the examination for the license of the College of Physicians. Hamilton devoted his rapidly growing practice to midwifery, an increasingly popular subspecialty. Queen Anne, whose own obstetrical problems were well known, knighted Hamilton in 1703; the College of Physicians recognized this distinction by naming him a fellow. He served Queen Anne as physician and confidante until her death in 1714.[20]

Hamilton had written his M.D. thesis on hysteria, and he ministered to Queen Anne not as an *accoucheur* or man-midwife, but as a "female doctor," a rubric covering a wide range of maladies. The queen's chief ailments by 1708 consisted of gout and "the vapors," which Hamilton defined as "a sinking of Spirits, and weakness of the Nerves." Radcliffe had earlier declared "That Her Highness's Distemper was nothing but the Vapours, & that she was in as good a state of Health as any woman breathing, could she but give into the Belief of it." Anne had promptly dismissed him.[21] Hamilton's greater sympathy earned him the queen's gratitude and trust. He attributed her case to a combination of physical illness and mental distress, and as his diary illustrates, much of his therapy consisted of conversation with her. The lesson of his success was not lost upon George Cheyne.

The varying career paths taken by three Scots of the post-1689 generation—John Arbuthnot, William Cockburn, and George Cheyne—demonstrate the increasing fluidity of London medical practice by 1700. John Arbuthnot (1667–1735) is remembered less as a physician than as a wit.[22] But he too served Queen Anne, and the government called upon his medical expertise during the plague panic of 1720–21. Four years after he graduated from Marischal College in 1685, his father lost his parish for refusing the Presbyterian oaths. His sons dispersed in the early 1690s: Robert followed the deposed King James to Paris, while John went to London, supporting himself as a mathematics tutor.

Intermittent tutoring, as Cheyne also found, was neither fulfilling nor lucrative, and in 1694 Arbuthnot obtained more regular employment when he entered University College, Oxford, as companion to the young and wealthy Edward Jeffreys. While Arbuthnot was still a tutor, this position, unlike his employment in London, gave him both a clear status and access to patronage. Arbuthnot did not pursue any particular course of study, but he made a number of important friends and connections, among them Arthur Charlett, the Tory master of University College. Arbuthnot's interest in mathematics naturally drew him to his fellow Scot David Gregory, and these three remained in close correspondence.

Edward Jeffreys left Oxford in 1696, and Arbuthnot, "resolved on some other course of life," decided to go into medicine.[23] Through the Jeffreys family he had met John Radcliffe, whose success could not have passed unnoticed. In 1696, at the age of twenty-nine, Arbuthnot took a degree in medicine from the University of St. Andrews. Within three months he prepared his theses and defended them before "solemn meetings of several Professors and Doctors of Medicine."[24] The topic of his theses, animal secretion, suggests Gregory's influence. Pitcairne protested to the university about the brevity of Arbuthnot's residence there and its acceptance of the recommendation of Dr. Thomas Burnet, an enemy from the Edinburgh College of Physicians, "who knows not Mr Arbuthnot" and in addition is an "ill-natur'd and ignorant curr."[25]

Armed with his degree and his new connections, Arbuthnot returned to London. By the following year he had entered the scholarly lists with his criticism of John Woodward's *Essay toward a Natural History of the Earth* (1695).[26] Arbuthnot's *Examination of Dr. Woodward's Account of the Deluge* brought him to the attention of the London scientific community. Perhaps also from Arbuthnot's pen came the *Essay on the Usefulness of Mathematical Learning*, published in 1701.[27] The *Essay* displayed Gregory's influence, who was at the time promoting the teaching of mathematics at Oxford. The *Essay* recommended mathematical study for its training of the mind in logical and objective thinking, as well as for its usefulness to a wide range of practical arts, including medicine. Once more the ideal of *mathesis*, of mathematics as a model for an ordered world, emerges.[28]

By the turn of the century Arbuthnot had built a medical practice as well as a circle of friends among the Tory intellectuals of London and Oxford: Humphrey Wanley, a Charlett protégé, described a 1698 dinner at the home of Samuel Pepys, whose guests included among others Henry Aldrich, Gregory, Arbuthnot, and Thomas Smith.[29] He distinguished himself from the mass of physicians surrounding Queen Anne by his chance cure of her husband, Prince George of Denmark, and was named one of the Royal Physicians Extraordinary in 1705. He had already been elected a fellow of the Royal Society.

William Cockburn (1669–1739), younger son of a Highland baronet, graduated from the University of Edinburgh and later studied in Leiden with Pitcairne, to whom he referred as "the great Ornament and Improver of our Northern Physick."[30] In 1693 he published in London an unauthorized translation of *De morbis acutis infantum* by Walter Harris. Cockburn dedicated his translation to the countess of Roxburghe, alluding to his "own particular Ties" to her.[31] Soon after, he, like Hamilton, took the examination for the license of the London College of Physicians, and the Admiralty Board chose him as one of its fleet physicians.[32] Such an appointment was a plum for a young doctor, and Cockburn must have had a powerful patron, possibly Lady Roxburghe's father, the marquis of Tweeddale, a privy councilor.

While he ministered to the fleet, Cockburn also sought to establish his authority as a learned practitioner. In his introduction to Harris's work he had defended the use of "Philosophy, h.e. [hic est] best informed Reason," in medicine against those mere empirics who "teach how to become Physicians by practising."[33] In his next two works, *Oeconomia corporis animalis* (1695) and *An Account of the Nature, Causes, Symptoms and Cure of the Distempers That Are Incident to Seafaring People* (1696, commonly known as *Sea Diseases*), Cockburn appealed to two constituencies: the navy, which valued practical results, and the upper-class public, who desired a learned consultant. In *Sea Diseases* he discussed practical therapies for seamen in the context of a fever theory that closely followed Pitcairne's recently published *De curatione febrium*.[34] The Royal Society affirmed his scientific credentials by naming him a fellow in 1696.

Cockburn attained medical success, however, by inventing a patent medicine, his "electuary," a specific for dysentery and other "loosenesses." Trials conducted among his patients in the fleet confirmed its efficacy, and the Admiralty promoted its use. Cockburn kept the formula a secret and made from it a vast fortune.[35] He attempted to distance himself from quack curemongers by obtaining an M.D. from King's College, Aberdeen, in 1697, but the London College remained unimpressed.[36]

Cockburn had already made his support of Pitcairne's "iatromathematics" clear in a paper he delivered to the Royal Society in 1699, "A Discourse of the Operation of a Blister When It Cures a Fever." By presenting this paper before the Royal Society rather than the College of Physicians, Cockburn acknowledged his strained relations with the College over the "electuary." He also brought the Edinburgh fevers dispute before an audience potentially more sympathetic to the "mathematical" approach. The "Discourse" was immediately published in the *Philosophical Transactions*. Cheyne and Pitcairne followed Cockburn's example, presenting the next phase of the fevers dispute, Cheyne's *New Theory of Continual Fevers*, before the Royal Society. In the larger picture, this is one more example of the dispersion of medical authority, which resided in no single institution, whether university, College of Physicians, or Royal Society, beyond the printed page. The Royal Society acted as one agent of the diffusion of power amid the chaos of medical practice.[37]

The practice of natural philosophy in Britain, like the practice of medicine or law, entailed membership in a group defined by special competence: a status group. Natural philosophy was not, in 1700, a profession from which one could make a living or even share common grounds and goals with other practitioners. "Natural philosophy" signified no single set of practices, and the Royal Society provided only the loosest of institutional frameworks.[38] As was true of other social groups, membership in the Royal Society had its basis less in a generally agreed-upon notion of merit than in rank and education; Michael Hunter has described the Society as "a high-class intellectual social club."[39] A non-university-educated "mechanic" such as Thomas Savery might be asked to demonstrate his ingenious steam engine before the Society, but he was not made a fellow. The organization of natural philosophy, like society itself, possessed many of the characteristics of a "court society," in which advance depended on membership in, and the patronage of, a particular status group that was itself hierarchically organized. Despite the inroads of market behaviors in this period, these traditional forms of social organization persisted.[40]

Although the Royal Society provided an institutional setting for scientific practice in London,[41] that practice in the 1690s appeared to be flagging badly. The ambitious experiments of the 1660s and 1670s had dwindled by the 1680s, and the *Philosophical Transactions* ceased publication in 1687. Even when the new secretary, Hans Sloane, resurrected the journal in 1691, its contents remained at the level of curiosities and antiquities, easily satirized by the author of *The Transactioneer* in 1700.[42] The secretary provided the strongest influence on the tone and day-to-day activities of the Society when presidents were chosen for their political rather than their intellectual value.[43] Natural history, antiquities, and anatomy reflected Sloane's own interests and those of many younger members such as John Woodward and the naturalist-apothecary James Petiver. Moreover, it accurately reflected the tone of learned culture in general.

Although the Royal Society's numbers declined from the 1660s, the proportion of members who were active was high, and from the mid-1690s recruitment increased. New recruits in 1696 included Woodward, Petiver, the natural philosopher John Harris, the anatomist William Cowper, and the physician John Hutton.[44] At the end of the decade, the members attempted to revitalize the Society's meetings, with regular programs of "Experiments or Observations in Natural knowledge," "observations" including the reading of reports of research by others.[45] As David Miller has recently suggested, the eighteenth-century Society's emphasis on reportage rather than research continued a central activity of the early Society; Steven Shapin has also pointed out that "the weekly meetings of the Royal Society required not trials but shows and discourses."[46] Hardly a moribund Society awaiting Newton's reviving touch, the Society Cheyne entered included active intellectuals who did not accept his pronouncements unquestioningly, no matter how closely he stood to Newton. In 1700 the triumph of "Newtonianism" was not yet a foregone conclusion; indeed, the definition of "Newtonianism" and of natural philosophy itself was fiercely contested.

The time was ripe for an intellectual take-off. In contrast to the Restoration, when the government strongly suppressed dissent, expression was much less restricted in the late 1690s. The Licensing Act was allowed to lapse in 1695, ending government censorship of the press. A flood of pamphlets, newspapers, and books followed. Already dominant in the book trade, London soon spawned the new industry of Grub Street. George Strahan, Cheyne's publisher, who like him had emigrated from Scotland around 1700, was one of a burgeoning number of printers and publishers.[47]

In 1696 Newton gave up his Cambridge professorship and moved to London to become warden of the mint, a position attained through the patronage of his friend and former student Charles Montagu, a Whig politician and president of the Royal Society. While not yet the "autocrat of science" he later became, Newton's reputation was sufficient to attract disciples from among the young natural philosophers coming of age in the 1690s. William Whiston later vividly described the heady atmosphere among those who were aware of "those sublime Discoveries which were then almost a Secret to all, but to a few particular Mathematicians."[48]

With knowledge came power. David Gregory had already used Newton's patronage to help win the Savilian chair of astronomy at Oxford in 1691; Newton may also have been among those who chose Richard Bentley as the first Boyle lecturer in 1692. As Warden, he placed his friend Edmond Halley in a post at the Chester mint.[49] Clearly, Newton was a man worth knowing.

Addison's *Spectator* complained in 1711 that medicine was "over-burdened with Practitioners, and filled with Multitudes of Ingenious Gentlemen that starve one another."[50] In 1722 John Woodward's satirical pamphlet *The Art of Getting into Practice in Physick, Here at Present in London* addressed the issue of competition, especially among "foreign Graduates and Country Physicians." He wrote,

And now as you are just arriv'd in Town, without having had the Benefit of establishing an Acquaintance at *Oxford* or *Cambridge* among the Nobility, Clergy &c. and an absolute Stranger here. . . . The first Thing then I am to advise you just now upon your Arrival, is to make all the Noise and Bustle you can, to make the whole Town ring of you if possible: So that every one in it may know, that there is in Being, and here in Town too, such a Physician.[51]

An anonymous commentator complained that the Royal Society was being overrun by "several young Physitians" whose "End was only to get a name for Extraordinary Men and procure a being taken Notice off [*sic*] and a large acquaintance for the increase of their particular Practice and advantage they give over participation."[52] Bernard Mandeville recommended that a budding physician "shew your self a Scholar, write a Poem, either a good one, or a long one; Compose a *Latin* Oration, or do but Translate something out of that Language with your Name on it. If you can do none of all these, Marry into a good Family."[53]

No poet, Cheyne chose the path of scholarship. He disingenuously declared in the preface to his *New Theory of Fevers*, "I neither expect nor desire any Reputation from these Papers." But his authorship, thanks to Pitcairne, was an open secret. The *New Theory* was an extraordinarily ambitious document, by which Cheyne intended to recast medical theory and practice. More immediately, he redefined the fevers debate: where Pitcairne had referred vaguely to mathematics, Cheyne appealed specifically to Newton, underpinning Pitcairne's assertion of certain rather than probable knowledge. He directed his treatise as much to physicists as to physicians, as much to the Royal Society as to the London College of Physicians. Who else would possess "the necessary Qualifications, of a moderate Attention, and a smattering of the Mathematicks" required to understand the text?[54] The *New Theory* was not for the faint-hearted; its "mathematical" format of postulates, lemmas, and scholia mimicked Newton's *Principia* as well as the more recent *Mathematical Principles of*

Christian Theology of his friend John Craig, and Cheyne immediately plunged the reader into geometrical demonstration.

Cheyne's opening "postulata" flatly asserted, "this Machine we carry about, is nothing but an Infinity of Branching and Winding Canals, fill'd with Liquors of different Natures."[55] Cheyne defined "postulata" not as hypotheses but, as John Harris defined them in 1704, "such easie and self-evident Suppositions as need no Explication or Illustration to render them Intelligible."[56] His second postulate extended the machine analogy: if the adjustment of a "particular Part" righted a "disordered" machine, then one may justly assume that the disorder lay in that part: a mechanical restatement of Newton's third hypothesis. At the outset, therefore, Cheyne claimed to be able to find the causes of disease—the mark of the rational or "philosophical" physician—and not simply to describe symptoms and signs.[57]

He demonstrated geometrically the quantity of fluid flowing through a canal in a given time to support Pitcairne's contention that a disturbance in the circulation caused a fever.[58] Pitcairne had hypothesized that an obstruction in the glands would cause the same effects on the blood vessels as if the quantity of blood was itself augmented or diminished, and could be calculated accordingly. Cheyne's elaborate proofs—which dealt with proportions, not absolute quantities—led to his "general proposition" echoing Pitcairne: "The general and most effectual Cause of all Fevers, is the Obstruction or Dilatation of . . . the Glands." This obstruction of the glands in continual fevers "will necessarily augment the Quantity of the Blood and Liquidum Nervorum."[59] He went on to explain the various symptoms of a continual fever in terms of suppressed secretions.[60] His theory could account for all symptoms of fever, a "considerable Argument" in its favor; and "the ceasing and dissolution of Fevers by Purging, Sweating, Vomiting, and Abscesses, is wonderfully accounted for from this Theory." Cheyne did not recognize that this conclusion amounted to begging the question, and he supported it with an uncritical mixture of secondhand evidence. He himself obtained no experimental proof and did not seek anatomical confirmation for his claims, and his work was devoid of even Pitcairne's minimal anatomical demonstration.

Cheyne described the critical function of secretion within the frame-work set up by Bellini and Pitcairne, but with the vocabulary of Newtonian physics, though in Cheyne's typically verbose style:

Separation or Secretion is perform'd by the Composition of two Motions in the Fluid; one propagated through the Length of the Canal; another transversely through its Sides. . . . in a mixt Fluid, consisting of greater and lesser Cohesion of Parts . . . That which has the least cohesion and greatest Fluidity, is first separated (i.e. separated in the *Glands*, whose compounding *Artery* is shortest, or at least Distance from the Heart, or Foundation of Motion) And these of the next Cohesion, and next greatest Fluidity is next separated; and so on: The Distances from the Heart being in a compounded Proportion of these. . . . The Quantity separated in every *Gland*, is in a compound Proportion of the Celerity of the Fluid at the Respective Orifices; and of the Orifices themselves, of the separating Canals.[61]

Here was Pitcairne's ideal of "iatromathematics," mathematized physi-ology; one needed simply to insert the numbers. The cohesion of the fluid particles was presumably a Newtonian chemical cohesion as in "De natura acidorum." To Pitcairne's references to the laws of hydraulics Cheyne added the apparently telling detail: "the Insertion of the separating canal ought to be at an Angle of 45 degrees with the *Artery*." He recommended to his readers the "admirable Book" of that "great Man" Newton, a book con-taining a "vast number" of "most Charming and useful Truths." Few of Cheyne's medical brethren so appreciated the *Principia's* charms.[62]

After a discussion as long and convoluted as the glands he described, Cheyne concluded, along with most other practitioners, that vomiting and sweating, preceded by copious bleeding, were the proper cures for fever. As the quotation above illustrates, he narrated the body's struggle with fever in deliberately difficult "mathematical" language. But the denouement was not new. The bad matter that caused the fever had to be eliminated in some way. Nor was the mathematics so forbidding. While Cheyne sprinkled his text with calculations and geometrical diagrams, his descriptive account employed no real quantities. For example, he deter-mined the operation of mercurial medicines in a fever by a chain of reasoning based on a series of proportions and estimates rather than exact quantities.[63] Cheyne wrote in English rather than Latin to reach a wider audience of potential patients, but his youthful brashness overcame his desire to be understood. The *New Theory* was a difficult book, and professional success did not follow on its heels.

Cheyne may not have demonstrated his claim that the human body was an analogue to the Newtonian universe, but his message reached at least one of its intended constituencies. Cheyne justified Pitcairne's confidence in him with his election to the Royal Society in March 1702, barely six months after his arrival in London. At the same time, Cheyne wholeheartedly entered London social life; as he later lamented, "I found the *Bottle-Companions*, the *younger Gentry*, and *Free-Livers*, to be the most easy of *Access*, and most quickly susceptible of *Friendship* and *Acquaintance*."[64] He loved to talk, and he found the taverns and coffeehouses of London to be the perfect places to display his wit. One purpose of this socializing was to drum up a medical practice. The strenuous program required for self-promotion demanded an endless round of coffeehouse attendance, lengthy dinners, and learned and witty conversation. Cheyne obtained employment by this means, though of a humbler sort than medicine. Like Arbuthnot, he again tutored mathematics.

Among the "younger Gentry" with whom Cheyne socialized was the earl of Roxburghe and his younger brother, the Hon. William Ker, then about twenty years of age. The Roxburghe account books note several payments to Cheyne between 1702 and 1704 for teaching mathematics to William Ker. This appointment apparently commenced in February 1702.[65] Pitcairne was well acquainted with the Roxburghe family, as patients and as friends; his letters to the earl are familiar and joking, and the Ker brothers shared his taste for Edinburgh tavern life. Pitcairne made use of the patronage of Roxburghe and other Scots nobles to place his chosen candidates in various university posts, and Cheyne acted as his intermediary with Roxburghe on these matters.[66] Moreover, Lady Roxburghe's resident advisor on the education of her children, who paid and probably hired Cheyne, was a certain James Gray. Gray, a Scottish Episcopalian minister ejected for nonjuring, may have been related to Pitcairne's London friend Dr. Robert Gray.[67]

Although the earl of Roxburghe was soon to prove himself an astute politician, he and his brother, Will, were two wealthy young men on their own in London, leading a predictably helter-skelter existence. Letters to their friend William Bennet in Scotland detail a life of drink and sex, punctuated by bouts of gonorrhea. Will wrote, "I am within these two or three minutes com'd down stairs from proffering my prick and my purse to the housemaid, which she has positively refused."[68] With such companions, Cheyne seems to have repeated the pattern of his life in the Wallace household in Edinburgh, though on a grander scale.

As in Edinburgh, he nonetheless managed to continue his scholarly endeavors, publishing two short books in 1702. Although both of these responded to the fevers debate, Cheyne directed them, like the *New Theory*, to an audience beyond Edinburgh. In 1701, following publication of Cheyne's *New Theory*, Pitcairne had published in Holland a Latin edition of his medical "dissertations," including his Leiden essays and the 1694 essay on fevers. Charles Oliphant soon replied with his own Latin dissertation, which proceeded from fevers to a general attack on Pitcairne's ideas. Another flurry of pamphlets followed between Oliphant and Pitcairne's advocate, his Edinburgh protégé James Johnston.[69] Cheyne particularly drew the wrath of Oliphant, who referred to him as a "little Pedant." Jealous of Cheyne's apparent success, Oliphant denied that Pitcairne had helped him in his own career (although Pitcairne probably had) and sneered at those who "impertinently brought in" Newton's doctrines to the theory of medicine. Pitcairne's "Club" had done this only "to show, how deep they are, in that great Man's Doctrine."[70]

Judging simply by the number of works invoking his name that were published in 1702, Newton had become a cultural force. He was named master of the mint in 1699, culminating his steady social progress in London since his arrival three years earlier. In addition, in the decade and a half since the publication of the *Principia*, a new generation of natural philosophers had emerged. Trained by such men as David Gregory, this group of young men—which included John and James Keill, William Whiston, Samuel and John Clarke, John Freind, and John Harris—was thoroughly trained in mathematics and had read and understood the *Principia*. The fruits of their studies now began to appear.[71]

In 1702 David Gregory and his student John Keill each published summaries of Newton's natural philosophy. Gregory's *Astronomiae physicae et
geometricae elementa* was the first astronomy textbook based on the Newtonian
system. Newton included with it the first publication of his lunar theory,
and he contributed to the preface, which discussed the ancient forebears of
his theory of gravitation. Gregory dedicated the work to Prince George of
Denmark, husband of the newly crowned Queen Anne; through the
patronage of Newton and Gilbert Burnet, Gregory had in 1699 been
appointed tutor to their son, the young duke of Gloucester, whose early
death severed this promising tie to the court.[72]

John Keill's *Introductio ad veram physicam* reproduced the lectures he
delivered as deputy to the Sedleian professor of natural philosophy at
Oxford. Keill's lectures introduced the *Principia* to students with a modest
knowledge of mathematics. In fact, he barely mentioned the *Principia* and
concentrated instead on basic principles of mechanics.[73]

Cheyne perhaps intended the *New Theory of Fevers* to follow these works
as introductory texts in Newtonian ideas, but it missed its mark. While
the book, along with Pitcairne's machinations, transported Cheyne from
obscurity in Edinburgh to a fellowship of the Royal Society, fame and
fortune did not immediately follow. Representative of the reception
afforded Cheyne's work by other physicians was a letter written in 1701 by
Martin Lister to the *Philosophical Transactions*. Lister, a physician and
naturalist, was an active and longtime fellow of the Royal Society as well
as a friend of Pitcairne.[74] Lister began his letter with praise of this "most
ingenious little Tract of Fevers." While he had read the treatise "with
delight" and agreed with its premises (not surprisingly, since the obstruction theory was a standard argument), Lister admitted that "for want of
Mathematicks, I could not well enter into some of his reasonings."[75]

He objected to a reference to an experiment he had performed some
years earlier of injecting a colored fluid into the intestines of a dog,
which eventually showed up in the animal's lacteal glands. Cheyne cited
Lister's experiment as proof of the *lack* of absorption of intestinal fluid
by the lacteals. Lister charitably attributed this error to the irregular
appearance of the *Philosophical Transactions*, in which his experiment had
been reported. With disingenuous courtesy, he pointed out another error

also due to ignorance of recent research, for Cheyne had used Richard Lower's figure for the quantity of blood of twenty pounds rather than more recent smaller estimates.[76]

Lister put his finger on the speculative nature of Cheyne's entire enterprise. Cheyne's use of mathematics as a methodological model followed Pitcairne's example. Although he extended it by including actual equations and geometrical models, these remained models and did not refer to any real quantities. Cheyne's neglect of experiment, particularly animal experiment, reflected not only Pitcairne's emphases but the tenor of the times. While public anatomical demonstration continued to be popular, demonstrations of animal research at Royal Society meetings had ceased by the late 1670s, and reports of animal experimentation elsewhere had dwindled by the 1690s, disappearing altogether for a period after 1700.[77] Cheyne's work, therefore, was an example of *mathesis* rather than mathematics, and as such fit well into Sloane's program of the 1690s.

Cheyne did not respond to Lister's criticism, and the offending phrases remained unchanged in later editions of the *New Theory*. Theodore Brown has argued that these criticisms indicated the ambivalence of the Royal Society toward Newtonian ideas; but Lister was notoriously conservative in his medical ideas and may not have represented general opinion.[78] The lack of response on either side could also be viewed as evidence of the inchoate quality of "Newtonianism" itself.

Cheyne reissued the *New Theory of Fevers* in the first half of 1702, still anonymously. He extended the work by applying his theory to acute and "hectick" or consumptive fevers as well as continual or chronic ones. He prefaced the new edition with *An Essay Concerning the Improvements of the Theory of Medicine*, which outlined an all-encompassing Newtonian theory of medicine. This essay remained the touchstone for all of Cheyne's subsequent work. He indicated his continued confidence in its statements when he reissued it, with the *New Theory*, in 1722, with his name at last on the title page, at a time when he had supposedly repudiated his early works.[79]

The *Essay*'s tone echoed Pitcairne's inaugural lecture at Leiden, and its content echoed as well both his profound social conservatism and his absolute faith in Newtonian physics as the basis of authority in both medicine and society. Cheyne ranked medicine among the "Liberal Arts"; but unlike the other arts, which "are reckoned necessary Qualifications for a *Gentleman*: but few study *Medicine*, save those who design to live by the Practise thereof." He set out to rescue medicine from the empirics and reestablish its gentlemanly standing by relying on the "genuine and true" Newtonian theory, which would regain for physicians the status and respect lost by their espousal of "precarious, absurd and often contradictory" theory. Correct theory would, moreover, so much improve therapeutics as to remove the empiric from contention as a rival. Medical practice would perforce be limited to those of sufficient learning in natural philosophy—to gentlemen, among whom Cheyne included himself.[80] Like Pitcairne, he used mathematical learning to buttress the traditional order of society against the sectarian mob. Yet his emphasis on the gentlemanly standing of physicians also betrays his anxiety about his own anomalous social status as simultaneously both employee and drinking companion of the Kers. Cheyne's father, after all, though he classed himself as a gentleman, was merely a tenant farmer.

Did Cheyne intend his program to appeal to the London College of Physicians, who might have welcomed such support in their struggle to control medical practice? Brown has argued that Cockburn had thoroughly burned any bridges between the College and Newtonian ideas by 1700, and this appears to be the case, since the College ignored Cheyne's work.[81] In redefining medicine as a branch of natural philosophy, Cheyne may have intended to bypass the College's influence on obtaining a medical practice in favor of that of the Royal Society. Lacking the status or medical training of Hamilton or Cockburn, Cheyne may have believed the College too formidable a bulwark to breach; Pitcairne's sponsorship would there have availed him little.

Like Pitcairne, Cheyne reacted to Sydenham's disdain of theory by linking the progress of medicine to that of the physical sciences, comparing the undeveloped state of medicine to exact sciences such as astronomy. Although, he wrote, one might by chance discover successful therapies empirically, medicine would remain unscientific without proper theory. Scientific medicine would build upon true postulates such as his own on fevers to indisputable conclusions and invariably successful cures, unlike the hit-or-miss techniques of contemporary therapeutics. The ancients, who had empirically discovered many treatments, had "done tolerably as to the Practical Part," but had made little progress in discerning the causes of disease.[82] Foreshadowing a major theme of his mature works, Cheyne added that ancient remedies were in any case not effective against the diseases of a less than golden age: the "Intemperance, Indiscretion and Lewdness . . . of our Days" (of which Cheyne had firsthand experience) increased the virulence of old maladies and led to the birth of "plaguy new ones."[83]

Cheyne criticized theories that did not conform to the true and certain laws of physics and geometry. Human function was not unique and could be understood by the same means by which astronomy and terrestrial mechanics had been comprehended. He praised Harvey, Steno, Borelli, Bellini, and Pitcairne as well as "several Gentlemen of the *Royal Society* at *London*" for their contributions to the true theory of medicine. Finally, he listed four requirements for medicine's improvement: a more thorough knowledge of anatomy, a "Compleat History of Nature," a "Compleat System of Mechanick Phylosophy," and the composition of a "Principia medicinae theoreticae mathematicae."[84]

Cheyne acknowledged that "a compleat System of Mechanick Phylosophy, i.e. an Account of all the Visible Effects of Nature upon Geometrick Principles" had been formulated by "that stupendiously Great Man, Mr. *Newton*." Newton's theories and mathematical method could therefore be applied to medicine to hasten its reform, as Pitcairne had foreseen; and Cheyne placed himself in the role of medicine's Newton. "I am perswaded," he wrote, "that from the same Principles the grand Appearances of Nature have been accounted for, these more minute ones [i.e., physiological phenomena] may be so too." For this purpose, he added, "We want to know the Mechanical Account of Chymical Operations."[85] Thus he emphasized the substructure of matter as the key to physiology rather than Borellian mechanics of motion. Two events would, he thought, "mightily conduce" toward the goal of a medical *Principia*: the publication of a general account of fluxions (Newton's system of the calculus), and an end to the secrecy among "the great Geometers of this present Age." While Cheyne brought these events to pass, the result was not what he had hoped.[86]

The Edinburgh fever debate continued, and in 1702 Cheyne contributed *Remarks on two late Pamphlets written by Dr Oliphant*.[87] In his *Essay* Cheyne had referred to "that Enemy to all Schemes, Figures, Sense and Demonstrations." Oliphant quickly replied to Pitcairne's "Bully under pay." He was sorry

> to see the study of Physick dwindle to that of a piece of Abstract Geometry, and every little Pedant that could talk of a Curve, a Quadrature, or a Series, and pretend to the understanding a little of *Borelli* and *Bellini*, set up for a Physician, and without either time or Education sufficient to qualifie him for so weighty an Employment.

Oliphant denied that the mechanical philosophy or even a knowledge of the "animal Oeconomy," that is, the system of the body, was necessary to a physician. Far from assuring the gentlemanly status of medicine, such learning would open it to upstarts such as Cheyne.[88]

Cheyne was compelled to reply, although at the end of the *Essay* he had foresworn further comment on the fever dispute.[89] Moreover, he replied in kind: a move he later regretted, less in contrition than because he thereby gave Oliphant an opening to make the damaging account of Cheyne's Edinburgh career in his next response. In his own reply, Cheyne indicated the content of a *Principia medicinae*. He acknowledged the limits of his approach, in response to Oliphant's taunts: "It is very hard to apply *Geometry* to *Physiology*, with such accuracy and Niceness, as to exclude all possibility of Wrangling: We must make some Allowances, & assume some *Data*." But if one then reasoned logically, even from flawed data, "all ingenious Men" would be satisfied.[90] So Pitcairne had argued.

To Oliphant's criticism that mathematical theories were of little use to medical practice, Cheyne countered that correct practice would necessarily follow from correct theory. Pitcairne's works, like the best treatises of natural philosophy, demonstrated "the *Infinit* wisdom of the CONTRIVER of the *Universe*." The Boyle lectures, now in their tenth year, purveyed a similar message, and Cheyne's introduction of this theme signaled his awareness of its importance to Newton himself. The "Infinit wisdom" of God justified his use of analogical argument, providing that "the same laws of *Mechanism* are observed in the lesser, as in the greater Bodies of this *Systeme*." He would elaborate on this theme a few years later in his *Philosophical Principles of Natural Religion*.[91]

In the remainder of his lengthy reply Cheyne defended the image of the physician as theoretical scientist (and therefore gentleman) over empirical craftsman. Empiricism alone could not produce invariably correct results. Even if new theories did not have immediate practical benefit, medicine could not survive as a science without them. Harvey's discovery of the circulation was a new theory that did not significantly alter therapy but was nonetheless valuable. Similarly, knowledge of mathematics may not be immediately useful. But in difficult cases, "A *Mathematician*, who besides the *Practice*, understands the *Theory*, will find *Expedients* for all *Emergencies*. . . . this is one principal *Difference* . . . between a meer *Mechanick* and a true *Philosopher*, who can both think and act." A *Principia medicinae* was needed: "The true Reason, why we do not at present reap all the Advantages in Practice from Mechanick Theories . . . is, that as yet . . . The whole *Animal Oeconomy* is not perfected." The perfection of the "oeconomy" entailed the reduction of medicine to a few laws of mechanics and of medicaments to "a few simple ones."[92]

Yet could Cheyne's reductionist program also serve to justify empirical practice? The old academic medicine of humors and temperaments saw illness in terms of the unique imbalance experienced by the individual patient, but Cheyne took an ontological view of diseases as entities, each with a single cause that was the same for each patient. If the causes were known, the same remedy should work equally well for each patient. Such reasoning could also allow empirical practitioners to promote their single cures for single diseases; William Cockburn's "electuary" was a successful example.[93] But quacks and their cures had flourished long before "scientific" claims to medical knowledge. Both responded to the demands of the medical marketplace. Cheyne pointed out that Pitcairne's treatises had "acquired him a mighty reputation which has hugely encreas'd his *gains by practice*," a success that Cheyne hoped to emulate in London.[94] He intended not to democratize medicine but to found a new academic medicine outside the traditional networks from which he was excluded.

Cheyne did not gain a medical practice from his writings, since he continued to work as a tutor. But his reputation among aspiring young Newtonians was sufficient to merit speedy imitation. Among the first was Richard Mead's *A Mechanical Account of Poisons*, also published in 1702. A dissenter, Mead had studied briefly in Leiden under Pitcairne; having obtained a medical degree in Padua, he practiced in Stepney, in East London. Mead's ambitions far outstripped Stepney, and the timely appearance of the *Mechanical Account* was no accident.[95]

In the *Mechanical Account* Mead credited Bellini, Pitcairne, and Cheyne with putting medicine on the new track of mechanical and mathematical reasoning. Soon, he said, "*Mathematical Learning* will be the Distinguishing Mark of a Physician from a Quack"; Pitcairne's dissertations, he added, gave "convincing Proof" of the value of mathematical method. Mead described his own work as a small contribution toward Cheyne's *Principia medicinae*. He referred to Cheyne as a "*Genius*" and eagerly awaited the appearance of his "*New Animal Oeconomy*."[96]

A Mechanical Account of Poisons contains very little mathematics; Cheyne's equations and geometrical diagrams are entirely missing.[97] In his first essay, for example, Mead used microscopic evidence to show that the venom of vipers consisted of acid salts that were sharp pointy crystals. When these crystals entered the bloodstream, he reasoned (following Bellini), they would literally tear up the blood. Like Pitcairne, he believed that the blood was a chemical mixture of various atoms that cohered in globules. This cohesion was by an attractive force "which is indeed, though express'd in other Words, the very same thing with the *Attraction* of the Particles one to another; this Mr. *Newton* has demonstrated to be the great Principal [*sic*] of Action in the Universe."[98] By this bold statement, Mead staked his claim among the medical Newtonians. The effect of the pointy acids, therefore, was not simply mechanical. Their extreme reactivity— owing to their strong attractive power, according to Newton in "De natura acidorum"—caused the observed physiological effects of venom.[99]

In other essays in *A Mechanical Account of Poisons* Mead discussed tarantulas, mad dogs, mineral and plant poisons, and "venomous exhalations," and concluded in each case that poisons operated by inducing some sort of chemical change in the blood, much as morbific matter acted in fevers. The particles of the blood cohered or separated irregularly, causing a wide variety of physiological effects.[100]

Mead soon gained admittance to the circle of Newton's young admirers. He was mentioned three times in the January–February 1703 issue of the *Philosophical Transactions*, including a long and favorable summary of the *Mechanical Account of Poisons*. Soon after, Mead was elected a fellow of the Royal Society and assumed the position of physician-in-ordinary to St. Thomas's Hospital in Southwark.[101]

Despite such citation, Cheyne's future was hardly secure. Oliphant's devastating portrait of Cheyne in his *Short Answer to Two Lybels* effectively terminated the fevers dispute and Cheyne's medical soapbox. The competition among young natural philosophers for Newton's favor steadily heated up. Gregory's protégé John Keill and his brother James were only two of a great number of potential rivals.[102] Sloane apparently asked Cheyne to give the Gulstonian lecture at the Royal Society, but he refused. In a letter to Sloane, Cockburn asked him not to be offended by Cheyne's refusal but to continue his patronage.[103]

Cheyne's next move seemed cleverly designed to put him in front of the pack of aspirants while also giving him a modern cachet among physicians. He would demonstrate his mathematical talents, so praised by Pitcairne: a topic, unlike medicine, that clearly interested Newton. Cheyne followed one of his own suggestions in his *Theory of Medicine* and published a general account of "fluxions," Newton's method of calculus. But his bold plan, while indeed displaying Cheyne's considerable talents, resulted in shipwreck and demonstrated how little Cheyne really knew about navigating the shoals of patronage.

The second issue in 1703 of the *Philosophical Transactions* included an account by John Craig of a method of quadratures in the form of a letter to Cheyne. He noted that Newton's method of fluxions "may be revealed by you [Cheyne] in your book, which you wrote to Dr. Archibald Pitcairne, that ornament of our country and age."[104] In November 1702 Newton had declared to Gregory and Halley his intention of publishing his treatise "De quadratura" along with his treatise on light. Both had long existed in manuscript, and Gregory had known of the work on quadratures in the early 1690s.[105]

Newton had not yet taken that step by January 1703, when Cheyne wrote to Gregory about his own "Mathematical paper," claiming that Pitcairne had "press'd" him to write and publish his book, *Fluxionem methodus inversa*. Pitcairne, he said, sent the manuscript to Arbuthnot to show to Newton, who "thought it not intolerable," though Cheyne was not certain that Newton had bothered to read it. Cheyne asked Gregory to read and comment on the work—he had also consulted Craig and Bower—noting that the work included methods from both Gregory and Newton. Gregory may have read Cheyne's manuscript, but his copy of the published work, which appeared in the summer of 1703, is barely marked.[106] Did Gregory tell Cheyne of Newton's own plans to publish?

Despite his precautions, Cheyne succeeded in offending the easily offended Newton. According to a later story, Newton, introduced to Cheyne by Arbuthnot, offered money to help pay for the publication of the *Fluxionem*; Cheyne refused the money and Newton was insulted.[107] A. R. Hall adds, "Though Newton had been obliging to Dr. Pitcairne's friend, he was not pleased to be thus published despite himself by a hand inferior to his own."[108] Gregory, Charles Oliphant's brother-in-law, fomented this disagreement, promoting his own student John Keill at Cheyne's expense. Cheyne seems to have been extraordinarily naive in asking Gregory for advice, although Gregory and Pitcairne remained close friends. Pitcairne commented to another friend, "take notice that Dr Gregorie & Dr Cheyne are not indissoluble friends, tho both are mine." He added in a postscript, "Also take notice that Mr Craig is very far from being a friend to Dr Gregory. [T]his for the politics. I am great with all."[109]

Fluxionem methodus inversa brought Newton's developing controversy with G. W. Leibniz over the invention of the calculus into the open. Cheyne credited only British sources of his methods, although he was undoubtedly familiar with continental work. He closed his book with the claim that Newton had discovered the method of fluxions twenty-four years ago. As Johann Bernoulli pointed out to Leibniz, if this were true, both he and Leibniz were merely "Newton's apes." Leibniz was furious that Newton should have allowed such a patently unjust claim to be made, and in his review of Newton's *De quadratura* in the *Acta eruditorum* in 1704 he slyly referred the reader to the work of Craig and Cheyne for further details of Newton's theory. Newton had prudently asked Cheyne to omit this claim, but Cheyne, ever eager to please his yearned-for patron, kept the passage.[110] In this he was no doubt abetted by Pitcairne, who complained that Newton had been "barbarouslie, orangically, & Hanoverianlie abus'd" by Leibniz and his cronies.[111]

Cheyne foolishly worried more about his reputation as a mathematician than about Newton's reaction to being scooped. Although he acknowledged that his work was an exposition rather than an original work, he agonized over its reception. Bernoulli described the work to Leibniz as "a most remarkable little book, stuffed with very clever discoveries," but he also pointed out several errors.[112] Cheyne attempted to forestall criticism by asking Sloane to report any comments on his book submitted to the *Transactions* so that Cheyne could publish a simultaneous reply. Early in 1704 Gregory reported the publication of a refutation of Cheyne's book by the Huguenot mathematician Abraham de Moivre, precisely the critic Cheyne most feared.[113] De Moivre, a skilled mathematician and later one of Newton's bulldogs in the calculus dispute, accused Cheyne of misunderstanding Newton's method. He only showed the method, said de Moivre, but did not derive it. De Moivre then enumerated in devastating detail the "many errors" in Cheyne's book.[114]

Moreover, in the "Advertisement" or preface to his *Opticks*, dated 1 April 1704, Newton himself implied that Cheyne had plagiarized his work. Referring to the manuscript "De quadratura," Newton commented that he had lately "met with some Things copied out of it." Newton's biographer R. S. Westfall comments, "Cheyne must have been startled to read the extent of Newton's resentment of his assertion of independence."[115] Cheyne attempted to pick up the pieces of the disaster by responding to de Moivre. Gregory gleefully recounted his frantic consultations with Bower and Pitcairne in the spring of 1704.[116]

Cheyne's response, published in 1705, masterfully covered his retreat. He acknowledged de Moivre's criticisms, and with breathtaking impudence referred de Moivre to Newton's treatise on quadratures—now, of course, published—to support his claims. In a lengthy preface, he further obscured the issue of his mathematical skills by accusing de Moivre of an "unpolished style" and an arrogance and lack of politeness "unworthy in a man of gentlemanly education."[117]

Although Cheyne got in the last word, his venture into mathematics can only be called a fiasco. Later in life he embarrassedly referred to it as "brought forth in Ambition and bred up in Vanity." More to the point, he added, "these barren and airy Studies . . . [are] only proper for publick Professors, and those born to Estates, and who are under no outward Necessities."[118] Worst of all, his show of mathematical learning failed to have the desired effect on his career. It had taken him far afield from his original program of reforming medicine and set him up to be ridiculed by Gregory and his allies. In comparison to Gregory's physician protégés such as John Freind and James Keill, Cheyne fared badly. Keill had recently established a lucrative medical practice in Northampton through the agency of Hans Sloane, and Freind, having lectured as Oxford Professor of Chemistry, was about to travel to the continent as the earl of Peterborough's physician at the battlefront. Mead and Cockburn had already established practices. In 1704 Cheyne was still a mathematics tutor and had little to show for two years of unremitting effort to establish himself in London.

Newton was elected president of the Royal Society at the end of 1703, and soon after published his *Opticks*. Publication of the *Fluxionem* had a serious impact on Cheyne's relations both with Newton and with the Royal Society: they ceased. Cheyne's name appears only twice in the Society's Journal Book, and the *Philosophical Transactions* failed to mention his book.[119] Cheyne had failed dismally in every way, and everything about him, from his size to his broad Aberdeen accent, revealed him as a country bumpkin. Unlike Gregory or Arbuthnot, he had failed to reinvent himself to fit his environment. Although no written evidence survives, he undoubtedly poured out his woes to Pitcairne.

4

PHILOSOPHICAL PRINCIPLES

In the wake of the disasters of 1704, Cheyne turned not to writing the medical *Principia* but to an altogether different project. Gregory described him in February 1704 as working on a book "on the existence of God as displayed by his works."[1] This work, the *Philosophical Principles of Natural Religion*, may have been an attempt to reingratiate himself with Newton.[2] Gregory noted its similarity to Richard Bentley's 1692 Boyle lectures (published in 1693), in which Newton's influence had been evident, and Cheyne clearly imitated Bentley's narrative format and even some of his subject matter. He may also have gained more recent inspiration from the 1704 Boyle lectures of Samuel Clarke, another Newtonian protégé.

In this book Cheyne addressed concerns about religion and society that were central to a number of his contemporaries. In their theological concerns Pitcairne, Craig, and Newton responded to the atmosphere of crisis at the turn of the century by steering a middle way between the extremes of atheism and enthusiasm. The purpose of the Boyle lectures was to "prove" Christianity against its foes, to convince unbelievers of the correctness of Christian doctrines. Cheyne knew Craig's work especially well. In his 1699 *Theologiae christianae principia mathematica*, Craig had attempted to apply Newton's calculus to religion and moral philosophy. As we have seen, he calculated a date for the Second Coming (based on the rate of decay of historical evidence for the truth of Christianity), and he also attempted a "Calculus of Pleasure" designed to quantify moral philosophy. Craig concluded, by means of mathematical proof, that "The true Christian is the wisest of all wise men. That atheists and deists are the most foolish of all foolish men."[3] In the *Philosophical Principles of Natural Religion*, published in 1705, Cheyne presented the latest facet of this project: the proof of the existence of God in the works of nature, or, more specifically, a demonstration of the immanence of God in the world by means of an exposition of Newtonian natural philosophy.

Cheyne continued to present Pitcairne's confident arguments that certain (not merely probable) knowledge could be obtained by means of mathematical method, that is, Newton's method. As Craig had applied it to biblical chronology, so Cheyne would apply it to the microcosm, and particularly to the animal economy, which he believed offered a uniquely convincing example of providential action. His main resources for this undertaking included the works of Pitcairne and Newton (particularly "De natura acidorum" and the queries to the recently published *Opticks*), as well as those of Borelli and Bellini. Craig, Arbuthnot, and John Freind offered criticisms, and Gregory, mollified by the intervention of Arbuthnot, proofread (he claimed to have found 429 errors in the printed version, mostly typographical).[4]

Cheyne repeated some of the cosmological and cosmogonical arguments of Bentley's Boyle lectures. Cheyne's emphasis on the body echoed Bentley's middle three Boyle lectures, which had refuted atheism "from the Structure and Origin of Humane Bodies."[5] Yet the body was in many ways the least amenable entity to the kind of analysis Cheyne now attempted. While, as Carol Flynn observes, "Ideally, the body discloses harmonious, divine proportion, matter made in God's image," by 1700 "the idealized human frame was breaking down to become fixed in its infirmities." Cheyne and his work therefore stand at a turning point in the history of the body, particularly in terms of its theological significance. In this era, Flynn adds, "Christian contempt for the body was giving way to a secular concern for the fate of the bodily container."[6] In the *Philosophical Principles* Cheyne attempted to bridge secular and religious concerns by means of a "natural religion" explainable in Newtonian terms. Cheyne added to Bentley's exposition new arguments from matter theory, optics, and medicine. He abandoned the "mathematical" style of exposition of his medical works in favor of a straightforward narrative. Yet ultimately, he believed, this attempt failed, and he turned, as we saw in chapter 1, to a mystical religion that embraced Christian contempt for the body, and which he described in the 1715 edition of his book. The two editions of the *Philosophical Principles* not only document his intellectual journey but also provide context for a broader view of the Enlightenment in Britain than the usual historiographical emphasis on secularization has previously allowed.

Cheyne dedicated the *Philosophical Principles* to Roxburghe, who had recently been named a secretary of state for Scotland. Cheyne claimed Roxburghe's patronage for his project, since his work was "undertaken in obedience to Your Commands, and contain[s] part of those Discourses, I had with your Lordship, when you allow'd me the Honour, to talk with you on *Philosophical Subjects*."[7] Cheyne emphasized the value of natural philosophical learning in creating the gentlemanly persona, which would include, in Roxburghe's case, public service.[8] While Cheyne's employment with the Kers had ceased by 1705, he continued to act as Pitcairne's intermediary with the earl on matters of patronage. In November 1704 Gregory mentioned "the intrigue betwixt My Lord Roxburgh, Dr. Pitcairn, Dr. Cheyn, &c. of reforming Colleges, &c. in Scotland" and Cheyne's "constant dining" with Roxburghe as part of this plan.[9]

Cheyne attributed to Roxburghe the opinion that "God had reserv'd to this last Age, those great Advantages by which the Secrets of Nature have been more happily unravell'd than in any former Times, on purpose to expose the Folly of a corrupt Generation of Men, who from their vitious Practices, being prone to *Atheism*, have vainly pretended, the *Oracles* of Reason to be on their side." Reason, in other words, proved religion and not its opposite. However unlikely it may seem that such sentiments emanated from the rakish Roxburghe, their millenarian tinge was unmistakable: this was the "last age" before the rule of the saints. Cheyne's references to the millennium remain, however, on this allusive level.[10] Yet Cheyne's association with Roxburghe also put him squarely amid the corrupt generation against which he wrote; were not his friendships based solely on "sensual Pleasures and mere Jollity"?[11] Did he write the *Philosophical Principles* as an act of contrition? Or was he simply buying into the program of latitudinarian apologetics established by Bentley and Clarke?

Cheyne argued in the *Philosophical Principles* that the amazing contrivance of the Newtonian cosmos could not have arisen by chance. The laws of nature revealed by Newton demonstrated the existence of a wise creator. In part 1 Cheyne distinguished between the laws by which the world had been created and the laws of nature by which it currently operated; God could suspend the latter laws at will, a clear statement of the voluntarist position detailed by Bentley and Clarke. Because Newtonian gravity was not essential to matter, it "must be a Principle annex'd to Matter by the *Creator* of the World"—a law of nature. While Newton had not stated this conclusion in the *Principia*, he had made this point privately, and both Bentley and Clarke reiterated it.[12]

Since attraction was the "great Law of Nature," it must account for all of nature's appearances. Because God initially impressed this force on matter, the universe and its motion were therefore sustained without the continued interference of God; Cheyne strongly opposed the notion of "occasionalism," which claimed that God continued to intervene. His model of God's role in nature was also a model for the conduct of natural philosophy. Closely echoing Pitcairne's inaugural lecture at Leiden, Cheyne wrote, "The whole Difficulty of Philosophy seems to lie in investigating the Powers and Forces of Nature, from the Appearances of the Motions given, and then from these Powers to account for all the Rest." Cheyne adopted an atomistic model of nature, duly modified by Newton's example in "De natura acidorum" and more recently in the queries to the *Opticks*. Cheyne concluded that the particles of matter cohered with a force "derived from nothing in Nature, but that *Universal Law* of Attraction."[13]

But Cheyne did not believe that short-range attractions were caused by the same force as long-range gravitation. He proposed an analogy, based on Newton's "Third Rule of Philosophizing," between the microcosm and the macrocosm, the organic and inorganic.[14] The inverse-square law was not universal. He cited the *Principia* in favor of his argument that at contact or at very small distances, such as would exist between two corpuscles, the universal power of attraction would diminish very quickly.[15]

Cheyne argued that gravity itself could not be explained mechanically. He rejected ethereal explanations for gravity, as well as such "subservient Divinities" as More's hylarchic principle and Scaliger's "plastick virtue" in favor of the direct action of God, recognizing, like Newton, that any

other explanation would render matter autonomous and God super-
fluous. The action of gravity, said Cheyne, was analogous to sensation:

> We know the manner of *Thinking*, and *Reflection*, of *Remembering* and *Sensation*, are
> things not easily to be explain'd, and yet we must admit them . . . [other
> phenomena] are not to be accounted for, and yet there is no denying, that such
> things really are, and when we are capable to explain how our Souls and our
> Bodies act mutually upon one another, we may come to be able to conceive how
> Matter acts at a Distance.

As bodily organs acted as mediators between sensation and the mind, so
gravity "is the effect of the *Divine Power and Virtue*, by which the Operations of Material Agents are preserv'd." These "Agents," which Cheyne
did not further identify, acted as intermediaries between God and matter.
Like Newton, Cheyne sought a middle way between voluntarism and
atheism, between God's direct and constant intervention and God's
absence, either total or, in the views of Descartes or Leibniz, only immea-
surably distant. Later, Cheyne would follow Newton's lead in identifying
the "Agents" with the ether.[16]

Cheyne's insistence on the centrality of gravity in God's operation of
the universe conveyed a pessimistic view of the future. The regularity of
natural law and its actions led inevitably to dissolution. He asserted that
"the Quantity of Heat and Light in the *Sun* does daily decrease," absorbed
by "Vegetables, Metals and Minerals" and scattered over the earth, never
to return to its source.[17] "Naturally and of itself," he added, the world
"tends to Dissolution," and not even the tails of comets (a theory attributed to "a *very great* Man") could entirely renew its diminishing resources.[18]
Cheyne's rejection of the renovating qualities of comets perhaps indicated his equivocal belief in the imminence of the millennium, since for
Newton the cyclical quality of comets provided a parallel to the millenarian cycle of decay and renovation of the universe.[19]

While others in 1700 were arguing that the end of time was soon,
Cheyne described a time frame almost infinite in extent. The universe, he
said, had been deliberately created by God and was neither eternal nor
the result of a chance occurrence of events. Opposing Aristotle's argu-

ment for an eternal universe, Cheyne contended that an eternal world, operating by the same laws of nature, would long ago have expended its resources; the light of the sun, for example, would be much dimmed, whereas in fact it had not sensibly diminished. All the particles of light emitted by the sun since the creation "may not be greater than a cubical *Inch*, or even a grain of sand."[20] Dissolution, therefore, was not yet at hand. Moreover, had humankind always existed, it would surely have reached a higher development of the arts and sciences than its present state.[21] Samuel Clarke, on the contrary, had argued in his Boyle lectures that the recent augmentation of human knowledge of nature foreshadowed the increase in human knowledge of God that would bring about the millennium. The decay of nature was a result of the moral decay of society and could be prevented.[22]

Cheyne's refutation of materialism borrowed heavily from both Bentley and Pitcairne, who may himself have borrowed from Bentley. The belief in material causes was, they believed, a direct road to atheism. "Not only [could] this Universe . . . not have been produc'd by the Laws of *Mechanism*, but there is scarce a single *Appearance* that can thence adequately be accounted for," he declared; matter and motion were, *contra* Descartes, insufficient causes to explain natural phenomena. In particular, "the Production of an Animal is altogether *immechanical.*" Geoffrey Bowles has pointed out that the term "immechanical" meant "not merely non-mechanical but totally opposed to all forms of mechanism and material causation." Like Pitcairne, Cheyne contended that the complexity of animal form and, especially, of function precluded mechanical causation: "when the *complications* are infinite the Machin is altogether above the Power of *Mechanicks*, and quite impracticable by the Laws of Matter and Motion." Moreover, the motion of such "Machins" could not be merely spontaneous; and "we shou'd be strangely surpriz'd if by any combination of material Organs, we shou'd produce the smallest part of their Actions and Passions."[23] Bentley had argued solely from complexity of design, but Cheyne added both the machine analogy (thereby turning the materialist argument on its head) and the production of motion and "passion."

Cheyne concluded that Newtonian natural philosophy, which he described as "a juster *Philosophy*, and a more genuine Explication of Nature, than was known till of late," proved the existence of God as convincingly as Euclid had proven the principles of geometry. Once more, Cheyne characterized Newtonian physics as certain, not merely probable, knowledge. While design was a convincing argument for a deity, only the certainty of mathematical demonstration guaranteed God's imprint upon the world. Cheyne drew specific examples from anatomy and physiology, emphasizing such Pitcairnean themes as secretion and muscular motion. He chose this mode of argument, he added, "because our Modern *Atheists* have taken *Sanctuary* within the Bounds of *Natural Philosophy*."[24]

Cheyne ended his work with a section "Of the Nature of Finiteness and Infiniteness and the Limits of Human Knowledge." Although in the 1715 revision of the *Philosophical Principles* the notion of infinity would be central, this earlier discussion of infinite numbers and infinite series seems intended merely to reassert Cheyne's mathematical credentials in the face of the criticisms he had recently received. Shuttleton has suggested that Cheyne here attempted to emulate the work of Craig. The mathematician Brook Taylor argued in 1714 that this section bore little relation to the rest of the book.[25]

Despite its extensive borrowings from other authors, the *Philosophical Principles* was a strikingly original work. Cheyne's understanding of fluxions had been proven faulty, but he understood very well many other implications of Newton's work. In particular, his emphasis on the analogy between the microcosm and the macrocosm seized upon a central Newtonian principle. Analogical reasoning in general, and the microcosm-macrocosm analogy in particular, had long been essential precepts in natural philosophy.[26] If Newtonian attraction was truly a universal principle of matter, it must necessarily operate not only on the large scale but also on the minute, illustrating the regularity of nature and the foresight of God. Cheyne was the first of the self-proclaimed Newtonians to provide an account of short-range attractions. He had gained much of his understanding from "De natura acidorum" via Pitcairne. Another channel of influence was the Neoplatonism of the Garden brothers, and a Platonic view of nature also underlay Pitcairne's work.[27] Cheyne's attention to matter theory foreshadowed his later obsession with the relationship between matter and spirit. Already he was pushing at the boundaries of what would become for him a critical continuum.

Cheyne harbored great expectations for his work's reception. He was obviously on a postcomposition high in January 1705, when Gregory reported that Cheyne "braggs that next summer he is to goe to Scotland, and together with Dr Pitcairne settle all the Practice of Physick, and publish unalterable Principles there of."[28] Pitcairne's friend Colin Campbell thought highly enough of the work to copy it out, as he had done with Newton's *Principia*.[29] Cheyne presented a copy to the Royal Society in June, but it was not reviewed in the *Philosophical Transactions*. Apart from Gregory's scurrilous comment that many thought it "stoln" from Bentley's Boyle lectures, it appears to have been largely ignored.[30] Despite his best efforts Cheyne remained outside the charmed circle of fame and success. This latest failure would have devastating consequences for his psyche, leading to his physical and spiritual crisis of 1705, described in chapter 1.

Following the crisis of 1705–6, Cheyne lived quietly for a decade, assiduously avoiding controversy. He settled into family life with his marriage to Margaret Middleton, daughter of a nonjuring Scottish Episcopalian clergyman, Patrick Middleton (1662–1736). Middleton was related to George Middleton (1645–1726), principal of King's College, Aberdeen, from 1684 to 1717, when he was removed for Jacobitism. The Aberdeen Middletons were also related to the Gardens, whose mother was Isobel Middleton; George Middleton was probably their first cousin. Margaret Middleton migrated to England with her brother John, a physician who settled in Bristol. Another brother, George, was a London goldsmith. The Cheynes had three surviving children: two daughters, Frances and Margaret (known as Peggy), and the youngest, a son, John, born about 1717.[31]

Cheyne stopped attending meetings of the Royal Society and published nothing. Although the 1707 union of the Scottish and English Parliaments promised some relief to Scottish Episcopalians, the correspondence of Garden, Keith, Ramsay, and their circle continued unabated and progressed to the importation and exchange of books on mystical topics.[12] Cheyne remained an active correspondent of this group as his spiritual quest continued. Although he asked Ramsay about George Garden's Rosehearty colony in 1708, he did not propose to join them.[13] But despite the strong Jacobite leanings of this circle, and his own numerous Jacobite connections, Cheyne also remained resolutely apolitical. Burned by his professional disasters, he did not intend to expose himself to further criticism.

Cheyne's correspondence with his close friend Ramsay shows his continued spiritual exploration. Despite his conversion, he continued to feel deeply sinful: "I wou'd fain hope that I shall be sometime delivered from the devil the world & my self, I will wait with patience till the joyfull day." Nonetheless, by 1709 Cheyne was being consulted in a dual capacity as physician and spiritual advisor. That summer, James Cuninghame (?1680–1716), a Scottish gentleman and member of Garden's circle, consulted Cheyne in Bath. His illness is not known, but Cuninghame soon found himself "recovered to a miracle."[14] Cuninghame was well read in mystical literature, and he and Cheyne conversed on religious topics. They probably discussed the recently published *Fides et ratio collatae*, a book examining the bases of religious belief (which, the author argued, lay in faith and not in reason). Among the authors treated in this work was Jacob Boehme, the German mystic whose doctrines had so influenced the Philadelphians. Cuninghame confided to Cheyne a resolution he had made to devote his life to God's service.[15] Cheyne was deeply inspired by Cuninghame's piety, which, he told Ramsay, made him feel all the less worthy himself; his public face masked his continued spiritual turmoil:

I hope I have only my masters image in him which indeed grows more pure & bright dayly, but I ought to suspect every thing that proceeds from so impure a fountain as my heart. Oh Ramsay I find an infinit source of uncleanness there, all my exteriour & interiour is meerly the effect of a broken constitution, but enough of this. . . . my health of body & mind [is] as ever I was. . . . my spirits are allwaies for one reason or another so turned & unsettled & it seems more out of my power to compose 'em but I fear it is all in my will. Pity me & pray for me, for Ramsay I will never fail you if I am not left by my Heavenly fa[the]r.[16]

Upon his return to Scotland, however, Cuninghame soon crossed the line between personal religion and enthusiasm, which Cheyne so carefully trod, and became involved with the French Prophets, who had descended upon Edinburgh in the spring and summer of 1709. The Prophets were a group of French Protestant millenarians who came together in southern France in 1688. A few of them migrated to London in 1706 and immediately attracted followers in that millenarian-ridden city, among them Newton's disciple Nicolas Fatio de Duillier, a Swiss mathematician. The Prophets lauded not silence and resignation but loud and vocal preaching against the established church and prophesying of imminent millennium, often accompanied by violent physical agitation.[37] George Garden tried to dissuade Cuninghame; in the previous year, he had warned against the Prophets in his preface to Bourignon's 1671 anti-Quaker work, arguing, as had Bourignon against the Quakers, that the Prophets were a mere sect and opposed to her quiet, passive reception of God's will.[38] Nonetheless, several members of Garden's circle joined the French Prophets; Ramsay commented in November 1709 that "there is not one person in or about Edinburgh that read the Writings of A.B. but what are more or less under the agitations."[39]

There is no evidence that Cheyne was sympathetic to the Prophets, although they were prominent in Bristol, near Bath. Back in London in the spring of 1710, however, Cheyne would have witnessed another manifestation of the evils of sectarianism. The trial of Henry Sacheverell, a violently Tory and High Anglican clergyman charged with preaching a seditious sermon, had ended with a declaration of guilt and a sentence so light as to be an embarrassment for the Whigs who had brought him to trial. The verdict sparked weeks of anti-Whig and antidissenter rioting throughout England. Even while the trial was taking place, London had exploded in one of the worst civil disorders of the century.[40]

Sacheverell's sermon, delivered at St. Paul's on Guy Fawkes Day 1709, used the old Tory cry of "the Church in danger" to attack all whom he perceived as enemies of the true church, ranging from Arians such as Whiston to latitudinarians such as Gilbert Burnet and the Boyle lecturers, "whosoever presumes to recede the least tittle from the express word of God, or to explain the great crescenda of our Faith in new-fangled terms of modern philosophy." All dissent, all toleration, presented unconscionable compromise with the true principles of the Church of England. The "False Brethren" of the state had similarly endangered the nation by failing to uphold the principles of obedience and nonresistance to the state.[41]

The Sacheverell Riots were directed particularly against dissenters. But to Cheyne, the riots gave yet more evidence of the evil of factionalism. At the same time, Sacheverell's words, which were widely distributed, would have struck another blow to an already tender conscience.

Around this time Cheyne became acquainted through the Garden circle with the works of another quietist author, Jeanne de la Mothe Guyon (1648–1717). Pierre Poiret had already begun to oversee the publication of her works as he had done for Bourignon. Andrew Michael Ramsay left Britain in 1710, visiting Poiret in the Netherlands and then seeking out Guyon's sponsor Bishop Fénelon in France. Ramsay remained with him as a secretary, later serving Guyon in that capacity, and converted to Catholicism. Garden also traveled to the continent in 1710 to visit Guyon, and thereafter actively disseminated her works.[42]

Owing to Fénelon's sponsorship, Guyon is a much better known figure than Bourignon.[43] The lives of the two women diverged widely. Guyon, a daughter of the nobility, had been married and had children. Widowed young, she was left a considerable estate, which she later renounced. Her quietism led to a furious public debate between two of the most prominent clergymen of the day, Bossuet and Fénelon. Unlike Bourignon, who was accused of sorcery and hounded for much of her life, Guyon garnered considerable public support. Nonetheless, she was imprisoned in the late 1690s. After several years she was released and allowed to settle in Blois in 1705, where she lived with a group of disciples until her death in 1717.

Guyon's mysticism developed gradually, reaching fruition only after she was widowed in the late 1670s. While Bourignon's call for spiritual passivity did not exclude the exercise of free will in daily life, Guyon prescribed a radically passive quietism that, taken to its logical ends, would exclude even desire for salvation from its goals. Guyon argued that the perfection of the soul in this life or the next was a state of love, *pur amour*, that excluded all other considerations. The ideally contemplative soul was completely indifferent to its state or to that of the body; it rejected all reason and even all thought. Guyon's ideas, first expressed in her *Moyen court et trés facile de faire oraison* (*Short and easy way to prayer*, 1685), bore some resemblance to those of the contemporary Spanish mystic Miguel de Molinos (1628–96), whose *Spiritual Guide* was very popular. Like Molinos, Guyon's ideas were viewed as morally questionable by the Catholic Church, because her complete passivity precluded the active pursuit of virtue and rejection of temptation.

Through Poiret, Ramsay, Keith, and Garden, Guyon's doctrines were disseminated through the Gardens' Scottish circle.[44] Both Bourignon and Guyon influenced Cheyne's continuing spiritual odyssey, and by the end of the decade he again began to write. Even in the throes of his illness and conversion, a second edition of the *Philosophical Principles* had been a goal. In 1706, describing himself as "being low in my Health, and otherwise engaged," he asked Craig "to write me down his Thoughts on, correct or alter" the section on infinites at the end of the book.[45] Apparently Craig had accomplished this task almost immediately, and now Cheyne began the arduous task of rewriting.

Despite the public disregard of the *Philosophical Principles* at its appearance in 1705, a few natural philosophers noticed it. In the spring of 1714— possibly after Cheyne had already concluded his revisions for a second edition—the mathematician Brook Taylor, a secretary of the Royal Society, penned a detailed critique of certain aspects of the 1705 edition.[46] Taylor spent some time correcting Cheyne's always chancy mathematics, but his critique centered on the issue of occasionalism, the notion that the world continued to require God's active intervention. Although Cheyne had stated his opposition to this concept, Taylor found suspect evidence. Early in the *Philosophical Principles* Cheyne had asserted that since neither rest nor motion were essential to matter, the preservation of a body in either of these states "does absolutely depend on *Almighty God* as its cause." Taylor countered that although neither rest nor motion were essential states, a body was always in one or the other, and that causes such as Cheyne required "are only necessary when changes are to be produced. But to keep things in the same State there certainly needs no

Action." Taylor's model of the Newtonian universe, in other words, was a steady state, in which the initial causes of motion would not materially alter its operation, rather than a dynamic system in constant flux.[47]

Taylor also objected to Cheyne's arguments against the eternality of the world. Cheyne had stated that "it is altogether impossible [that] this present state of things shou'd have been from all Eternity *of itself*, since at present it cannot subsist in a regular and beautiful *System* without the perpetual influence of some superiour and *extrinsick* Power." Cheyne furthermore proposed that the chain of causation inevitably led back to the original design and contrivance of God, because no link in that chain could exist of itself. Taylor, in contrast, argued that "The order of the World, and the conspiring of all things to certain great ends, do fully convince us that all these things are govern'd by an overruling Being who makes things subservient to these ends; but it is no Demonstration of the beginning of the existence of any of these things consider'd seperately." In other words, "a body that is found to be in Motion may have been so from all Eternity," again emphasizing the consistency and stability of the Newtonian universe. Taylor believed that Cheyne's views smacked of millenarianism and enthusiasm, even though Newton himself, as Cheyne knew, believed that the system did lead to dissolution. Taylor's arguments for a cosmology of the steady state may also have been intended to counter the destabilizing influence of deists such as John Toland and Charles Blount, who contended that activity was inherent in matter and did not require an external cause.[48]

Taylor's comments remained unpublished. Cheyne may have seen them, since in the 1715 edition he removed the passage that argued that preservation of a body in rest or motion is directly dependent on God. But he ignored Taylor's other criticisms. Cheyne went through his great work line by line, word by word. The change in title indicated his new focus on revealed religion. In his preface to part 1, on natural religion, Cheyne listed as his principal sources the *Opticks* and the second edition of the *Principia*, edited by Roger Cotes, which had appeared in June 1713. William Derham's 1711–12 Boyle lectures, also published in 1713, provided further inspiration, and Gregory (before his death in 1708) and Craig had suggested corrections. Cheyne also cryptically referred to "a *Gentleman* at

Cambridge who conceals his Name" as a source of "some very Judicious Reflections." This gentleman may have been William Whiston, who by 1715 had reason to conceal his name, having been thrown out of his Cambridge professorship in 1711 for doctrinal unorthodoxy. Whiston attributed the powers of nature to the "constant Influence" of God in his 1716 *Account of a Surprizing Meteor*; however, it is impossible to tell which way the arrow of influence pointed.[49]

Although any reader of his text would recognize that Cheyne did not derive his conclusions from the very conventional Derham, he did not wish to advertise his departure from convention, nor any hint of Jacobitism. The change in policy toward the Scottish Episcopalians signaled by the 1712 Toleration Act proved to be short-lived. Geoffrey Holmes viewed the 1712 act as part of the post-Sacheverell Tory program, which did not survive the queen. George Garden had dedicated his 1703 edition of the works of John Forbes to Queen Anne, and the brothers were presented to the queen in the spring of 1714 and professed their adherence to the English Prayer Book. But her death later that year not only ended Episcopalian hopes in Scotland but reestablished and even widened the political divide between Jacobites and everyone else. Both Gardens supported the invasion of the pretender in 1715; George Garden escaped imprisonment by fleeing to Holland, while James was allowed to retire to the country. George Garden's Bourignonist colony at Rosehearty broke up. Though Roxburghe was a major political power in Scotland after 1715, his former drinking companion Cheyne received no preferment from him.[50]

Cheyne did not cite his principal sources—Garden, Bourignon, and Guyon—but his work showed their influence on every page. In place of Pitcairne's argument for the absolute certainty of mathematical explanation upon which he had relied in 1705, Cheyne now inserted words and phrases into his text that softened its assertions toward contingency rather than necessity. Following Pitcairne's death in 1713, perhaps Cheyne felt freer to deviate from his teacher's ideas. In this "lapsed" world, he commented, human faculties were perhaps not capable of attaining certain knowledge. Natural philosophy itself was limited, he added, reaching only "some of the grosser *Lineaments*, or more conspicuous *Out-lines* of the

Works of the Almighty."[51] Robert Leighton had argued that natural knowledge, even mathematical knowledge, is not certain and cannot prove that the soul is immortal.[52]

Although Cheyne had discussed the role of analogy in natural philosophy in 1705, a decade later this concept became the unifying principle between God and nature, a demonstration that natural and revealed religion were one and the same. He explained, "The whole Foundation of *Natural Philosophy*, is *Simplicity* and *Analogy*, or a Simple, yet Beautiful *Harmony*, running through all Works of Nature in an uninterrupted Chain of Causes and Effects."[53] Cheyne echoed the "Rules of Reasoning" in the new edition of the *Principia*, which labeled simplicity and analogy essential qualities of nature. But his heavily Platonized rendering of these views recalled also the words of a much younger Newton, who in his 1675 "Hypothesis of Light" had shown himself still to be under the influence of the Cambridge Platonists.[54] While Cheyne may have been acquainted with this work, he was by this time far better acquainted with the works of Leighton and Scougal, who had also read the Cambridge Platonists.

Cheyne took literally Newton's suggestion in query 20 (28) of the 1706 *Opticks* that nature was the sensorium of God. Newton's further comments about God's nature in the "General Scholium" of the 1713 *Principia* added details to Cheyne's description. But Newton did not provide Cheyne's 1715 explanation of gravity as analogous to God's love:

God being the sole *sovereign, self-existent* and *independent Being,* when he made Creatures partaking of himself, Images, *Emanations, Effluxes* and Streams out of his own *Abyss* of *Being,* could not but impress upon their most *intimate* Natures and Substances, a *Central* Tendency toward himself, an Essential Principle of *Re-Union* with himself, which in him is a Principle of *Attraction* of them towards him, *Analogous* to this Principle now mention'd in the Great Bodies of the Universe.[55]

Cheyne's argument in the *Philosophical Principles* had therefore two dimensions: the principle of analogy and a Platonic continuum between matter and spirit. In the second section of his work, he coupled the arithmetic of infinites with the "*Philosophick Principles of Reveal'd Religion.*" Here he recast his mathematical work from the first edition, not to rehabilitate his reputation as a mathematician, but to prove, by means of the mathematics of infinitesimals, the continuum between matter and spirit.

Cheyne's outline of his plan began with a reference to the chain (or "cone") of being, which he likened to the light of the sun. The farther one stood from the sun, the weaker its light; less perfect beings therefore dwelled farther down the chain. From this image, Cheyne drew his chief points:

I That there is a perpetual *Analogy* (Physical not Mathematical) running on in a Chain, thro' the whole *System* of *Creatures*, up to their *Creator*.

II That the Visible are Images of the Invisible, the Sensible of the Insensible, the *Ectypical* of the *Architypical*, the *Creatures* of the *Creator*, at an absolutely infinite distance. . . .

V That if *Gravitation* be the Principle of *Activity* in *Bodies*; that of *Re-union*, with their Origin, must by this *Analogical* Necessity, be the Principle of Action in *Spirits*.

VI That *Material Substances*, are the same with *Spiritual Substances*, of the higher Orders, at an infinite distance, or that *Material Substances* are *Spiritual Substances* infinitely condensed or contracted, since in the *Scale* of *Existence*, the *first* are supposed at an *infinite* distance from the *latter*.[56]

Analogy, then, governed the actions of both the universe and the soul, for gravity and the love of God were aspects of the same "great and universal *Principle*." Body and spirit occupied opposite ends of the chain of being, yet both were extended and therefore capable of changing into each other. This symmetry, which he perceived to be evident throughout the universe, was a sign of that analogy which proved the existence of God as certainly "as any *Mathematical* Demonstration infers its Proposition." All created beings were simply the visible representations of the archetype in the mind of the Creator, a literal transformation of thought into flesh. Again echoing Newton, Cheyne concluded, "Hence *universal Space* may be very aptly called the *Sensorium Divinitis*." This is a far cry from the argument from design employed by the Boyle lecturers.[57]

From this relationship Cheyne constructed an elaborate model of rational beings, who, he said, possessed three levels of consciousness: first, the five senses; second, the "rational soul" or mind; and third, the "supreme spirit," infinite in capacity, by means of which one communicated with God. In the "due *Subordination*" of these three levels humans could reach their fullest perfection, a true imitation of Christ in which the soul was united with God by the principle of reunion. Too often, however, the sensual overrode the other two levels, leading to corruption and depravity.[58] Cheyne drew an analogy between several sets of threes, including gravity, matter, and the universe, as proof of the divine Trinity of Father, Son, and Holy Spirit. He did not realize that here he parted with the Arian (antitrinitarian) Newton.[59]

Following both Newton and Bourignon, Cheyne attempted to steer a course between two physico-theological extremes: Toland's argument for the innate activity of nature and the voluntarism of Sacheverell and his followers. Newton acknowledged the necessity of intermediate causes when he reintroduced the ether in the "General Scholium" attached to the second edition of the *Principia* in 1713.[60] It served as an intermediary between God and nature, a means for divine action. Cheyne's Platonic continuum served the purposes of an ether. Like Newton, Cheyne ended his work with a General Scholium.

Craig's section on the arithmetic of infinites, which followed Cheyne's philosophical effusions, also provided their scientific underpinning, since much of Cheyne's argument was based on the nature of the infinite, which he believed proved the continuum between matter and spirit. In this manner Cheyne combined Pitcairne's arguments for the certainty of mathematics with Newton's calculus and ether and with Bourignon's mysticism. The incarnation of Christ himself provided the final proof. Christ's body, said Bourignon, "tho' material, [is] of the same Nature with Spirits."[61] The incarnation was literally the spirit made flesh, traveling down the scale of being for a time, only to return later.

Cheyne had finally resolved his decade-long crisis. His physical ills, only partially cured by medicines, had led him to a spiritual awakening. This crisis led him to recognize the interrelationship between body and spirit, matter and God. The ideas set forth in the 1715 *Philosophical Principles* would sustain him for the rest of his life. He had worked out to his satisfaction the vexed relationship among mind, matter, and spirit. This understanding would now guide him as he turned back toward the world and the practice of medicine.

5

A BATH PHYSICIAN
AND HIS PRACTICE

Cheyne's *Philosophical Principles of Religion, Natural and Revealed* had a mixed reception. According to the historian Frank Manuel, Newton found the work "too saturated with religious Neoplatonism for his taste."[1] While it was nearly ignored in England at its time of publication, it later found a place in the university curriculum. Cheyne wrote of it in 1724, "I thought [it] might be of Use to other young Gentlemen, who, while they were learning the Elements of natural Philosophy, might have thereby the Principles of natural Religion insensibly instilled into them. And accordingly it has been and is still used for that Purpose at both Universities."[2]

It was recommended reading at Cambridge in 1730 both in natural philosophy and in moral philosophy, and the Cambridge tutor Daniel Waterland had recommended the 1705 edition as a natural philosophy text as early as 1706. At least one Oxford tutor also recommended the book as a text in natural philosophy.[3] Cheyne did not include the Scottish universities in his assessment, and its use there is more difficult to trace. The Glasgow professor of moral philosophy Gershom Carmichael mentioned Cheyne as a source for the argument from design in his 1729 text *Synopsis theologiae naturalis*, and Cheyne is referred to in several graduation theses from Marischal College, Aberdeen, between 1715 and 1753.[4] The Edinburgh professor of natural philosophy in the 1720s, Robert Steuart, included works of Cheyne in his "Physiological Library," whose catalog was published in 1726. Michael Barfoot has described this as a "map or plan for Steuart's students to find their way around 'physiology,'" which term referred to the study of nature in general.[5] David Hume was among Steuart's students.

The Amsterdam philologist and theologian Jean LeClerc (1657–1736) devoted over one hundred pages to the 1705 edition in his journal *Bibliothèque ancienne et moderne* in 1715. LeClerc strongly approved of Cheyne's work, which was regrettably "little known on this side of the sea." He especially lauded the central role God played in Cheyne's system, in contrast to Descartes, "who believed that it sufficed that God had once given motion to matter."[6] The popularity of natural theology in the Netherlands is indicated by the translation of Cheyne's work into Dutch in 1716, and the natural philosopher Nicolaas Hartsoeker reviewed the 1715 edition in LeClerc's journal in 1717. LeClerc translated Cheyne's work into French, and an Italian translation followed in 1729. Thus the cycle of transmission from the Netherlands of Bourignon to Britain and back again continued.[7] In Germany, Leibniz noted the work to the extent of asking Cheyne for his opinion in his ongoing debate with Samuel Clarke.[8]

Cheyne seemed unconcerned with the reception of his book. He had resolved his intellectual crises and was now determined to get on with his life. He permanently settled in Bath in the summer of 1718, seeking the professional success that had so long eluded him.[9] If, as he claimed, conversion had diminished his desire for intellectual recognition, he nonetheless had a young and growing family to support.[10] A glimpse of Cheyne at this time appears in *The Gold-Headed Cane*, that fount of medical anecdotes first published in 1827. Early in 1715 Cheyne acted as physician to his kinsman Bishop Gilbert Burnet. An eyewitness described

Dr Cheyne, a Scotchman, with an immense broad back, taking snuff incessantly out of a ponderous gold box, and thus ever and anon displaying to view his fat knuckles; a perfect Falstaff, for he was not only a good portly man and a corpulent, but was almost as witty as the knight himself, and his humour being heightened by his northern tongue, he was exceedingly mirthful. Indeed, he was the most excellent wit of his time, a faculty he was often called upon to exercise, to repel the lampoons which were made by others upon his extraordinary personal appearance.[11]

Cheyne's witty conversation, delivered in his broad Aberdeen accent, had made him a popular figure in coffeehouses and taverns and was an

essential component of his bedside manner. His letters to Samuel Richardson, discussed in chapter 7, give some of the flavor of his conversation.
John Mullan, among others, has discussed the significance of sociability, of
conversation and correspondence "dependent upon the communication of
passions and sentiments," which was central to the evolution of eighteenth-
century culture.[12] By 1715 Cheyne had returned to his favorite conversational
haunts and his old indulgent habits.

This anecdote also hints at the extent of Cheyne's medical practice at
this time. Burnet had summoned Cheyne from Bath to London for care
in 1710 and again in 1713.[13] The physician Sir David Hamilton consulted
Cheyne about his own health in Bath in 1715 and 1720, and probably at
other times.[14] Hamilton had already referred some of his own patients to
Cheyne when they visited Bath, including the earl and countess of Loudoun in the spring of 1709.[15] James Cuninghame, laird of Barns in Fife,
visited Cheyne that summer.[16] The Baillies of Jerviswood, like Cheyne kin
to the Burnets, had met Cheyne in 1708, probably through Roxburghe.
They consulted "Dr Shien" in London in 1715; formerly Pitcairne's
patients, they almost certainly saw Cheyne during their numerous trips to
Bath.[17] In 1716 Cheyne wrote to James Keith's friend Robert Harley,
former lord treasurer and a member of the Scriblerus Club, about a
patient.[18] The Scriblerus Club included Arbuthnot as well as Pope and
Gay, both of whom consulted Cheyne in the 1720s.

By this evidence, many of Cheyne's clients at this point were Scots of
good family who were referred to him by a better-known practitioner.
Politically, they formed a diverse lot, from the Whigs Baillie and Burnet
to the Tory Hamilton, for publicly Cheyne distanced himself from the
shifting political boundaries of these years. Cheyne had not by 1715 established an extensive clientele on his own, however, and his success did not
approach that of his contemporaries Mead, Arbuthnot, and Freind.
Mead and Freind were elected fellows of the Royal College of Physicians
of London in 1716; Arbuthnot had already served a term as one of Queen
Anne's physicians.[19] Hans Sloane's position as arbiter of aristocratic medical
practice was codified by his election as president of the Royal College of
Physicians of London in 1719; he had already been created a baronet in
1716.[20]

After he chose to remain in Bath year round, Cheyne needed one or more London patrons who would regularly, rather than intermittently, refer patients to him. One candidate for this post was Hamilton, but he had fallen from power at Queen Anne's death and only partially recovered his reputation when he was appointed physician to the princess of Wales. Moreover, Hamilton was himself ailing, and his fame as a man-midwife may have made him less valuable as a patron than Sloane.[21] The value of Sloane's patronage had already been made apparent over a decade earlier to the Scot James Keill. More recently, Sloane had sponsored the career of another Scot, Alexander Stuart. Cheyne had called in Sloane and Mead to assist him with Gilbert Burnet's case in 1715, and he eagerly accepted his patronage when it was offered. But Sloane sprinkled his largesse liberally. As Bath became increasingly fashionable, competition among its medical practitioners heightened. As in London, Cheyne needed more than patronage to distinguish himself from the rest of the pack.

Cheyne's choice of Bath as the site for his professional aspirations may, as he claimed, have been influenced by his own state of health. But Bath had much to offer an ambitious younger physician. Although its hot springs had been known since antiquity, it came into its own as a spa town only in the first half of the eighteenth century. Despite royal visits, including one by Queen Elizabeth I (who was unimpressed), and the increasing popularity of mineral water therapy, Bath for most of the seventeenth century was another weaving town in decline.[22] Celia Fiennes in the 1680s found the houses there "indifferent," a far cry from the city of a century hence.[23] Yet her visit, preceded by that of Charles II's queen, Catherine of Braganza, and succeeded by his niece Princess Anne, signaled the beginning of Bath's heyday. While the waters remained the main attraction—now not only to be bathed in but to be drunk—the town's additional attractions as a center for leisure led to its astonishing growth and prosperity in the eighteenth century.[24] In the 1720s Defoe described it as "the resort of the sound, rather than the sick; the bathing is made more a sport and diversion, than a physical prescription for health; and the town is taken up in raffling, gaming, visiting, and in a word, all sorts of gallantry and levity."[25] Hamilton had more succinctly

commented to Sloane in 1715, "There are many here but I am of opinion
that ther are more haile than sick."[26]

The appearance of this "leisure town" was not an isolated event but
part of a larger phenomenon that the historian Peter Borsay has labeled
the "urban renaissance." The economic boom of the Restoration had not
only increased the wealth of the gentry but had greatly added to the
numbers and wealth of the trading and professional men of the cities
and towns, the so-called middling men. Recent studies of probate inven-
tories have demonstrated the dramatic increase in the number and quality
of goods possessed by these individuals, for a salient sign of the increase
in wealth was an increase in consumption. Borsay has distinguished
between towns that created wealth in this period and towns that attracted
surplus wealth with multiple opportunities for consumption. In the latter
category stood not only spas, including Bath, but such disparate sites as
Shrewsbury and Weymouth, which were reborn in the eighteenth century
as newly fashionable gathering places. Walks, theaters, assembly halls, and
booksellers provided cultured entertainment, and itinerant scientific lecturers added intellectual excitement, which Cheyne would appreciate.
Neoclassical architecture and widened, cleaned, and lighted streets provided aesthetic, safe, and salubrious surroundings. If local industry flagged,
the professional classes, including lawyers, physicians, bankers, and archi-
tects, flourished in these surroundings.[27] Cheyne's future publisher James
Leake moved to Bath in 1722; by 1740 many subscribed to his bookshop
at five shillings a season "for Pleasure or Amusement."[28] A new commerce
arose between visitors and the residents of Bath, who now sold services
as well as goods.

While other spas—Epsom, Tunbridge Wells, and later Scarborough
and Buxton—also flourished in this period, they did not enjoy the
remarkable popularity of Bath. Penelope Corfield has singled out accessi-
bility, amenities, patronage, and promotion as the cornerstones of its
success. Bath was only one hundred miles from London: close enough to
be accessible, but far enough away to remain exclusive. Improvements in
road and river navigation increased access not only to travelers but to the
goods that underpinned the life of leisure. During the course of the
eighteenth century the town enormously extended its medical and social

amenities. The first playhouse was built in 1705. The first Pump Room, to shelter those who came to drink the waters, was erected a year later.[29] In that year, stated the architect John Wood,

a Row of new Houses was begun on the South Side of the Gravel Walks; before which a handsome Pavement was then made, with large flat Stones, for the Company to walk upon. . . . In the Autumn, an Application was made to Parliament for a Power to amend the Principal Roads leading to Bath; to pave, cleanse, and Light the Streets, Lanes, &c of the Town; and to regulate and licence a sufficient Number of Chairmen, that nothing might be wanting for the publick Utility of the City.[30]

Assembly rooms and improved accommodations soon followed, and Wood commenced Bath's architectural renovation with his Queen Square in 1728.

Bath also benefited greatly from publicity. Royal patronage drew London society to take the waters, and both patients and physicians followed the new social "seasons": summer in the country or at the spas, winter in London. An anonymous observer of Bath in 1700 complained, "five Months in the Year 'tis as Populous as *London*, the other seven as desolate as a Wilderness."[31] Bath's particular popularity owed much to two factors: Richard Nash and the physicians. As master of ceremonies from 1705 until 1761, Nash maintained a schedule of activities and, more importantly, set standards for polite conduct. Although Nash's influence on Bath's success has lately been disputed, the spa's unique tone, if not its physical amenities, owed much to his presence.[32] He promoted the mingling of gentry and middle class at public assemblies while enforcing a decorum that kept these assemblies of strangers from degenerating into licentiousness. Even royalty was required to adhere to Nash's standards for dress and behavior, and to stop dancing promptly at 11 P.M. Licentiousness existed, but not in public; the 1700 observer nonetheless labeled Bath "a Valley of Pleasure, yet a sink of Iniquity."[33] Nude bathing, common in the seventeenth century, had ceased by 1700, but plenty of opportunities for dalliance remained. Nash also promoted "raffling," or gambling and card games, which proved to be both lucrative for him and entertaining for Bath's visitors.[14]

For the visitor, according to Defoe, "the whole time indeed is a round of the utmost diversion."[15] John Wood detailed the daily round in his *Description of Bath* (1749). The "Amusement of Bathing" was followed by a trip to the Pump House to drink the waters, where "the Intervals between their Drinking are made agreeable . . . by the Harmony of a small Band of Musick, as well as by the Conversation of the Gay and Healthy." From the Pump House the ladies returned to their lodgings for breakfast, while the gentlemen frequented one of the many coffeehouses to read newspapers and eat Bath buns with their coffee. Afternoon was the time for public display on Wood's Grand Parade and Queen Square, alternating with more serious exercise on foot, coach, or horseback or with visits to the bookshops or gaming tables. Dinner, later in the afternoon, was the main meal of the day. It was followed by another visit to the Pump House. Twice a week at 6 P.M. public balls commenced in the Assembly Rooms; on the remaining evenings, private entertainments were pursued.[16]

These diversions of course cost money. From a colonial outpost in 1709, the Hon. Thomas Pitt wrote his son, "it was a surprise to me to hear that all my family, who I left in a pleasant habitation, were removed to the Bath, and there spending my estate faster than I got it."[17] Cheyne's patients the Baillies spent eighty-eight pounds traveling from Scotland to Bath in the 1720s and eighteen pounds a month on lodging when they arrived. At the time, one hundred pounds per year was considered a decent income for a shopkeeper.[18]

This round of entertainment and consumption appeared to leave little room for medical care. Nonetheless, its physicians were as important to the life of Bath as its diversions. For centuries, bathing had been a recommended therapy, and various learned treatises from the 1570s onward expounded on the efficacy of Bath's waters in particular. It was extolled as a cure for infertility, and Catherine of Braganza sought its benefits. The infertility of her sister-in-law Mary of Modena was indeed relieved, making Bath responsible for the Glorious Revolution. The

Restoration fashion of drinking mineral waters, even waters as foul-tasting and -smelling as Bath's, redounded to its advantage, since those disinclined to bathe could come to drink the waters and enjoy the social life of the Pump House. While many Bath physicians argued that efficacy could only be guaranteed at the source, this did not prevent a flourishing industry in bottled water from Bath and other spas. Cheyne himself prescribed a variety of bottled mineral waters, both domestic and foreign, each with its own specific qualities.

By the 1720s Bath's physicians had produced an extensive body of literature, including a mass of case histories detailing the particular excellences of Bath waters. Robert Peirce's *Bath Memoirs* (1697) recited "many instances, that may be given of great Recoveries obtained here, by the use of these Waters, under my Directions, even when great Means and long Methods of *Physick* have failed."[39] When some physicians revived a fashion for cold bathing, the physicians of Bath quickly leaped to the defense of hot water. To a 1697 treatise on cold bathing, Edward Baynard responded in a letter extolling hot baths, particularly "The Wonderful Effects of the *Bath-Water*, drunk hot from the *Pump*."[40] John Quinton's *Practical Observations in Physick* (1707) "proved the Noxious qualities of Cold Mineral Waters."[41] Dr. William Oliver, who practiced in both Bath and London after 1702, appended a "Dissertation on the Hot Waters of Bathe" to his *Practical Essay on Fevers* of 1704, in which he argued that the hot waters might be beneficially drunk year-round, not just in summer. But, he added, drinking in the present unsheltered area could be dangerous. Soon after, construction began on the Pump Room. Oliver continued his promotion of Bath in his *Practical Dissertation on Bath Waters* in 1707, dedicated to Queen Anne. In this work he admitted that Bath waters could profitably be drunk cold as well: "'tis not absolutely necessary in all Cases to go to the Pump." But both modes of therapy together were most efficacious.[42] Both also increased Bath's clientele.

Popular medical treatises directed at the literate middle and upper classes, such as those of the Bath doctors, were not a new genre. Particularly in the era following the Civil War, when antimonopoly sentiment flourished, publication of vernacular treatises grew manyfold, and they continued to proliferate after the Restoration.[43] Elite physicians, even in

the London College, did not have the political or intellectual authority to
control the flow of medical information. Lucinda Beier has argued that
"there was no consensus in the general population that licensed healers
were the sole authorities in medical matters."[44] Therefore, a very wide range
of information was available, mirroring the range of healers, from members
of the London College to illiterate herb sellers. As Barbara Duden has
noted, "the choice of a healer was driven by a social logic whose dynamic
was controlled by the sick person."[45] Robert Peirce addressed, he said, not
the physician but the patient, informing them "where and how to seek for
remedy,"[46] with the knowledge that his was one option among many. Yet
Cheyne and his colleagues cooperated as well as competed. Christopher
Anstey's *New Bath Guide* (1766) described a patient in the clutches of
medical men:

> And so, as I grew ev'ry day worse and worse,
> The doctor advis'd me to send for a nurse,
> And the nurse was so willing my health to restore,
> She begg'd me to send for a few doctors more;
> For when any difficult work's to be done,
> Many heads can dispatch it much sooner than one.[47]

The social and economic changes of the Restoration had created, by
the early eighteenth century, a class of patients more demanding of
physicians. More people had more money. A middle class of tradesmen
flourished, and above them an upper middle class of professionals, both
increasingly sophisticated in the new environments of the "urban renaissance." Greater affluence meant that these people, as well as the gentry,
spent more on food, books, and medicines. Smollett's Matthew Bramble
complained, "Every upstart of fortune . . . presents himself at Bath . . .
men of low birth, and no breeding, have found themselves suddenly
translated into a state of affluence. . . . and all of them hurry to Bath,
because here, without any further qualification, they can mingle with the
princes and nobles of the land."[48]
These people were well informed about contemporary medical theory
and practice, a knowledge fed not only by popular medical treatises but

also by new periodicals such as the *Spectator* and later the *Gentleman's Magazine*, and they had decided ideas about what their physician should be doing. Correspondence and diaries amply illustrate the informed interest taken by the literate classes in their state of health, and the lengths to which they went to preserve it, including the expenditure of comparatively large sums. The Bethlem physician Richard Hale charged a guinea for a consultation, and Cheyne's London colleague Richard Mead charged two guineas.[49]

The extent of patient knowledge meant that, unlike in our time, the physician's explanatory model of illness largely coincided with that of the patient.[50] Patients and healers alike thought not in ontological terms of disease but of the individual experience of illness. As Barbara Duden has argued, following Gianna Pomata, the multiplicity of healers coincided with multiple views of the body; there was no one single "body" or "illness" that a single practitioner could master.[51] Physicians and patients both continued to discuss illness in traditional humoral terms of balance and imbalance, surfeit and deficiency. These terms were translated into fashionably mechanical language by 1700, but their meaning remained largely unchanged from Galenic times.[52] Gail Kern Paster has argued that "humoralism had broad and pervasive effects on the discourse, experience, and expression of bodiliness and on the enculturation process in general." As she points out, the humoral language of bodily fluids—translated by Cheyne and others into a discourse on hydraulics—continued to be the dominant discourse on the body.[53] The anthropologist Arthur Kleinman has defined "clinical reality" as "the social, structural, and cultural context of sickness and care." When social reality is changing and unstable, clinical reality reflects this instability, and beliefs about illness and healing change.[54] Galenic clinical reality was just beginning to erode in the first half of the eighteenth century. As social change accelerated, so too did medical thinking.

The values of the new urban culture included gentility and politeness, an ideal of behavior far removed from the sectarian passions of the previous century. As Lawrence Klein has argued, politeness served as a bridge between the older land-based gentry and the new urban elites who sought to be gentlemen.[55] Attention turned to the cultivation of the personal, to leisure, comfort, even luxury. Puritan stoicism gave way to an intolerance for suffering, and personal sensitivity became a sign of a highly civilized being.[56] G. S. Rousseau and G. J. Barker-Benfield, among others, have traced the course of "sensibility" over the eighteenth century from its original connotation of the nervous system to a much broader moral discourse, especially in the novel.[57] Yet as John Mullan has pointed out, in the eighteenth-century novel "it is the body which acts out the powers of sentiment,"[58] and Cheyne's life and practice provided a perfect example of the cultivation of the soul through attention to the body. In contrast to the low expectations Beier attributed to seventeenth-century patients, eighteenth-century medical consumers demanded relief of their symptoms, or at least the feeling that the physician was doing something, and physicians conformed to these demands.

Competition among physicians for patients spawned a variety of professional strategems, which gave eighteenth-century medical practice its peculiar character.[59] Some physicians cloaked themselves in Newtonian science in an effort to appear learned and therefore to gain or retain status. Bernard Mandeville referred to "those Braggadocio's, who . . . only make use of the Name of Mathematicks to impose upon the World for Lucre."[60] But therapies, while they may have been more aggressive, changed little in their essential character. Bloodletting, purges, and emetics, as they had since antiquity, remained central to medical practice.

The demand for effective therapy was therefore difficult to fulfill.[61] Such doubtful expedients as tar water and Mrs. Stephens's dissolvent for the stone were eagerly promoted by learned physicians, but their popularity was short-lived. Cinchona, "the bark," effective against malaria, was also used to treat other fevers against which it had little effect. In addition, it served as a general "astringent" drug; it was a great favorite with Cheyne, who thought it thinned the blood. These uses indicate only a fitful grasp of disease ontology. With little knowledge of the causes of disease, physicians continued to treat symptoms. Some physicians expressed their feelings of helplessness in correspondence and private musings. James Keill wrote his patron Hans Sloane of a patient, "the Medicines he has taken are almost innumerable"; and over the drawn-out case of Lord Leominster he despaired of his ability to do anything effective.[62]

Patients did not rest easy. At one point Lady Leominster asked Sloane to affirm in his own handwriting his approval of Keill's therapy; at another, she ordered Sloane to consult two other physicians, Drs. Upton and Mead, and specifically not to consult either Garth or Gibbon.[63] Lady Elizabeth Hastings, daughter of the earl of Huntingdon, dispensed medical advice to her sisters and sister-in-law and forthrightly gave her opinions of their physicians.[64] The duchess of Chandos rejected Cheyne's prescription of Jesuit's bark and Bristol water but requested his advice for taking the waters at Tunbridge.[65] The Baillies called in no fewer than four physicians for a single illness in January 1707. Cheyne complained to Sloane in 1720 of his patient Mrs. Barry, who "rail'd . . . most ludicrously" at her doctors and demanded that they obtain for her a certain medicine from a "Quack" in London. Her doctors, Cheyne and Charles Bave, complied.[66] In Anstey's *New Bath Guide* the doctors meet in learned consultation and prescribe "decoctions and syrups . . . pill[s], bolus, julep and apozem." The narrator's servant, however,

> seiz'd all the stuff that the doctors had sent,
> And out of the window she flung it down souse
> As the first politician went out of the house.[67]

Lucinda Beier has argued that during the seventeenth century "the most commonly used kinds of medical therapy were self-treatment and treatment rendered by lay-people."[68] This was true both of the poor and of the literate classes who read vernacular medical works. In the eighteenth century the concept of self-maintenance or self-regulation assumed equal importance both to the care of the physician and to self-medication in the minds of the middle classes both in England and elsewhere. The Enlightenment concept of hygiene in France, with its implications for the personal management of health, had its counterpart in England.[69] Norbert Elias has argued that the disciplining of the body was an important part of the "civilizing process" in the eighteenth century; yet as Gail Paster has noted, the continued medical interest in messy secretions complicated this process.[70]

Cheyne's later works, particularly the *Essay of Health and Long Life*, first published in 1724, contributed to this new concept of self-maintenance while retaining a basis in the physiology of fluids. These works emphasized obtaining a personal, individual equilibrium through judicious management of the body. While focusing on the Galenic concept of the "six things non-natural" (sleep and waking, exercise, the passions, food and drink, air, evacuations), self-help literature also emphasized the interrelationship between humans and their environment. The cleaning and renovation of nascent urban areas in this period were thus part of this overall project of personal management of health.[71]

While public health renovations could affect the poor, only those with sufficient leisure and capital could devote time to personal well-being. The interface between the new culture of leisure and its relationship to health was especially evident in the new spa towns. The maladies for which the waters of Bath were recommended were legion. Bathing had long been a remedy for skin afflictions; the fictional Matthew Bramble expressed his disgust at the sight of a "child full of scrophulous ulcers" being lowered into one of the baths.[72] It was also believed to tone or relax the body, depending on one's theory. Robert Peirce noted its effectiveness in "palsies" and various pains.[73] The advent of drinking mineral waters opened up a new realm of therapy, and very nearly every malady at one time or another was thought to benefit from it, particularly since many were thought to stem in some way from impaired digestion. Cheyne noted, "These Waters are beneficial in almost all chronical Distempers . . . and introduce a natural Warmth . . . into decayed, worn-out, superannuated Constitutions."[74] Bath waters were diuretic and purging. Cheyne claimed their effectiveness for the stone and other digestive ailments, to which Peirce added barrenness, diabetes, the king's evil, and the "greensickness," or chlorosis, a mysterious ailment that attacked young women and whose symptoms included a suppression of appetite and the menses.[75] Two maladies were especially prominent among eighteenth-century visitors to Bath: gout and various nervous afflictions.

Gout formed the topic of Cheyne's initial foray into popular medicine. Today gout is defined as a specific disease caused by an excess of uric acid and manifesting itself in characteristic swellings around the joints. In the eighteenth century, as Roy Porter has explained, "Gout is one of those rich disease labels . . . used to denominate a great diversity of pains striking different regions of the body—not just the joints, but also the inward parts, the stomach, and the head." It was closely associated with affluence and overindulgence, "a sort of success tax."[76]

Cheyne's next published work after the 1715 *Philosophical Principles*, completed in July 1719, was *Observations Concerning the Nature and Due Method of Treating the Gout: Together with an Account of the Nature and Qualities of the Bath Waters: Intended for the Benefit of Richard Tennison, Esq.*, issued by George Strahan in 1720. It reached a third edition within a year.[77] In this work Cheyne turned from theory to practice and to the exhortation of self-help. He departed drastically from his earlier works in both style and content and built instead upon the model of his Bath colleagues.

In the *Essay on Gout* (as it came to be known in subsequent editions) Cheyne established his new themes: mechanical physiological theory, practical self-help advice, and liberal doses of moral exhortation. Cheyne described gout in terms of the physical and chemical state of the fibers and fluids of which the body is composed, following standard mechanical accounts of physiology such as his own earlier works and those of James Keill. Gout, he said, was caused by "the Abundance of Tartarous, Urinous, or other Salts, introduc'd into the Blood by the Food."[78] Any treatment would involve widening and relaxing the blood vessels to prevent them from being clogged by these salts, and eliminating or diluting the salts themselves. A tendency to gout was inherited, and it attacked particularly those of robust body type, with "stiff and springy" fibers, which trapped the offending salts.[79]

While Cheyne's general description of the gout borrowed much from Thomas Sydenham's well-known 1683 account, it differed in several critical respects. Both agreed that some individuals possessed a temperamental disposition toward gout and referred its origins to the digestion. Sydenham blamed a defective system that allowed "crude and undigested humours" to rise to the surface in the form of gouty tumors. "Reckless and inordinate drinking" was often a factor in so disturbing the system.[80]

Cheyne acknowledged the role of systemic deficiency in the onset of gout, but he paid far more attention than did Sydenham to external causes, particularly diet and indulgence in alcohol. Sydenham acknowledged weak nerves as a consequence of the same "paucity of spirits" that produced gouty symptoms, but Cheyne went on to identify a distinct variety of gout that he termed the "*Nervous* or Flying *Gout*." It particularly attacked those whose robust appearance disguised their weak nerves, much like Cheyne himself. He neatly tapped into the second great category of Bath patients, those suffering from nervous disorders.[81] While Sydenham had admitted that gout "kills more rich men than poor, more wise men than simple," as a good Puritan he dourly acknowledged gout as a judgment of Providence. Cheyne elaborated on this theme in a manner highly flattering to his audience. The sensitive, Cheyne claimed, were particularly susceptible to gout; therefore the laboring classes were blessedly immune, as were most women, who possessed the requisite sensitivity but not the proper body form. Gout, sighed Cheyne, was a cross we sensitive types have to bear. Hamilton had reached similar conclusions in his treatment of the gouty Queen Anne.[82]

Like Sydenham, Cheyne himself suffered from gout. His patients could therefore find in him a sympathetic ear, though at his peak weight of thirty-two stone he could hardly have presented an example to follow. By the time he completed the 1715 *Philosophical Principles*, Cheyne had returned to his old bad habits of overindulgence, and his weight crept up to and beyond its former heights. Moderation consisted of "not above a Quart, or three Pints at most" of wine with his dinner, and since he ate virtually nothing until the evening, it is not surprising that "every Dinner necessarily became a *Surfeit* and a *Debauch*." By the late 1710s his legs "broke out all over in scorbutick Ulcers" and he could not walk any distance without "extreme Pain and Blowing." He traveled to his patients by coach; "if I had but an Hundred Paces to walk, I was oblig'd to have a Servant following me with a Stool to rest on."[83] The playwright John Gay referred to "Cheney huge of size" in 1720, an acknowledgment also of his increased public reputation following the publication of the *Essay on Gout*.[84]

The attractively intimate tone of the *Essay on Gout*—in contrast to Sydenham's stern Latin—stemmed from personal experience.[85] Like others,

Cheyne lamented that a cure remained elusive. The diplomat William Temple had tried the Chinese remedy of moxa, and the proprietary "Diaphoretic Compound Ipecacuanha Powders" of Dr. Thomas Dover—a violent emetic—remained popular, as did the exotic Goddard's Drops, distilled from human bones. Cheyne criticized Sydenham's advice against evacuations, recommending rhubarb, a mild laxative, as a remedy. He especially promoted the use of sulfur, defining its character and activity in a slightly garbled paraphrase of Newton's "De natura acidorum." Sulfur, said Cheyne, consisted of very small particles of strong attractive force; it could therefore break up obstructions in even the smallest vessels, and also attract and destroy the effects of the saline particles that caused gout's specific symptoms. Cheyne expected potential patients to understand these arguments.[86]

Since no certain and universal cure existed, the best treatment included many of Sydenham's recommendations: exercise, a change of diet away from red meat and distilled liquors, and the use of strengthening medicines such as cinchona bark. To this Cheyne added mild purging and the use of dilutants such as mineral waters. Contemporaries such as the physician and clergyman William Stukeley had come to much the same conclusion.[87] Cheyne's "Advertisement to the Reader" declared that Providence had wisely provided the waters of Bath "as the most *Sovereign Restorative* in all the Weaknesses of the *Concoctive Powers*," and Bath water figures prominently throughout the text. He even provided a chemical explanation of its effectiveness.[88] In this case, however, the waters were strictly for drinking, not bathing, and he recommended cold baths as a supplemental treatment.

Yet if Cheyne's patients took themselves to Bath to drink the waters and enjoy the doctor's conversation, they might not fully enjoy its other pleasures. Cheyne's originality lay not in his prescriptions but in the distinct moral dimension he added to them. He declared that "were there neither Sin nor Shame in it, as there are eminently both, a *Gouty* Person ought to avoid Intemperance, as he would avoid the Bite of a Snake or Mad Dog." Cheyne chastised himself as well as his patients as "the *Rich*, the *Lazy*, the *Voluptuous*," and he virtuously hectored his audience, "TEMPERANCE only, Divine, Innocent, Indolent and Joyous *Temperance* can

Cure or effectively Relieve the *Gout*."[89] One might think that these admonitions would sit badly with the consuming classes, whose reward for
experiencing the baths was the social life of Bath. But the *Essay on Gout*
went through eight editions in the 1720s, and in his revisions Cheyne
retained his moral exhortations while reemphasizing the importance of
Bath waters. In place of the literal providentialism found in the seventeenth
century, Cheyne's moral argument was both more subtle and more flattering to his audience.[90] The sensitive, he said, were more sensible of the
effects of sin; but like Bourignon, Cheyne rejected the sackcloth-and-
ashes approach to penitence in favor of moderation. He subtly altered
clinical reality to fit prevailing social reality, offering continued attention
to the spiritual as a bridge between the providentialist past and a secu-
larizing present.

The second major ailment among visitors to Bath was nervous disorders.
To be a man or woman of feeling was to set oneself apart from the
laboring population and their coarser emotions. The protean "spleen"
could emerge as melancholy, hysteria, hypochondria, or headaches; all were
symptoms of an excess of spirit as opposed to body, of mind as opposed
to matter.[91] These ailments were often expressed in terms of a vague malaise
involving vertigo, various pains, nausea, and gastrointestinal upset. A visit
to a spa, with its change of scene and undemanding regimen, along with
the benefits of the waters, was often prescribed in these cases. Women's
constitutions were naturally weaker, and Sydenham and other physicians
argued that they were especially susceptible to nervous disorders. While
Radcliffe had declared that Queen Anne's illness was "nothing but the
Vapours," that vaporous ailment refused to dissolve into thin air.[92] Instead
it became increasingly fashionable. In the years following the success of
the *Essay on Gout*, Cheyne increasingly turned toward "nervous" patients.
As his own case history demonstrated, he viewed such illness in the usual
somatic terms. As Roy Porter has pointed out, attribution of these ailments to the body skirted the question of the disordered mind, which
would indicate madness and not merely "the Hyp."[93] But at the same time,
Cheyne acknowledged a spiritual dimension that his contemporaries often
overlooked.

One cause of the increase in nervousness was the South Sea Bubble, which burst in the fall of 1720. In July, South Sea stock had reached a height of £1000 for a £100 investment; by 1 October, the stock had fallen to £290.[94] Both Cheyne and Hamilton had invested, and Hamilton was rumored to have lost as much as £80,000, while Newton's losses approached £20,000; he commented on "the madness of the people" in the affair.[95] Over the summer, James Keith in London had complained to Lord Deskford, "There is a strange Spirit gone forth both here and there of encreasing and multiplying money of a sudden. It has fill'd most people's heads and hearts." By September, he reported, "Many here of all ranks are ruin'd by that Fall and many more hurt in their temporal estate."[96] Jane Pitt wrote to her mother-in-law in early October,

We hope that you will . . . come to Bath this season very soon, for upon the fall of South Sea, the place emptys so fast that you may have your choice of lodgings at the winter price. . . . most peoples harts are so down that scandell is not entertained as usuall, and the wits have something elce to think of . . . which makes the bath more agreeable now than ever I knew it.[97]

Cheyne commented to Sloane in December 1720 that "the S.S. & other disappointments & passions of the mind" had kept him much occupied in his profession that autumn.[98] In 1721 a physician, John Midriff, wrote his *Observations of the Spleen and Vapours: Containing Remarkable Cases of Persons of Both Sexes, and All Ranks, from the Aspiring Director to the Humble Bubbler, Who Have Been Miserably Afflicted with Those Melancholy Disorders since the Fall of South-Sea and Other Publick Stocks. Applebee's Journal* reported in January 1721,

We are assured, that the Number of Distemper'd Heads is so strangely encreas'd for some Months past, by the sudden rising and falling of Men's Fortunes and Families, under the operation of South Sea Vomits . . . that there is not room to be had among the private BEDLAMS, or *Mad-Houses as they are call'd*, throughout the Town.[99]

Many viewed the South Sea crisis as a plague; Pat Rogers argues that Defoe's *Journal of the Plague Year*, published in 1722, was inspired as much by this crisis as by the actual plague looming in Marseilles.[100] The crisis jolted the investors, big and small, whose wealth had, since the 1690s, been tied to the fortunes of the national debt; it also revealed massive corruption in the upper reaches of government, many of whose members had accepted bribes in the form of South Sea stock. On the other hand, Richard Mead noted a number "whose heads were turned by the immense riches which fortune had suddenly thrown in their way" to the extent that they, too, were committed to Bethlem.[101]

Robert Walpole's actions during the South Sea crisis gave him the reputation of a statesmanlike distance from partisan politics. After two decades in politics, Walpole in 1720 neared the top of the Whig hierarchy. His scheme to save the day, involving the purchase of South Sea stock by the Bank of England, was never actually put into practice but gave him the political clout to assume the premiership by 1722.[102] As the South Sea crisis developed, however, his eldest daughter, Catherine, fell ill. Catherine was sent to Bath, and Walpole's physician, Hans Sloane, referred her case to Cheyne in April 1720.

Cheyne revealed his therapeutics in a series of letters he wrote to Sloane between 1720 and 1723 concerning Catherine Walpole. At about the same time Sloane also turned over to Cheyne the case of Lord Montrath.[103] Cheyne displayed his still-tenuous status by his extreme deference to Sloane, the senior practitioner, addressed in all seriousness as "you who move in superior orbits." Catherine's mother, exercising her free will as a patient, almost immediately called in Hamilton to consult with her daughter's new caregiver. Coupled with this evidence, Cheyne's brash references to Sloane of his dozens of cures sound more like bravado than truth.[104] In contrast, a decade later Cheyne addressed Lady Huntingdon directly in the confident tones of the experienced practitioner.[105]

During the South Sea crisis, Walpole thus also contended with the illness of his eldest daughter. It is difficult to determine what exactly was wrong with Catherine Walpole. Just sixteen at the time of her first meeting with Cheyne, she suffered from that commonplace but baffling complex of symptoms that often found relief in Bath. These included "fitts" and faintings and lack of appetite, coupled with an inability to retain food and complicated by a mysterious pain in her side. We might now label such symptoms "anorexia nervosa," but in 1720 the usual diagnosis was "the vapours" or "hysteria," and Cheyne referred to her "fitts" as "Hysterick."[106] Theories of anorexia speculate that the emergence of symptoms often occur at a time of family, especially fatherly, crisis, so that the timing of Catherine's illness may not have been wholly coincidental.[107] But retrospective diagnosis is a risky business, and it is not clear that Catherine's lack of eating was voluntary. Cheyne did not call her illness "chlorosis," which some historians have also identified as anorexia.

Contemporary theory argued that nervous disorders were somatic in nature, with physical causes and cures. But Cheyne also recognized from his own experience the intimate interaction between physical, mental, and spiritual states. Catherine Walpole's case allowed him to put into practice some of his insights, while he gained deeper knowledge of women and their illnesses. Like the female saints whose works Poiret had recommended, eating, or the lack of it, was at the center of Catherine's illness. Cheyne's gouty patients, and at times, the doctor himself, were, in Thomas Tryon's phrase, "digging their *Graves* with their *Teeth*,"[108] while waifish teenagers like Catherine starved themselves. To someone as acutely conscious of food as Cheyne, Catherine's case was revelatory. The sympathy with female nature (including his own female side) that he had already gained from Bourignon and Guyon he now applied to his patients. Catherine's case is also eerily reminiscent of the fictional Clarissa twenty years later.

Catherine's illness was not caused by excess. Cheyne commented to Sloane, "it was rumour'd disappointments had some hand in [her] original ail."[109] Nearly two decades earlier, Cheyne's mentor Pitcairne had encountered a similar case of a twenty-one-year-old woman: "she having been chagrin'd in some love affaire became obstructed. . . . She is now lean, pale, takes cold & then hot fits."[110] The obstruction was of her menses. While Pitcairne had prescribed such exotic substances as ass's milk and "an infusion of horse dung with juice of millipedes," Cheyne recommended a fairly standard array of medicines: bitters and cordials to aid and stimulate the digestion, along with the purgative hiera picra mixed with lavender, thought to be good for the nerves. These, along with drinking Bath waters, would have an "opening" effect that would remove any physical blockages in the digestive system and secondarily in the circulatory system.

Cheyne was greatly concerned about menstrual obstruction, "wherein, I take a great deal of her Distemper to Ly."[111] Although menstruation was a critical indicator of female health, theories differed about its purpose. Hamilton had taken it as a sign of health when the forty-five-year-old Queen Anne's "Menses happend to her as if she had been but 20 years old," noting too its effects in relieving her "Disquiet." Cheyne subscribed to the view that menstruation resulted from a plethora of blood, a view described in mechanical detail by his fellow Newtonian John Freind in 1703. Suppression of menstruation would result in the excess blood taking another course, possibly traveling to the brain, where it might result in hysteria, the so-called fit of the mother ("mother" being a common locution for womb). Freind claimed that men also "become plainly *Hysterick*" when analogous discharges such as nosebleeds or hemorrhoids were suppressed. The duke of Chandos reported his wife's nosebleeds, which "relieved her very much."[112]

Amenorrhea can be a result of fasting; the medieval female saints with which Cheyne was familiar often did not menstruate, which was an additional sign of sanctity. The psychological literature on anorexia points to amenorrhea as a desired effect of the subject's resistance to maturity.[113] Gail Paster notes, "Because menstrual blood was a form of plethora— even one recuperated into a narrative of biological providence—menstruation as a process took on an economy of impurity and waste, so that upper-class women who ate rich, moist foods were thought to flow more heavily than their lower-class counterparts."[114] Catherine's failure to menstruate was a transgression with multiple meanings.

Cheyne's initial conservative regimen with Catherine Walpole did not bear immediate results, and he was very soon anxious about his lack of success. Complicating the case was the pain in Catherine's side. Cheyne referred to "scrophulous tumors," but this was a broad term for any odd swelling (although he later described the side as depressed). Scrofula was a tubercular affliction of the lymphatic glands that caused hard swellings at lymph nodes. He wished to try Bristol water and flowers of sulfur, both "cooling" medicines as well as being cathartic, and in the case of

sulfur, diaphoretic, meaning it promoted sweating.¹¹⁵ If he pursued Sanctorius's arguments (scrupulously followed by Pitcairne) about the equivalence of discharges, then sweating could take the place of menstruation;
and Freind had argued that women of an overly hot constitution, such as
"*Virago's*," did not menstruate.¹¹⁶

As Cheyne frequently stated to Sloane and presumably to the Walpoles,
a lasting cure could take many months. Yet the traditional emphasis on
time and patience—the "age & Maturity" of Catherine, he said, would
help her as much as medicines—conflicted with his need to provide evidence of a cure. Catherine's mother attempted to speed the course of
recovery by calling in Hamilton. Much to Cheyne's relief, Hamilton concurred with his treatment, recommending rhubarb (another purgative)
and bitters. Catherine's appetite appeared better, and she at last menstru-
ated.¹¹⁷ In this era before X rays and stethoscopes, when the doctor
seldom touched the patient, bodily discharges were critical indicators of
internal activity. Cheyne felt the throbbing in Catherine's side not only
through her clothes but also through her iron stays. The seemingly obses-
sive concern with the eliminative functions had both practical diagnostic
meaning and theoretical import.

By July 1720 Cheyne sought a "more Active Medicine" than Bristol or
Bath waters. Although some of Catherine's symptoms had abated, the
pain in her side remained, which Cheyne now attributed to a "sharp
serum . . . like the Humour that breeds the Rickets in Young Children."
He therefore added to her regimen castor (presumably castor oil),
another purgative, and "steel" or iron, thought to be strengthening and,
in some preparations, to stimulate menstruation (it was thus used in
chlorosis), along with an "emmenagogic and aromatic bitter" to promote both digestion and menstruation. This was still a fairly conservative regimen, relying heavily on mineral waters, including the Belgian Spa
and the German Pyrmont. He was still optimistic of recovery because
he felt her illness was not due to a "mala configuratio partium," which
would indicate that it was congenital and therefore incapable of cure.
Catherine's "natural faculties," he said, were intact, meaning both her
mental functions and, in the Galenic sense, the functioning of her
various bodily organs.¹¹⁸

The stalemate in the case continued, for by the end of July Sloane ordered Catherine to leave Bath and spend some time in Bristol. Bristol was not noted as a resort; another of Cheyne's patients later commented that Bristol was reckoned "a very Dull place . . . & indeed I think so too."[119] Its water was said to be cooler and less powerful than that of Bath, and Catherine had already been drinking it for some time under Cheyne's care. But by the end of August her father wrote to Sloane, "Her severall symptoms are rather worse than better since she went to Bristoll." Cheyne concurred with this estimation, but Walpole awaited the opinion of Sloane. In a postscript, however, Walpole revealed the patient's prerogative: "Since I wrote the accounts from Bristoll are so bad that the girl is coming back to Bath w[i]th out waiting for orders." And back to Bath she went.[120]

"She looks miserably bad," wrote Cheyne to Sloane a few days later. Catherine suffered from continual fainting and ate scarcely a thing; she had experienced "a severe Hysteric fit of four houres Last night." In contrast to his conservative therapy, Catherine's Bristol physicians took much more vigorous action, prescribing opiates to relax her and strong "Emmenagogic Pills" to counteract the constipating effects of opium. "She told me her self," wrote Cheyne, "that . . . she cou'd not have liv'd had she stay'd another Month."[121] The use of opiates was much debated in this period. Cheyne's use generally concurred with the advice of his mentor Pitcairne, who, following Thomas Willis, advocated restraint in its use, particularly in cases involving the nerves. In contrast, advocates such as John Jones, in his well-known *Mysteries of Opium Reveal'd* (1700), touted it as a cure-all.[122]

By October 1720 Catherine's symptoms were considerably relieved under Cheyne's care: "she has had none of the Great fitts (which I call Hysterick) these 12 or 14 days. Her faintings are less frequent . . . [her] only Complaint . . . is her Sickness after eating, which indeed is terrible, she is confin'd to her bed for 3 hours after dinner." For this symptom, Cheyne suggested she try bathing, recommending the Cross Bath, the coolest (and most popular) of the hot baths. He supported his suggestion with learned citation, ancient and modern. "The Antients," he noted, recommended "warm fomentations," and he referred particularly

to Pitcairne's favorite Sanctorius on the dangers of "obstructed perspiration," which bathing would relieve.[123] William Oliver had observed that in
the Cross Bath "Hysterical Women, and Hypochondriack Men, Bathe
often with good Success." It was, he said, "peculiarly famous for Shrinkings,
and Contractings of the Nerves, and Tendons."[124]

A few weeks later, Cheyne reported that bathing and "pumping"
(pouring) water onto her stomach had greatly relieved her symptoms:
"She has Lost at Least two hours of her Sickness after dinner. . . . She
has misst her Hysterick Fitt 17 days, & has not above 3 or 4 faintings a
day." With evident relief, Cheyne announced that she would indeed
recover, although probably not as quickly as she wished.[125] By late
November, Catherine was sufficiently recovered—or sufficiently bored,
since by this time most of Bath's visitors had left for London—to
become restless. Cheyne described Catherine's recovery as "much at a
stand." She was down to one fainting fit and a half-hour of sickness a
day, and one hysteric fit a month, and patient and doctor regarded this as
a satisfactory cure; only the pain in her side, said Cheyne, remained
resistant to therapy. To be cured in this era did not necessarily mean
perfect health, but only the ability to get through everyday life. Cheyne's
tone is almost conspiratorial; he seems to be scheming with Catherine for
her release to the London season and her friends.[126] A disappointment, he
reminded Sloane, could undo all their efforts. But Cheyne the physician
prudently relinquished all responsibility for possible negative
consequences.[127]

Catherine went to London in December 1720 "most miraculously
recovered."[128] Alas, this recovery was short-lived, and Cheyne soon urged
her return to Bath. Catherine's case would not be as easily resolved as that
of Lord and Lady Carmarthen, who were "subject to the infirmity of
too much Good nature, & so of being tempted to drink more wine than
water."[129]

Cheyne's last three letters to Sloane chronicle Catherine's slow decline.
In August 1721 Cheyne stated that she had not again reached the state of
health she had enjoyed the previous winter. Although he was "convinced"
that the case was "a Scrophulous Taint," he did not dare risk those
stronger medicines, "the Mercurials & Sulphurs." "I shall venture

Nothing new with her," Cheyne wrote, referring responsibility for her care to her family; "It was unlucky she left Bath last winter for she never recovered it tho it was none of my fault, she wou'd go."[130] In September, however, Cheyne described Catherine as improved: "I had allwaies Observed that Low Valetudinary Persons get up a Little after Midsummer. . . . The Sun it seems by that time gets the better of the Sizeness of the juices & raises & exalts them as it does those of the vegetables." He also took the opportunity of observing Catherine's symptoms over several hours by having her spend an afternoon at his house. By his description, her symptoms were still much as they were in winter; but his postscript betrayed the seriousness of her case when he admitted that she was too weak to bathe. He wished to prescribe strong mercurial purgatives to "plump . . . up the Habit," optimistically estimating that another course of Bath waters in the spring would complete her cure.[131]

A year later, Cheyne finally admitted he had "but faint hopes of her Recovery." All her other symptoms "are all together or allmost gone, she is more active, & her Spirits more free. But what can be expected from one, who lives all most on air & water, two thin Elements; she eats not food Sufficient to Maintain a Parrot." Cheyne described her as "emaciated" and also "totally obstructed," probably referring once more to her menses, "& her Legs so constantly swell, that they threaten a confirm'd phthisis." A "confirmed phthisis" meant incurable pulmonary tuberculosis, but medical terminology was so loosely employed that it is impossible to determine if Catherine really suffered from what we would call tuberculosis. In Cheyne's anxiety to force a cure, he now deluged Catherine with medicines: steel, vitriol, elixir proprietatio, hellebore, all of them varyingly purgative. But even his optimism failed him. "In a word my opinion is, to let her do just as she pleases, to attempt nothing . . . & wait till Nature has releas'd her, or indicated some thing that may effectually relieve her."[132] Catherine died at Bath on 9 October 1722, aged not quite nineteen.

Cheyne's failure in this case did not prevent Sloane from recommending more patients to him, including one "Mistris Smith," with remarkably similar symptoms to Catherine Walpole; and judging from the names he cited to Sloane, many of his patients were women. Yet

Catherine Walpole was in many ways atypical of the patients he would address in his next publication, the *Essay of Health and Long Life*. Her symptoms were quite the opposite of those cases of overindulgence. In addition, Cheyne apparently did not recommend to Catherine those spiritual works that had so helped him. But the letters to Sloane give evidence that Cheyne's therapy was not merely pharmaceutical. He attended Catherine several days a week and spent much time in conversation with her. This obese middle-aged physician empathized with the needs and fears of the frail teenager as few other physicians of the time attempted. In stark contrast stood the practice of Mead and other London physicians, who notoriously prescribed for patients they had never seen on the basis of an apothecary's description of their symptoms. Cheyne's use of conversation differed from Radcliffe's bedside manner, or even from Hamilton's role as confidante to Queen Anne. More than his patients' physician, Cheyne was their friend. By the time he treated the countess of Huntingdon a decade later, Cheyne had perfected his techniques, and his letters to and conversations with Lady Huntingdon constituted an essential part of her therapy. Cheyne's "talking therapy" may be viewed as an anticipation of the "moral therapy" for the insane employed later in the eighteenth century; from our perspective, it also anticipates modern counseling therapies.

Cheyne's participation in the foundation of Bath's hospital indicated his increased status in the Bath community and perhaps also contributed to that status.[33] Queen Elizabeth I had, by a 1597 act of Parliament, given the sick poor free use of the baths of Bath. Parishes took advantage of this opportunity to unload their indigent on the city, and by 1700 the "Beggars of Bath" had become a byword. Such individuals clashed with Bath's increasingly fashionable image, and local pressure led to the repeal in 1714 of the Elizabethan act.[34] Yet the poor remained, legally or not. As elsewhere in Britain, an enlightened few in the community began to realize that a hospital could serve multiple functions both for the poor and for the community. In the words of the 1737 public statement of the hospital's organizers, the sick poor were at present "a burthen to themselves and their Neighbours and dragg on an uneasie life, which by Gods blessing on the charity here proposed might be render'd comfortable to themselves and profitable to the Publick."[135] A hospital would allow the sick poor to receive systematic care while removing them from the public gaze and sequestering their diseases from public contact. In addition, during the time of convalescence, the patient's moral health no less than his physical health could be ameliorated.[136] An additional benefit, the Bath organizers noted, would be the number of clinical observations a hospital could afford of the benefits of Bath's waters: "surely if the knowledge of the nature & Efficacy of these Waters could be rendered still more extensive & certain, it would be doing a great Service to every individual Person in any Country or age." This combination of what Roy Porter has called "the heart of generosity with the brain of utility" made the voluntary hospital a particular focus for Georgian charity.[137]

In 1716 Henry Hoare and Lady Elizabeth Hastings proposed to found a hospital in Bath for the sick poor. Lady Betty Hastings (1682–1739) was a frequent visitor to Bath and was well known for her piety and philanthropy; Richard Steele had praised her in the *Tatler* in 1709 as "Aspatia," a "Female Philosopher." Among other projects, she sponsored Mary Astell's Chelsea charity school, opened in 1709 and connected with the Society for the Propagation of Christian Knowledge (SPCK), a high-church voluntary society founded during the "church in danger" days of 1697. Lady Betty's father, the seventh earl of Huntingdon, had been a stalwart Tory who was at times suspected of Jacobite sympathies.[138] She, her half-sisters Frances, Ann, and Margaret, and her sister-in-law Selina, wife of her half-brother the ninth earl, were all Cheyne's patients by the late 1720s.[139]

Lady Betty's partner in the Bath scheme was her banker, Henry Hoare (1677–1725), a member of a prominent Tory banking family and an active supporter of the SPCK. He was one of four members of the Charitable Society founded in London in 1716, which led eventually to the founding of London's Westminster Infirmary. Another member of the London society was the Anglican minister Patrick Cockburn, a son of George Garden's antagonist John Cockburn.[140]

The instigators of the Bath scheme were thus a distinctly Tory and high-church pair with which Cheyne would feel both familiar and comfortable. It is not clear how far Hoare and Lady Betty pursued their plans, however, and the next step in the enterprise was taken by Sir

Joseph Jekyll (1663–1738), master of the rolls and a frequent visitor to Bath, who initiated a subscription for the hospital in 1723. Jekyll's participation indicates, as Roy Porter and others have argued, that hospital foundations were intended to be nonsectarian, even antisectarian.[41] Jekyll was a stalwart Whig, educated at the Dissenting Academy in Islington, a longtime M.P. who had been one of the prosecutors at Sacheverell's trial in 1710.[42] He too was Cheyne's patient.

At the first general meeting of the hospital's organizers in October 1723, Cheyne was one of thirteen named to manage the charity. He had not, as yet, made a contribution. The group included Richard Nash; Henry Hoare; six medical men including Charles Bave, John Quinton, and the surgeon Jerry Peirce; and a few merchants. As the membership indicates, this was very much a community effort by those with a direct interest in Bath's success as a spa and in the increased prestige that charitable acts accrued to the giver.[43] The £270 that had been collected was invested in South Sea bonds, and the income was to be used to support deserving paupers. The committee of thirteen was to meet monthly to consider applications for its funds. But the scheme apparently never got off the ground, although the committee continued to meet and even to add members to its ranks.[44]

The hospital plan also languished, in the face of what the committee called "surprizing disappointments." By the time it opened in 1742, Cheyne and Peirce were the only surviving medical members of the original committee. Debate over a site for the hospital raged for well over a decade, and although Cheyne continued to be listed as a member of the managing committee, there is no evidence that he played a major role as an organizer. A site was finally found in 1737, and fund-raising again began in earnest; at this time Cheyne and three of his fellow physicians, including the younger William Oliver, each contributed fifty pounds to the scheme, an indication of their prominence in the community, since the remaining members of the committee contributed twenty pounds each. Nash, Oliver, and Cheyne's Bath publisher James Leake solicited the donations that now began to pour in. Cheyne continued among the committee members (now numbering thirty-two) but did not attend any of the weekly organizing meetings that now began to

be held. He was not named as one of the governors of the hospital when
it opened in 1742.[45]

By the early 1720s Cheyne had reached moderate success as a physician. He was happily married, the father of three children, an author of
minor renown. If he had died at the age of fifty—as did many of his
contemporaries—his passing would have caused barely a ripple outside
Bath. But Cheyne's life was about to take another turn.

6

THE PASSIONS
OF THE SOUL

The popularity of the *Essay on Gout* revealed an audience eager for Cheyne's advice. The wealth of clinical experience he now had gave him material for a more ambitious guide to health. He sought advice on a manuscript of "some rules of Health" from his patient Sir Joseph Jekyll in March 1724.[1] Jekyll approved, and Cheyne dedicated to him *An Essay of Health and Long Life*. Jekyll, he said, "desired of me to draw up some Instructions in writing to direct him in the Conduct of his Health for the future, and in the Manner of supporting his Spirits free and full, under the great Business he is engaged in."[2]

Published in 1724, *An Essay of Health and Long Life* reached nine editions in Cheyne's lifetime. It was translated into several European languages and reprinted as late as the 1820s.[3] Cheyne crafted a finely honed model of illness and therapy, of the roles of doctor and patient. He stated, "I have consulted nothing but my own Experience and Observation on my own crazy Carcase and the Infirmities of others I have treated."[4]

In the *Essay of Health and Long Life* Cheyne further revealed himself to his patients as a fellow sufferer. Carol Flynn calls him "a physician who repeatedly attempts to heal himself to heal his age."[5] In uncovering the interweaving of bodily, mental, and spiritual illness, Cheyne took another step toward his own healing, begun nearly two decades earlier. This healing was urgent, for Cheyne believed he had little time left. His "crazy Carcase" continued to plague him as he paid the price of increasing success. While his medical practice grew, he also composed the *Essay of Health and Long Life* and continued to revise the *Essay on Gout*, which reached a sixth edition by 1724, while the *Philosophical Principles* was rereleased the following year. His weight again crept upward. In his 1733 autobiography he wrote that in midsummer 1723 "I was seiz'd with a severe *Symptomatic Fever*, which terminated with the most violent *Erysipelas*" (an inflammation of the skin). Having seen two of his "full-bodied" patients die of "*Mortifications* from that Distemper," Cheyne was anxious. He decided to return to his "*old Friends, Milk* and *Vegetables*," but he would not have relief for several years.[6]

Cheyne's preface therefore had an elegiac tone. "This being probably the last Time I may trespass on the Publick," he reviewed his past works and controversies, apologizing for "personal and peevish" remarks; he retracted all "malicious and unmannerly Turns, all false and unjust Representations."[7] But he never repudiated the works themselves or their Newtonian content. In 1722 George Strahan issued a third edition of Cheyne's first two works, *A New Theory of Fevers and An Essay Concerning the Improvements in the Theory of Medicine*. Although the title page proclaimed the volume a revision "with many Additions," it was identical to the second edition of 1702, except that Cheyne's name now appeared on the title page.[8]

The *Essay of Health and Long Life* fell into the well-known medical genre of commentary on the Galenic "non-naturals."[9] Cheyne transformed the six non-naturals into the seven deadly sins. Reflecting his patients' priorities, he devoted nearly half the text to diet and evacuations, and the passions occupied a substantial portion of the remainder. His "hyppish" patients suffered often from headaches, stomachaches, and "colick," the effects of "Repletion, or living too fully"; from drinking too much wine, or worse, "Punch"; from abusing coffee, tea, chocolate, and tobacco. Cheyne lectured his patients on the page much as he must have lectured them in person on the dangers of overindulgence: "There is nothing more *ridiculous*, than to see tender, *hysterical* and *vapourish* People, perpetually *complaining*, and yet perpetually *cramming*; crying out, They are ready to *sink* into the Ground, and faint away, and yet *gobbling* down the *richest* and *strongest* Food, and highest Cordials, to oppress and overlay them quite."[10]

Health was the responsibility of the individual, a physical and moral imperative: "He that *wantonly* transgresseth the *self-evident* Rules of Health, is guilty of a Degree of *Self-Murder*," a crime against God as well as nature. Here he echoed Calvinist descriptions of the body as "God's workmanship."[11] The biographer of the pious Lady Betty Hastings noted, "her Body she knew was the Temple of the Holy Ghost, and . . . her Support of it by Meat, Drink, and Sleep, was ever bounded by Necessity."[12]

Cheyne noted wryly that the only individuals who might take umbrage at this advice were "my Brethren of the Profession, for endeavouring to lessen the *Materia Morbifica*." He added with characteristic bluntness, "'tis easier to *preserve* Health than to *recover* it . . . for the Knowledge of [diseases] the far greatest part of Mankind must apply to others, of whose Skill and Honesty they are in a great measure ignorant, and the Benefit of whose Art they can but conditionally and precariously obtain." Doctors were a risky proposition at best. Far better, advised Cheyne, to "*bear and forbear*" and thus preserve one's own health.[13]

His general advice was simple, and from the perspective of the 1990s, both intelligible and sensible. He emphasized moderation, a light diet of white meats and vegetables, and drinking water (especially Bath water) rather than alcoholic beverages. Cheyne described the most suitable foods in considerable detail, noting that young fruits and vegetables and those that appear earliest in the spring are most easily digested, "because they have less of the *solar* Fire in them." Similarly, young animals and those of lighter flesh have parts more easily digested than larger, redder-fleshed animals, whose juices contain more salt and fat; both of those substances, according to Newton in "De natura acidorum," possessed greater attractive power. "*Strong, poignant, Aromatick*, and hot" tastes—either naturally occurring or as a result of preparation—were to be avoided, both for their abundance of noxious salts, and for their excessively stimulating effects on the appetite. "*Rich Soop, high Sauces*," and other elaborate modes of cookery were "the Inventions of *Luxury*, to force an unnatural *Appetite*."[14]

This protest against "foreign" food was a common trope. Defoe claimed that luxurious foreign foods fueled sexual appetites, while John Woodward's 1718 *The State of Physick: And of Diseases* blamed rich foods for all the illnesses of civilization, both physical and moral.[15] Yet the English were victims of their own success. The growth of trade and the expanding empire not only fueled the growth of London but weighted ever more heavily the English dinner table. The public virtues of commerce, as Mandeville claimed in the *Fable of the Bees*, could only lead to the private

vices of luxury and gluttony. Cheyne would elaborate upon this theme in
The English Malady.

Cheyne later told his friend Samuel Richardson that women were
especially susceptible to the attractions of luxury; most women "I fear
would rather renounce Life than Luxury."[16] Defoe's Roxana, who sold her
body for food, displayed the voracious female appetite. But so too did
Bourignon and the medieval saints she imitated, who restrained their
bodily desires and achieved saintliness by refusing to eat.

With regard to sleep, Cheyne claimed, "Nothing can be more
prejudicial to *tender* Constitutions . . . than lying long a Bed, or *lolling* and
soaking in *Sheets,* any time after one is distinctly awake."[17] His advocacy of
exercise included coach riding, cold baths, and the use of the flesh brush,
all of which led to the desired effect of increased circulation and
perspiration. This sort of exercise, which involved the body's being
moved rather than moving itself, could appeal only to a class that could
afford servants to do the moving. Such a regimen would keep the
hydraulic machine of the body in operation, the pipes flexible and free of
obstructions, while avoiding the coarsening effects of vigorous exercise.[18]

Cheyne's book was quite unlike the multitude of books produced by
his Bath colleagues such as Robert Peirce, the two William Olivers,
Edward Baynard, John Quinton, and John Wynter, all of whom extolled
Bath's virtues but gave little practical advice. Their books advocated
patient autonomy only to the extent that the patient could choose to go
to Bath and be treated by the author. The *Essay of Health and Long Life*
harked back, instead, to the self-help manuals of the seventeenth century
(which were often written by laymen), allowing the patient to control his
or her own health by active preventive measures. His models included
Luigi Cornaro's long popular *Trattato della vita sobria* (1558), which similarly
recommended temperance as the key to long life. Cornaro's work, along
with the equally popular *Hygiasticon* (1611) of Leonard Lessius, had first
been translated into English in 1634 and had been reprinted most recently
in 1722.[19]

Unlike many other physicians, Cheyne did not merely recite cures, or
in the manner of Bernard Mandeville offer general advice as a rhetorical
aid to chastise physicians and patients alike. Cheyne instead followed

popular practice in giving specific instructions the patient could follow. He placed them, moreover, within a compelling moral framework: "The infinitely wise *Author* of *Nature* has so contrived *Things*, that the most remarkable RULES of preserving LIFE and HEALTH are *moral Duties* commanded us, so true it is, that *Godliness has the Promises of this Life, as well as that to come*." Our lives are God's, and we must therefore use them properly. Calvin had said this, and so had Henry Scougal; in addition, the first principle of natural law was that life is to be preserved. The hard-won lessons of Cheyne's life now instructed his patients. "He who lives *physically*," he wrote, "must die miserably." Yet he did not advocate the valetudinarian's excessive solicitude for his health; this was "*to die for fear of Dying*." Over-physicking was worse than neglect, as Mandeville had argued in 1711: his hypochondriacal patient Misomedon ruined his health when he turned from "quacking" himself to consulting more and more physicians and apothecaries. The bluestocking Elizabeth Montagu commented in the 1720s, "I have swallowed the weight of an Apothecary in medicine, and what I am better for it, except more patient and less credulous I know not. I have learnt to bear my infirmities and not to trust to the skill of Physicians for curing them." Philosophy and a cheerful disposition, said Montagu, were the best allies. Cheyne would add religion to this formula, but the message was the same. He knew his audience well.[20]

Moderation was the key. The rules of health were "*self-evident*," given by God; Cheyne was only the Moses who conveyed those rules to the populace, much as Bourignon had seen herself as the instrument through which God delivered his instructions for salvation. Cheyne preached, "To die *Martyrs* to our *Luxury* and *Wantonness*, is . . . beneath the Dignity of *human Nature*, and contrary to the *Homage* we owe to the *Author* of our being." As Bourignon had recognized, the body as well as the spirit must participate in the work of attaining salvation, and the tyranny of the body over the spirit was not inevitable.[21]

Regulation of the passions was a particularly relevant theme, and Cheyne revealed the therapeutic insights of his experience of conversion. He found the passions at the root of many ailments. Sensitive, intelligent, imaginative people were most liable to their influence: "The *Indolent* and the Thoughtless, suffer *least* from the Passions: The *Stupid* and Ideots *not at all.*" He addressed, therefore, not the Hogarthian eater of roast beef, but the "*tender* and *valetudinary,* who lead "*sedentary* Lives, or indulge *contemplative* Studies." The implications for status in this description fed into the desire of the upwardly mobile middle classes to differentiate themselves from the less sensitive orders immediately below them. In addition, this description was particularly applicable to women, or at least to those who cultivated the feminine emotions.[22]

Sydenham had noted that the majority of hysterical complaints were suffered by women; indeed, he claimed, rarely was a woman wholly free from these ills.[23] Yet sensitivity or "sensibility" held fashionable appeal to both genders, and Cheyne's imagery in the *Essay of Health* is not as specifically feminine as it would be in *The English Malady*, composed a decade later. The more masculine images in the *Essay of Health* emphasized the "*springy, lively,* and *elastick* Fibres" of "Men of *Imagination.*" The sensitive were also sensual, and more given to the pleasures of the flesh. By nature, therefore, they were also more susceptible to its ravages.[24] The philosopher David Hume in 1734 described himself as suffering from "the Disease of the Learned," whose symptoms included a "Weakness. . . of Spirits"; yet for a time he also possessed a "very ravenous Appetite."[25] In the 1730s Cheyne characterized both himself and Samuel Richardson as "serious, virtuous Valetudinarians," whose sufferings were a necessary consequence of a "fine and lively Imagination."[26]

As we have seen, hypochondria and hysteria were not in this period distinguished as masculine or feminine illnesses but were, in medical terms, largely interchangeable, and this fluidity of definition was essential for Cheyne's sympathy with his patients, both male and female. He defined "the Hyp" to Richardson simply as "every Distemper attended with Lowness of Spirits." At the same time, he assured his patient the countess of Huntingdon that he had himself "felt and gone through" all the ills she suffered, although he elsewhere acknowledged that those ills were a result of noble blood and frequent childbearing. "I know no Difference between the Sexes but in their Configuration," he told Richardson. "They are both of the same Species and differ only in Number as in Number two is after one." Sensibility could take many forms; as both sufferer and healer,

Cheyne the physician assumed a Christ-like stance of taking on the suffering of his patients. Bourignon had cited the ability to heal as a sign of grace.[27] How far had Cheyne traveled, from the masculine culture of the turn of the century to a recognition of his own androgynous nature.

In the *Essay of Health and Long Life*, Cheyne divided the passions into two varieties, animal and spiritual, corresponding to the Cartesian division between body and mind. Cheyne's animal passions or soul governed bodily functions, while the spiritual passions existed only in intelligent beings and, said Cheyne, was "the Foundation of *Liberty*, or *Freewill*." This was an old concept, now given a new twist. Returning to the language and imagery of the 1715 *Philosophical Principles*, he drew an analogy between spirit and Newtonian gravity, both motive principles bestowed directly on passive matter by God. Laws of nature govern the actions between bodies, and laws also govern the interaction of body and soul. Since the body—matter—is wholly passive, we must assume the existence of an "*active, self-motive, self-determining Principle*" that acts upon it as gravity acts upon matter. On the topic of passive matter, Cheyne referred the reader to various works of Samuel Clarke, including his exchange of letters with Leibniz.[28]

Yet spirits interact not only with the body but also with each other: bodies and spirits both gravitate toward one another, and as the planets tend toward the sun, so do souls tend toward God, impelled by love. He defined spiritual passions as the "*Sentiments* produced on the *Soul* by *external Objects*," and the animal passions were such effects produced on the body. In both cases the bodily organs were the immediate cause of sensation; therefore, these two sorts of passions were closely linked. Cheyne's complex schema outlined four possible varieties of interaction: between bodies (governed by gravity); the influence of body on soul; the influence of soul on body; and the influence of soul or spirit on soul (each governed by the passions). The material body was passive in principle, but closely bound up with the spirit in its actions. The interaction between mind and body was a two-way street: as Locke had argued, external sensation (including physiological changes in the body) influenced the mind; but Cheyne also asserted that the mind, possessing a self-motive principle, equally affected the body. Lester King has noted some similarity between the concept of "spiritual substance" and the *anima* of the German pietist physician Georg Ernst Stahl (1660–1734), but it is not known whether Cheyne read Stahl.[29]

Sensitivity could easily cross the line to madness. Uncontrolled, the passions wrought havoc on the nervous system. Grief, melancholy, and hopeless love all wore out parts of the nervous system, and continued strong emotion could so pattern the nerves that the emotional state became habitual. Violent emotion would "*screw up, stretch and bend*" some nerves, while others would "*rust*" from disuse.[30]

From his own experience, Cheyne described "that kind of *Melancholy*, which is called *Religious*, because 'tis conversant about matters of *Religion*; although, often the Persons so distempered have little *solid Piety*." Manifested in physical symptoms, this was indeed a physical disease, although arising generally from "a *Disgust* or *Disrelish* of worldly *Amusements* and *Creature-Comforts*." Therefore physical regimen, which he had recommended and employed in his own case, was the first resort. But if this was inadequate to quell the "tumultuous, overbearing *Hurricanes* in the Mind," then the sufferer must turn to God and drown all other passions with the love of God.[31]

Cheyne endeavored to demonstrate scientifically the influence of "*Spiritual Love*" on the animal economy with his analogy between this love and Newtonian attraction. Like gravity, love is a principle, an "inherent *Power* in the *Soul*." But as a stone mortared into a wall cannot act upon its natural gravity and fall to the ground, so the soul, being "*drowned* in Sense . . . drawn and hurried away by the *Devil*, the *World* and the *Flesh*," is prevented from exerting its natural tendency toward God. Since body and soul were inextricably linked, both the proper physical regimen and the desire for spiritual reunion were necessary to tame the wayward passions and lead the sufferer toward God and health.[32] In the poem "Platonick Love," attributed to Cheyne, the same thought is expressed: "Who crys this Love down, must needs oppresse/Nature's first law, and Man's last happiness."[33]

His account of the passions applied to both sexes, but it was especially relevant to the contemporary perceptions of the dual female nature: animal-like and sensual on the one hand, sensitive and otherworldly on the other. Much of Cheyne's imagery, as well as his specific therapy of taming the passions through diet and God, were based on an essentially feminine idea of spirituality derived from his reading of Bourignon and other mystics. Cheyne's repetition of the words "drowning" and "love" echo Jeanne Guyon's radical quietism; two decades later, John Byrom claimed that Cheyne "was always talking in coffeehouses about 'naked faith, pure love,'" a juxtaposition of place and word that is utterly Cheynean.[34] With regard to diet, he had the example of the many women mystics catalogued by Poiret in 1708. As Caroline Bynum has pointed out, the connection between food and spirituality was peculiarly female, related to the role of food in women's social function. Gail Corrington has further noted that the self-control exhibited by fasting can be seen as an assertion of autonomy by women who have had few other opportunities for such an assertion.[35] As we have seen, the female appetite seemed especially to require restraining.

Cheyne's dietary guidelines and their relationship to the passions suggest a continuity of ideas and images between the most-studied mystics of his era and the life of the early eighteenth century. Cheyne required a renunciation of meat eating or at least a shift from red meat to white. Meat eating, and red meat in particular, had long been viewed as distinctively masculine and associated with passion and violence. The radical hatter Thomas Tryon had argued in the 1690s that the blood of beasts was "endued with all kinds of Beastial Passions," which would be conveyed to the eater of meat.[36] Cheyne replaced meat with milk, a food associated with women and motherhood.[37] The idea of renouncing food, or choosing some foods over others, also had a distinct class bias, since only those of a comfortable level of income could choose not to eat or what to eat, and these individuals composed Cheyne's audience. His patients, like the doctor himself, grew in spirit as they wasted in flesh.[38]

But Cheyne, like the Church of England, emphasized not the extreme of asceticism but moderation in all things. Thus had Garden interpreted the life of Bourignon. The best cure was prevention, and the best prevention was a moderate regimen and a serene religion. True pleasure and happiness, he said, consisted in loving God, and a true devotion would keep the less desirable passions within check. He translated the language of mysticism into everyday life. His patient Lady Betty Hastings "sanctified" her body by attending to its necessary wants and occupied the intervals between with "pious meditations."[39]

The *Essay of Health and Long Life* was reprinted six times in the next year and translated into French and, for the benefit of the learned, into Latin. Dutch and Italian translations soon followed. Cheyne's modification of the extremes of asceticism and enthusiasm greatly appealed to those who frequented Bath, enabling them to ameliorate both their bodies and their consciences under the rubric of a fashionable sensitivity. Not everyone had high expectations of the work. Dr. William Stratford, canon of Christ Church, Oxford, wrote to a friend, "I shall enquire for my friend Cheyney's book; I should be glad to meet with anything that may contribute to health whilst we live. As to short or long life it is not much worth while to be very solicitous. I expect some nostrums."[40] But a few months later, an undergraduate at the same college named John Wesley wrote to his mother, "I suppose you have seen the famous Dr Cheyne's Book of Health and Long Life. . . . He refers almost everything to temperance and exercise . . . and recommends for drink two pints of water and one of wine in twenty-four hours . . . [the book] is chiefly addressed to studious and sedentary persons." By 1726 Cheyne's book was being read aloud at dinners and, no doubt, at coffeehouses.[41]

The *Essay of Health and Long Life* immediately spawned both imitators and detractors. The Bath physician John Wynter lavishly cited Cheyne in his *Cyclus Metasyncriticus* (1725). Wynter vigorously denied any opposition to Cheyne in his preface. Despite a few passages disagreeing with aspects of Cheyne's *Essay on Gout*, Wynter relied heavily on his ideas, arguing that "the remote Causes of *Chronical Diseases* are, no doubt, *Inactivity* and *Intemperance . . . Sloth* and *Luxury*."[42] Wynter again cited Cheyne in his 1728 *Of Bathing in the Hot Baths, at Bathe*, dedicated to Freind, and the publisher's catalog printed at the end reinforced the message, listing several of Cheyne's works.[43] However, Wynter also wrote the following satirical poem in the 1730s:

Dr. *Wynter* to Dr. *Cheyne*, on his Books in Favour of Vegetable Diet

> Tell me from whom, fat-headed Scot,
>   Thou didst thy system learn;
> From Hippocrate thou hast it not,
>   Nor Celsus, nor Pitcairne.
>
> Suppose we own that *milk* is good,
>   And say the same of *grass*;
> The one for *babes* is only food,
>   The other for an *ass*.
>
> Doctor! one new prescription try,
>   (A friend's advice forgive;)
> Eat *grass*, reduce thyself, and *die*;
>   Thy *patients*, then, may *live*.

Cheyne exercised his famous wit in his reply:

Dr. *Cheyne* to Dr. *Wynter*, in Answer to the Foregoing

> My system, Doctor, is my own,
>   No tutor I pretend:
> My *blunders* hurt myself alone,
>   But *yours* your dearest friend.
>
> Were *you* to milk and straw confin'd,
>   Thrice happy might you be;
> Perhaps you might *regain* your *mind*,
>   And from your *wit* get *free*.
>
> I cannot your prescription *try*,
>   But heartily "*forgive*;"
> 'Tis nat'ral you should bid *me* die,
>   That you yourself may *live*![44]

Wynter's Bath colleague John Quinton criticized Cheyne's doctrines in his 1726 pamphlet *De Thermis*, claiming that those who "propose a Water-Course instead of Malt Liquors . . . may be good Men and have Grace in their Hearts, but no Blood in their Faces." Had he ever met Cheyne? Quinton claimed to have been free from illness for twenty-four years, "[and] I drink at least a Quart of Strong Drink every day." Yet by 1733 Quinton listed Cheyne among his authorities—and subscribers—in his *Treatise of Warm Bath Waters*, a new edition of a work first published in 1707.[45]

Outside Bath, several pamphlets and a few longer works critical of Cheyne's doctrines quickly appeared. Many of them expressed dismay at Cheyne's omission of the physician from the daily regimen of health. A "fellow of the Royal Society" defended physicians in his *Remarks on Dr Cheyne's Essay of Health and Long Life* (1724). Such works as Cheyne's "may please such as will flatter themselves, but can never save them from death." The author sneered at "Dr *Diet*" and claimed he would show that "the Trick for making Men Immortal upon *Asparagus* and *Parsnips*, will not deserve a Patent." More tellingly, the author noted that unlike the doctor, he could cite two hundred books on the topic. He went on to defend not only ale, punch, and fat but mathematics, expressing dismay at Cheyne's apparent retreat from his scientific principles.[46] A broadside declared, "O Cheyne! O Cheyne! If ere thy Health fails/They'll surely dispatch thee for telling of tales."[47]

Rather more serious was the anonymous *Letter to George Cheyne*, also published in 1724, which brought up the old and vexed issue of professionalism. Mankind, said the author, "cannot enough detest those who set up for the *Art of Healing*, without any other Qualification, but their *Diploma*, to recommend them; and having nothing in their view, but making or mending their Fortunes, neglect that Knowledge, which is absolutely necessary, to make their Practice Honourable and Successful." By prescribing general rules for health, Cheyne undermined the physician's claim to expertise; for "so infinite is the variety of Diseases and Constitutions, that the best Physician in the World, can only determine, [those] he is intimately acquainted with." Once again was posed the issue of distinct diseases versus distinct constitutions. Even though Cheyne

claimed to prevent illness rather than cure diseases, the whiff of the proprietary nostrum, in this case Bath water, arose from his work. Echoing
Cheyne's own words of two decades earlier, the author thundered, "the
Practice of Physick SIR, is a sharp Edged-Tool, and seldom or never fails
of having very ill Consequences when put into unskillful Hands." He
invited Cheyne to reply, but the doctor had learned his lesson well and
remained silent.[48]

The physician Edward Strother (1675–1737) made similar criticisms, at
considerably greater length, in his 1725 *Essay on Sickness and Health*, dedicated to Sloane and Mead.[49] While admitting that "Sobriety, Abstinence,
and Moderation" were powerful preventives against illness, Strother decried
Cheyne's advice as being far too general. "It would be equally just," he
claimed, "to prescribe one Remedy for every Disease, as one diet for
every unhealthy Person." Strother defended too that joyous potion Punch,
which he claimed was valuable as a diuretic.[50]

More trivial was "Pillo-Tisanus," who published his verse *Epistle to
Ge——ge Ch——ne* in 1725. The author called Cheyne's work "extrav-
agantly extraordinary . . . (especially coming from one of his Profession)." He added, "Could one of *Galen's* sons so meanly think/To save
Mankind, and let the *College* sink?" "Pillo-Tisanus" chided the doctor for
his dietary advice:

> O, Doctor, Doctor!—who wou'd with you dine?
> When your whole Bill of Fare is one starv'd Line,
> *Mutton six Ounces!—and a Pint of Wine!*
> . . . For my Physician I accept your Book;
> But, by the *Gods!*—you ne'er shall be my *Cook!*

However, Pillo-Tisanus noted a curious gap in Cheyne's account of the
passions; for as he pointed out, Cheyne did not discuss sex: "To regulate
our *Passions* you presume,/But ne'er touch that, from whence all others
come." Pillo-Tisanus did his best to fill this gap himself.[51]

Cheyne responded to his critics by authorizing a Latin translation of the
Essay, "expanded and made more elegant." The translator, John Robertson
(1690–1761), was a physician in nearby Wells and a fellow Aberdonian.[52] A

Latin translation would expand the audience for his work to non-English speakers and increase its scholarly aura. Cheyne noted in his preface (dated 23 August 1725) that he had recently been named a fellow of the Edinburgh College of Physicians.[53]

Cheyne answered charges that he had abandoned natural philosophy with a new book. Bound with the Latin translation of the *Essay* was his first work on medical theory since the 1702 *Essay Concerning the Improvements in the Theory of Medicine*. This short treatise (only ninety-eight pages) was simply titled *De natura fibrae* (On the nature of fibers). Here Cheyne detailed his mature medical theory and mapped his future course. The chapter on the passions in the *Essay of Health and Long Life* served as a preface to an intensive study of the nerves and nervous diseases now embarked upon in *De natura fibrae* and completed seven years later in *The English Malady*. In these works Cheyne helped define the ongoing discourse of passion and sensibility in terms of the nerves.

His audience in *De natura fibrae* consisted of his peers rather than his patients; but still seeking patronage, he dedicated the book to Archibald Hutcheson (ca. 1659–1740), a Tory M.P. of Jacobite sympathies, probably a patient.[54] Cheyne returned to the debates on the value of natural philosophy to medicine, asserting that medicine could approach certainty only by the use of correct scientific theory. That theory was, as the title page proclaimed, that a "looseness" or "slackness" of the fibers ("laxae sive resolutae") caused illness.[55] He applied this theory particularly to nervous disorders.

Cheyne adopted the aphoristic style of medical works rather than the "mathematical" style of his earlier works on theory, and the calculations and diagrams of those works are entirely absent. Also absent was the usual multitude of classical references common to learned medical works. Cheyne's lack of deference to texts continued to infuriate his critics but was entirely in keeping with his persona of the natural philosopher whose knowledge was largely empirical. In fact, Cheyne's aphorisms were more axiomatic than empirical. "The bodies of animals," he declared in his first sentence, "are ultimately fibers." He distinguished muscle fiber, dense and full of blood, from soft, white nervous fiber, "undulating and vibrating."[56]

Nervous fibers were moist but solid. Their function could be impeded in four ways: by too much or too little surrounding fluid, which made them unnaturally dry or moist; by "insinuating salts," which interrupted their branching structure; by "viscid juices," which distended the surrounding vessels and pressed on the nerves; or by a looseness and lack of elasticity in the fibers themselves.[57]

Cheyne classified ordinary diseases of the nerves into three general types. Those in which the senses ceased to function, such as apoplexy, were caused by sluggish or tenacious fluids in the body, which obstructed nervous function. This category included hypochondria and hysteria. The second category, paralysis, resulted from a lack of proper elasticity in the nerves and other solids, which retarded circulation and other functions. The third category included epilepsy and convulsions and resulted from an excess of acrimony in the ambient fluids, which caused the solid nerves to erode.[58] These categories constituted a continuum: "All Nervous Distempers whatsoever from Yawning and Stretching, up to a mortal Fit of an Apoplexy, seems to me to be but one continued Disorder, or the several Steps or Degrees of it, arising from a Relaxation or Weakness, and the Want of a sufficient Force and Elasticity in the Solids in general, and the *Nerves* in particular."[59]

By reducing all nervous diseases to a single uniform cause, he could also reduce the number of necessary remedies. Therapy, he stated, had three purposes: to dilute the thick, sluggish humors, to remove their acrimony, and to return elasticity to the fibers. Although he noted that intemperance often played a role in the onset of nervous disorders, he emphasized medicines rather than regimen to the doctors who would read *De natura fibrae*: mercurial cathartics such as Aethiops mineral and cinnabar to remove acrimony, "dilutents" such as mineral water to attenuate the humors, chalybeats and astringents such as Peruvian bark to tighten the loose fibers.[60]

While physicians and their patients shared the same explanatory model of disease, the same "clinical reality," they did not necessarily respond to illness in the same way. Cheyne recommended regimen to his patients, but as the case of Catherine Walpole revealed, he did not hesitate to use the full armamentarium of the early modern apothecary to bring about a cure. In the *Essay of Health and Long Life* he spent several pages detailing the usefulness of opium; but don't, he warned, try this at home.[61] *De natura fibrae*, therefore, also responded to those critics who complained that his popular works undermined the physicians' claim to expertise. He returned to Pitcairne's arguments that the only true expertise was Newtonian natural philosophy.

The historian of medicine Theodore Brown has argued that Cheyne's attention to the solids of the body over its fluids owed much to the theories of Herman Boerhaave.[62] Like Pitcairn and Cheyne, Boerhaave envisioned the body as a hydraulic system of tubes, postulating that the fiber, formed by the union of invisible particles, was the basic unit of composition.[63] Cheyne, however, asserted that the nerves were not tubular, as the common belief held, but solid. In *The English Malady* Cheyne cited Leeuwenhoek's microscopic observations of the nerves as evidence of their solidity.[64] The ultimate source for Cheyne's description was not Leeuwenhoek but Newton, who had described the nerves as composed of "solid, pellucid and uniform Capillamenta" along which "the vibrating motion of the Aetherial Medium" was "uniformly . . . propagated" in query 24, added to the 1717–18 edition of the *Opticks*.[65]

Cheyne had already used Newton's ether theory, first introduced in the 1713 *Principia*, in his *Philosophical Principles of Religion, Natural and Revealed*. He did not reveal his debt to Newton's query 24 until the appearance of *The English Malady* in 1733. But in an appendix to *De natura fibrae* Cheyne reaffirmed his Newtonian credentials in a short commentary on contagion, particularly the plague. During the 1720 plague scare, Richard Mead had written a *Short Discourse Concerning Pestilential Contagion*, in which he argued that contagion was caused by inorganic chemical particles that were a product of the "Fermentation" caused by the disease. This fermentation in the body caused the emission of "a Volatile active Spirit, of Power to agitate, and put into intestine Motions, that is, to change the Nature of other Fluids into which it insinuates it self."[66] Mead's book, which reached an eighth edition by 1722, sold even more briskly than Cheyne's *Essay*. Cheyne reiterated Mead's explanation but added material from queries 30 and 31 from the 1718 *Opticks*. He identified the contagious particle as a salt, recalling Newton's definition of salt as the most active and volatile substance. Cheyne boldly stated, "The *Active Principles* of all bodies, animal, vegetable, & mineral (nearest after that universal agent, which is either Light or a certain more subtle Aether to which Light owes its action) seem to be due to pure, simple, innate & incorruptible *Salt*."[67] Cheyne's tentative identification of the "universal agent" with light followed Newton's own hesitations and prevarications on this topic. In query 30 he had rhetorically asked, "are not gross Bodies and Light convertible into one another, and may not Bodies receive much of their Activity from the Particles of Light which enter their Composition?" In the next query, however, the "Powers, Virtues or Forces" which acted on the particles of bodies acted also on light.[68]

Cheyne pondered the mysteries of matter amid an increasing consciousness of his own materiality. As if to remind himself of his spiritual duties, he reissued the 1715 *Philosophical Principles* in the same year of 1725. The price of success was heavy, for his health continued to decline, as he recounted in his 1733 autobiography. A "full, tho' (commonly accounted) *temperate Diet*" along with little exercise had made him "*Heavy, Dull, and Lethargick*," and the onset of illness in the summer of 1723, particularly a severe attack of erysipelas, in turn led to renewed depression. The doctor found his blood to be "one continued *impenetrable Mass* of *Glew*," with "every *Vein* and *Artery* . . . like so many *Black-Puddings*," and he endeavored to thin it out with a light diet and Bristol water, reducing his alcohol intake to a pint of wine a day.[69]

This regimen helped but did not entirely cure Cheyne, who for the next two years endured periodic attacks of fever and erysipelas as well as gout. At the end of the summer of 1725, however—a month after he had sent *De natura fibrae* to the press—"I was seiz'd with such a perpetual *Sickness, Reaching* [retching], *Lowness* [weakness], *Watchfulness* [insomnia], *Eructation* [belching], and *Melancholy*, continuing six or eight Months: that Life was no longer supportable to me, and my Misery was almost extreme." This was his usual postpartum illness with a vengeance; yet unlike in 1705, when his career lay in shambles, two decades later he was famous. Whence came this "*melancholy Fright* and *Pannick*"?[70]

Melancholy could result from success as well as failure; this illness, which endured for four more years, points to an underlying emotional cause found in his deep sense of sin. He had already chastised himself in *An Essay of Health and Long Life* for the weakness of his faith; now his body once again manifested his spiritual shortcomings. Cheyne's success, like his failure, led to excessive weight. He had apparently remained at thirty-two stone (448 pounds) since shortly after settling in Bath in 1718. A life-and-death struggle ensued between the spirit and the despised flesh, that "putrified overgrown Body from Luxury and perpetual Laziness, scor-butical all over."[71] To be fat was not only aesthetically and medically undesirable, it was morally reprehensible. Cheyne viewed his body, in Susan Bordo's words, "as animal, as appetite, as deceiver, as prison of the soul and confounder of its projects." Although mechanical physiology viewed the body as morally neutral, Cheyne could only see his body as a site for sin, requiring moral control.[72]

Having reasserted his expertise in natural philosophy, Cheyne suddenly found, as he had in 1705, that his reason was "of no Use to me"; he could barely look at his friends and patients, yet could not abide being alone. He followed his standard regimen with growing terror, drinking quantities of Bath water, riding in his coach for hours. Soon he needed to resort to vomits for relief from the intolerable bloated pains in his stomach; and then, increasingly, the Pandora's box of medicines opened before him. From "*Foetids, Gums,* and *Volatiles*" he turned to opiates, "which I knew were a slow *Poison.*"[73]

Cheyne tried to rationalize his illness, pinpointing its causes in "*Gouty* and *Erysipelatous* Matter," but to no avail. His sickness ran more deeply. His family urged him to consult his fellow physicians in London, but London was more frightening than illness, another temptation for his weakened spirit: "I might be teized to change my *Regimen,* and sneer'd at by the Free-livers." Finally convinced, he traveled "with great Difficulty" to London in December 1725. There he consulted half a dozen of his professional rivals and friends: Arbuthnot, Mead, Freind, Noel Broxholme, and his fellow Scots James Douglas and James Campbell.[74] They counseled him to give up opium, drink mineral water, and take a "chalybeat Electuary." Cheyne also continued his light diet and gave up meat entirely, though not without criticism from his colleagues. He supplemented this, however, with a daily gill (four ounces) of port. His flesh exploded in a final act of rebellion against the spirit, a paroxysm of erysipelas: "the whole *Leg, Thigh,* and *Abdomen* being *tumified, incrusted,* and *burnt* almost like the skin of a *roasted Pig.*" The self-hatred expressed in this phrase is startling. To Cheyne, the ugliness of his body represented the darkness of his soul. The roasted pig seemed to melt, discharging "a Quantity of *Ichor,*" echoing the gallons of choler discharged in 1705. It is perhaps significant that "ichor" could refer not only to a discharge from a wound but also quite commonly to a "spirituous fluid," the "blood of the gods."[75] The wretched flesh finally yielded, and his health began to improve.

Cheyne later told Richardson that he had lost "16 or 18 Stone Weight of my rotten Flesh before I stopped wasting"—that is, as much as 250 pounds—but then gained some back to "the just Mediocrity of neither too fat nor very lean." In the end Cheyne had lost about a third of his weight—leaving him at a still-hefty 300 pounds—undergoing, he said, "a State of entire bodily *Purification,* a true *Cyclus Metasyncriticus.*" The "cyclus metasyncriticus" was the turning point in the progress of a disease, signified by the evacuation of morbid matter, particularly through the skin. Recognizing the spiritual implications of this purification, he told Richardson,

I have often thought *Low-living* . . . has a great Analogy and Resemblance to the Meanest Purification and Regeneration preserved in Holy writ. . . . [The] *Cyclus Metasyncriticus* or the Transubstantiating Round and Circle . . . [will] throw off the old corrupted Mass, representing Repentance, Self-Denial, avoiding the Occasions of Sensuality and Sin, and throwing off the Old Man with his Works of Darkness.[76]

His symptoms recurred for some time—which he attributed to "craming" (*sic*)—compelling him to refine his diet yet further. He finally gave up all meat and wine and lived on milk and vegetables.[77]

Cheyne did not cease activity while undergoing this crisis, although he did not write anything for several years. By the late 1720s he had many patients and a wide circle of friends and correspondents. Keith's letters to Deskford show that Cheyne continued to be closely associated with the Garden circle. By the end of the decade, however, that circle was disintegrating: Poiret, the center of the distribution of mystical literature upon which the group depended, died in 1719; Keith and James Garden died in 1726; and George Garden's health was failing.[78] Keith had served as the nerve center of the circle, distributing books, writing letters, and bringing people together. Although both Rousseau and Shuttleton have argued that Cheyne played a major role in the distribution of mystical literature, I have found little to support this claim; Cheyne seems to have been more of a consumer of literature than a distributor.[79]

His involvement with the circle is indicated by his patronage of the translator Nathaniel Hooke in the late 1720s. Nathaniel Hooke (d. 1763) was the nephew and namesake of a notorious Jacobite colonel. Hooke the younger entered Lincoln's Inn in 1702 and apparently was a victim of the South Sea Bubble, for in 1722 he wrote Harley seeking his patronage. "At that instant," he wrote, he was "just worth nothing."[80] With Harley as patron, Hooke translated Andrew Michael Ramsay's *Life of Fénelon* and began a career as a man of letters. He often frequented Bath and resided in Cheyne's house in 1727 while translating Ramsay's allegorical novel the *Travels of Cyrus*, which had just been published in Paris.[81] Ramsay himself visited England in 1729–30 and was made a fellow of the Royal Society; he probably saw Cheyne during this time.[82] William Warburton (1698–1779), bishop of Gloucester and antideist, referred to Hooke as a "mystic and quietist, and a warm disciple of Fénelon."[83]

Cheyne's circle of friends gradually expanded after he settled in Bath. Although he visited London infrequently (his 1725 visit was the first, and the last, for several years), he maintained his contacts there, often employing as intermediary his brother-in-law George Middleton, a goldsmith in the Strand.[84] These contacts were essential for his medical practice, and London was also the center of publishing. Cheyne's kinsman George Strahan continued to be his publisher despite his crusty manner, which, Cheyne complained, "would rust even Gold."[85] He also acquired a local Bath publisher, James Leake, whose name appeared with Strahan's on the title page of the *Essay of Health and Long Life* and subsequent works.[86] Leake (1686–1764) had moved to Bath in 1722; he was later an active member of the Bath hospital committee. Strongly Tory in his politics, he had printed several of Archibald Hutcheson's anti-Walpole pamphlets in the early 1720s. His family business in London was taken over by Samuel Richardson, who later married Leake's sister Elizabeth. Cheyne met Richardson, his patient and correspondent in the 1730s, through Leake.[87]

Cheyne introduced several of his friends and patients to his Oxford friend William Stratford, dean of Christ Church.[88] The doctor was also well acquainted with the London wits. John Gay had satirized him in 1720, and Arbuthnot continued to be a good friend. He wrote his *Essay Concerning the Nature of Aliments* (1731) in response to the success of the *Essay of Health and Long Life*, by "my learned and worthy Friend Dr. *Cheyne*." Cheyne's work "became the Subject of Conversation, and produced even Sects in the dietetick Philosophy"; Arbuthnot intended to give a scientific basis for dietetics, a *"Physiology* of *Aliment."*[89] Gay and Arbuthnot had both been members of the Scriblerus Club, which had also included Robert Harley (who died in 1724), Swift (in Ireland during most of the 1720s), and Alexander Pope. Pope advised Gay when he visited Bath in 1722 to consult with Arbuthnot and "Dr Chene" concerning "those regions about the *Abdomen* . . . to what exact pitch yours may be suffer'd to swell, not to outgrow theirs, who are, yet, your Betters."[90] Pope often consulted Cheyne during visits to Bath in the 1730s.[91]

Religion continued to be a common thread in Cheyne's friendships. The Bath-Bristol area was a hotbed of religious activity. Bristol continued to have a sizable Quaker community. It had been one of the strongholds of the French Prophets, and the Methodists later made inroads there.[92] Cheyne's translator John Robertson and his brother-in-law, the Bristol physician John Middleton (?1710–60)—both Aberdeen men—were active in evangelical circles in the area. Middleton, the Wesleys' physician, was later described as an "awakened man."[93] Middleton knew John Heylyn, D.D. (1685–1759), known as "the Mystic Doctor" and one of the executors of Cheyne's will. Heylyn, mentioned in the Keith-Deskford correspondence, was named vicar of the church of St. Mary-le-Strand in London in 1724.[94] In the same year, he published *Devotional Tracts Concerning the Presence of God and Other Religious Subjects*, a collection of mystical writings, including Cheyne's favorites Brother Lawrence, the Baron de Renty, and Ramsay's mentor Fénelon.[95]

Heylyn's one-time curate was William Law (1686–1761), whom he may have nudged toward mysticism.[96] By the early 1720s, when he was appointed tutor to the young Edward Gibbon (father of the historian) and moved to a cottage in Putney, Law was well known on several fronts. He had been chastised at Cambridge in 1713 for a thinly veiled pro-Jacobite speech.[97] He refused to take the required oaths to church and state at the accession of George I, ending his Cambridge career, and published several sermons making clear his high-church Tory principles. He intervened in the Bangorian controversy in the late 1710s and responded to Mandeville's *Fable of the Bees* in 1723. Although his 1726 attack on the theater won him few friends, his next work, also published in 1726, *A Practical Treatise upon Christian Perfection*, was widely admired.

Christian Perfection was a manual for Christian behavior. This, he declared, was not a mere "polishing our manners. . . . it implies an *entire change* of life."[98] The imitation of Christ must be the model for every Christian life. Law's Christ is austere, even puritanical: everyday entertainments such as the theater or light reading were "vain and contemptible," distractions from the work of attaining salvation.[99] At the center of Law's message was self-denial in clothing, in luxury, and especially in food and drink. As the seat of earthly corruption, the body was most in need of Christian discipline. "A constant course of full feeding," wrote Law,

is the death of the soul. . . . When a man has rejoiced himself with full eating and drinking, he is like any other *animal*, dispos'd only to *play* or *idleness*. . . . abstinence or self-denial . . . is as necessary for a Christian, that would get rid of the disorders of his nature, and lessen the weight of sin, as it is necessary for a man in a *dropsy* to abstain from *drink*, or a man in a *fever* to refrain from such things as *inflame* his blood.[100]

While Law and Cheyne had probably not met by 1726, numerous parallels between *Christian Perfection* and Cheyne's comments on physical and moral regimen in the *Essay of Health and Long Life* point to common sources: various Catholic mystics, Bourignon, Guyon. Cheyne's description of the relationship between the corrupt body and the troubled and sinful soul in his autobiography also show signs of Law's influence, although Cheyne disdained light reading only in this instance, since he recommended it to his patients and was himself addicted to French novels.[101]

An anonymous benefactor gave Law one thousand pounds after the publication of *Christian Perfection*, which Law used to open a charity school for girls in his native Northamptonshire. This benefactor may have been Lady Betty Hastings, who supported several such institutions and individuals.[102] Lady Betty may also have served as the model of Christian womanhood for Law's next work, *A Serious Call to a Devout and Holy Life*, published at the end of 1728.[103]

Like Cheyne, Law in *Christian Perfection* and *A Serious Call* addressed an audience of a certain status. His illustrative characters included the wealthy businessman Calidus, for whom "every hour of the day is . . . an hour of business," the honest tradesman Negotius, who "hears of the pleasures of debauchery, and the pleasures of piety, with the same indifference," and the "maiden sisters" Flavia and Miranda, who each inherited two hundred pounds a year, a comfortable middle-class income.[104] He contrasted the fashionable Flavia, who spent her time in "eating, drinking, dressing, visiting, conversation, reading and hearing Plays and Romances, at Operas, Assemblies, Balls and Diversions," to her saintly sister Miranda, ascetic, spiritual, and self-sacrificing, who spent her income to help others. Flavia was "so over-careful of her health, that she never thinks she is well enough; and so over-indulgent, that she never can be really well."[105]

Miranda, who "renounced the world to follow Christ," "eats and drinks only for the sake of living, and with so regular an abstinence, that every meal is an exercise of self-denial, and she humbles her body every time that she is forced to feed it." Unlike her peers, Miranda "will never have her eyes swell with fatness, or pant under a heavy load of flesh."[106] While Flavia's library contained "books of wit and humour, and . . . an expensive collection of all our English poets," Miranda read only "the lives of pious persons" and other uplifting works.[107] Lady Betty, who like Miranda spent no more time or effort on personal maintenance than was necessary, was quoted as saying that "she never read but one tale of fiction, and that she deeply regretted." Lady Betty mentioned Law's book with approval to her friend Bishop Thomas Wilson in 1730, another author of devotional works.[108]

At about this time Lady Betty introduced Cheyne to her new sister-in-law, the former Selina Shirley (1707–91), daughter of Earl Ferrers. Her sisters were already under the doctor's care.[109] By 1730 Selina, Lady Huntingdon, consulted Cheyne in Bath, and although she hated the spa (she wrote to her husband in 1732, "I think if possible this place grows more disagreeable every hour"), its benefit to her health seemed worth the trouble. Although she lived to the age of eighty-four, Lady Hunt-ingdon's health was usually described as delicate, and in the 1730s she lurched from one crisis to the next. Her "distracting, sinking, nervous complaints" were compounded by her almost continuous state of pregnancy.[110]

Cheyne prescribed his usual regimen for Lady Huntingdon, with particular emphasis on diet. He complimented her,

I extremely approve and rejoice at your ladyship's courage in your diet, not to make you a hugeous compliment. Do you know many ladies of your rank, quality, youth and necessary high living that has sense, virtue, or indeed faculties capable of a conviction, resolution, and courage to enter upon such a course of self denial for these poor disregarded low things (such as they are commonly reckoned), of good spirits, cheerfulness, health, and long life; and pray what is all the grandeur and glory of the world without them?

This regimen would help Lady Huntingdon heal both her body and her soul.[111]

By the early 1730s Cheyne appears as a link in another network that included Lady Betty, William Law, and a young Oxford don named John Wesley (1704–91) as well as Heylyn and Middleton.[112] Wesley, educated at high-church Christ Church and a stalwart Tory, had already read several of Cheyne's works, including the 1715 *Philosophical Principles*, and he may have met Lady Betty in the fall of 1729 on a visit to York, near her home at Ledstone. In November of that year he and his brother Charles (1707–88) initiated their "Holy Club" in Oxford, which emphasized "practical Christianity" in the manner of Law. A hostile observer in 1734 wrote,

"They imagine they cannot be saved if they do not spend every hour, nay minute, of their lives in the service of God." This service included preaching, fasting, praying, and visiting jails; "God deliver me from a half Christian" Wesley wrote his father.[13] The Wesleys would have agreed with John Byrom, who wrote in 1729 that "Christian religion [is] mightily out of fashion at present . . . people . . . agree with one another in nothing but rejecting many received opinions. . . . they have established a nominal Christianity and forsaken the practical Christianity."[14]

The occasion of Byrom's remarks was his purchase of Law's *Serious Call*, and this book also appeared on John Wesley's reading list in 1730. Byrom was so inspired that he soon sought out Law at Putney. By 1731 Cheyne knew Law well enough to recommend to him a favorite work, *Fides et ratio collatae*, that summary of mystical tenets which includes reference to, among others, Jacob Boehme.[15] Law then read Boehme's own writings, which, he said, "put me into a perfect sweat."[16] In the same year he published his antideist work *The Case of Religion and Reason; or, Natural Religion Fairly and Fully Stated* in response to Matthew Tindal's *Christianity as Old as the Creation; or, The Gospel a Republication of the Religion of Nature*, a work known as "the Bible of the deists." Law's work launched a renewed antideist campaign in the 1730s.[17]

Law in turn recommended mystical works to Wesley, who visited him at Putney in the summer of 1732. Wesley had already spent an afternoon with Lady Betty a few months earlier.[18] In that year a crisis occurred in the ranks of the Holy Club with far-reaching effects. During the summer, one of the founding members of the Holy Club, William Morgan, died of an unknown affliction. Toward the end he became raving mad, to the extent that he was threatened with confinement in an effort to jar him back to reason: "by the direction of the physicians he was threatened with ropes and chains, which were produced to him and rattled." He had exhibited symptoms of religious melancholy. Morgan "used frequently to say that enthusiasm was his madness, [and] repeated often 'Oh religious madness!' that they had hindered him from throwing himself out at the window."[19]

An extended criticism of the Wesleys' role in Morgan's demise appeared in December 1732 in *Fog's Weekly Journal*; among its contentions was that the

Holy Club's rigorous fasting had hastened Morgan's demise. A few months later a pamphlet appeared in response. Titled *The Oxford Methodists*, it contained the first extended account of Methodist views and has been attributed to William Law.[120] The author of *The Oxford Methodists* concluded that Morgan's melancholy was a case of religious deficit, not surfeit, resembling Cheyne's case in the *Essay of Health and Long Life*.

Cheyne's new religious connections influenced his decision to take up his pen again in the early 1730s.[121] At the age of sixty he needed to look back on his life, to give form and meaning to his bodily and spiritual transformation. His new insights into nervous disorders required expression, and he also wished to reestablish his authority as an interpreter of Newton. Most importantly, in keeping with Law's program, he felt compelled to steer Newtonianism away from the abyss of deism toward which it approached ever more closely. In the eight years that followed *De natura fibrae*, a second wave of self-consciously "Newtonian" works on physiology, especially nervous physiology, appeared. Equaling the first wave of the 1700s in quantity, these newcomers responded to the new Newtonian orthodoxy of ethers in ways that seemed clearly materialist.[122]

Like Cheyne, John Hutchinson (1674–1737) argued against the deist tendencies of Newton's doctrines in his *Moses's Principia* (1724–27). Hutchinson's intent, however, was to repudiate rather than to defend Newton. Newton's emphasis on God as the final, immaterial cause of gravity, Hutchinson contended, was contrary to Scripture and undermined the transcendent power of God. He argued that fire, light, and air were the material causes of motion by direct contact. Hutchinson's doctrines found some favor among high-church Anglicans from the 1730s onward, making Cheyne's task all the more urgent.[123]

In *The English Malady*, published in 1733, Cheyne elaborated upon his earlier accounts of the relationship among mind, body, and spirit. He joined together the theoretical framework of *De natura fibrae* (often translated verbatim from the Latin) with therapeutic recommendations and moral and spiritual exhortation, providing the fullest expression of his medical philosophy. Cheyne concluded *The English Malady* with a number of case histories, including his own autobiography.

He dedicated his book to his friend and patient William, Lord Bateman (?1695–1744), M.P., son of the London financier Sir James Bateman.[124] Bateman recommended Cheyne to Lady Huntingdon and is frequently mentioned in Cheyne's letters to her. He described Bateman to her as one of his success stories who, owing to a low regimen, "is so full of life, gayety and spirits" that he hardly resembled his former "cross, peevish" self.[125]

Cheyne defined the English malady to include "*nervous* Distempers, *Spleen, Vapours,* and *Lowness of Spirits.*" He would not talk about madness as such, although his methods would apply to that as well, but rather about the more common ailments suffered by his readers.[126] He entered a century-long discussion of the English propensity to "spleen," from Robert Burton to Thomas Sydenham to Bernard Mandeville, Sir Richard Blackmore, and Nicholas Robinson.[127] The historian Andrew Scull has argued that these physicians "attempt in thoroughly entrepreneurial ways to legitimize as authentic diseases new and milder (and presumably more treatable) varieties of 'nervous' disorders—the spleen, hypochondria, the vapours, hysteria—which apparently afflicted a more fashionable and desirable clientele than most of the Bedlam mad."[128] Yet the spleen was not merely an invention of the physicians, for the fashionable who flocked to Bath truly suffered, as Cheyne's case histories detailed, and the novelty of these disorders could be directly attributed to the progress of society. All was not well in the buzzing hive.

Cheyne claimed that such illnesses attacked as much as a third of the population, encompassing therefore not only the aristocracy but also the middle ranks. The infamously depressing English climate contributed to the malady, but its root causes were English wealth and success, which led to town life and too much leisure, especially among "the better Sort."[129] "Since our Wealth has increas'd, and our Navigation has been extended, we have ransack'd all the parts of the *Globe* to bring together its whole Stock of Materials for *Riot, Luxury,* and to provoke *Excess.*"[130]

That prime symbol of English success, London, the greatest city in the world, was also the site of the "most frequent, outrageous, and unnatural" nervous disorders. The very air of the city was unhealthy from smoke, animals, and rubbish dumps, not to mention "the Clouds of stinking

Breaths and Perspirations" the city dweller was forced to inspire. The
stresses of urban life, including its fast pace, crowded living, and multiple
entertainments, also contributed to the English malady.[131] Cheyne echoed
an earlier pastoral tradition and also prefigured the idealization of country
life so characteristic of the "age of sensibility"; he himself left London
and retired to the country to be cured. It was, to be sure, the English
malady and not the British malady, a disease of the crowded streets of
London and the fashionable haunts of Bath, not of the Highlands or even
of Edinburgh or Aberdeen. A Scot to the last, Cheyne excepted his
birthplace from the stigma of melancholia. In his own case, he did not
experience symptoms until he left Scotland for the sinfulness of London,
and he was cured only by going home to the piety of his childhood.

However, geography and circumstances were no excuse. Cheyne
bluntly declared, "If *Nervous* Disorders are the Diseases of the Wealthy,
the Voluptuous, and the Lazy . . . and are mostly produc'd, and always
aggravated and increased, by *Luxury* and *Intemperance* . . . there needs no
great Depth of Penetration to find out that *Temperance* and *Abstinence* is
necessary towards their *Cure*."[132] Cheyne nonetheless spoke to the patient
in sympathetic tones: "of all the Miseries that afflict Human Life . . . in
this Valley of Tears, I think, *Nervous* Disorders . . . are the most
deplorable." An "erected Spirit," however, could bear many miseries. His
own experience, the doctor added, would guide the reader. Cheyne
advised those anxious for relief to skip the "merely *Philosophical*" sections
that followed and go straight to the remedies; the patient need only have
the barest notion of the body as "a Machin of an infinite Number and
Variety of different Channels and Pipes, filled with various and different
Liquids and Fluids."[133]

For those who would read on, Cheyne was only too happy to expound
upon theory, and much of the first section of *The English Malady* repeated
De natura fibrae. In response to the flurry of treatises on Newton's ether,
however, Cheyne extended his discussion and contributed to the ongoing
antideist campaign by countering interpretations of Newton's ether that
minimized the role of God. For example, Nicholas Robinson's *New System
of the Spleen, Vapours and Hypochondriack Melancholy* (1729) defined the soul as a
"self-moving principle" that animated the "organiz'd Machines" of the

body, much like the deists' God who initially animated the universe. Individual thoughts, intelligence, and personality were all caused by the mechanical arrangement of the parts, not by differences in souls; both madness and idiocy were caused simply by a "clog of matter" in a particular part. Robinson postulated a material "animal aether" that received motion from the brain and transmitted it to the animal spirits, but he did not detail how it differed from the animal spirits.[134]

The Irish physician Bryan Robinson (1680–1754) in his 1732 *Treatise of the Animal Oeconomy* identified "a very Elastick Aether" with the animal spirits. Like Cheyne in *De natura fibrae*, he denied the notion of the hollow nerve, citing Newton's query 24.[135] In the *English Malady* Cheyne denied the identification of the ether with animal spirits; indeed, he discarded animal spirits altogether, arguing that any material fluid would be too dense to cause muscular motion. "The Notion of *animal Spirits*," he declared, "is of the same Leaven with the *substantial Forms* of *Aristotle*, and the *coelestial System* of *Ptolemy*." He reasserted his views on the structure of the nerves, citing Leeuwenhoek and the 1724 treatise on muscular motion of the Newtonian Henry Pemberton (1693–1771).[136] Impulses or vibrations were transmitted along the solid nerves by the action of an ambient subtle fluid, in a manner analogous to music: the brain acts as the musician and the musical vibrations flow along the nerves.[137]

Cheyne continued the discussion of Newton's ether theory begun in the 1715 *Philosophical Principles*. Such actions in nature as cohesion and elasticity may be caused by an "infinitely subtil, elastick Fluid, or Spirit," a suggestion "made not improbable by the late *sagacious* and *learned* Sir Isaac Newton."[138] A material ether whose parts were themselves elastic and repulsive held an inherent contradiction; since we cannot postulate another ether and another in an infinite regress, "we must suppose these Qualities innate to them, and to have been impress'd on them immediately by the *first* and *supreme Cause*." But the split between material and spiritual was not therefore abrupt. As in 1715, Cheyne proposed a Platonic hierarchy of "Intermediates between *pure, immaterial Spirit* and *gross Matter*." Using Newton's format of queries, he tentatively identified Newton's ether as an "intermediate material Substance," the "*Medium* of the Intelligent Principle," which may, among other functions, "make the

Cement between the human Soul and Body." Cheyne's concept of the ether called for the direct and active involvement of God in contrast to the deistic concept of a self-moving soul, which only implied God's action.[139]

Cheyne then returned his discussion to the standard ascription of nervous disorders to the body. Just as a musician cannot play on an imperfect instrument, so the musician of the soul could not act effectively on an unfit body. Loose and relaxed nerves, said the doctor, were the true cause of melancholy. His detailed physiognomic description of the weak-nerved patient emphasized feminine qualities: the nervous tended to be small-boned and white-skinned, with "soft and yielding" flesh, fat rather than muscular, low and soft in voice. Such individuals were also "quick, prompt, and passionate . . . have a great Degree of Sensibility; are quick Thinkers, feel Pleasure or Pain the most readily, and are of most lively Imagination."[140] Cheyne compared the spasms of hysteric fits to the "*Throws* and *Convulsions*" of childbirth.[141]

Many physicians claimed that women were physically and temperamentally far more susceptible to nervous disorders than men. Moreover, their weaker bodies more easily and visibly displayed its symptoms. Nicholas Robinson confined his observations to "the Fair Sex" for this reason.[142] Yet Cheyne's use of feminine imagery can also be viewed as an early manifestation of what Terry Castle has called "the feminization of human nature" during the eighteenth century, when "feminine" characteristics such as sensitivity came to be applied to both sexes.[143] Cheyne's practice was about evenly divided between men and women, and he did not explicitly direct his comments to one or the other. His dietary advice in the *Essay of Health and Long Life* had distinctively feminine characteristics, yet Cheyne did not intend it to apply only to women. Diet continued to form the center of his therapy.

Cheyne argued that the basis of "the hypp" was to be found in "ill-condition'd Juices," and could be remedied by the proper regimen, including diet, exercise, and medicines. First the fluids would be diluted from their "glewy" state, then restored to sweetness; and finally, the fibers would regain at least some of their "*Tone* and *elastick* Force."[144] Cheyne initiated a course of treatment with the standard evacuations, recom-

mending preparations of mercury and antimony both for their eliminative effects and for their usefulness in unclogging the small tubes of
the body. Sweeteners included *"foetid* and *volatile"* substances such as
asafoetida, garlic, and horseradish, though these may be "offensive to
delicate Persons." Best, however, were mineral waters, particularly those of
Bath. Strengthening and astringent medicines to tone the fibers included
"Bitters, Aromaticks, and *Chalybeats"* such as cinnamon, wormwood, and
camomile and Cheyne's favorite, cinchona bark.[145] Cheyne's recommendations, not much changed since his treatment of Catherine Walpole
twelve years earlier, lay well within the bounds of standard practice.

As he knew, Cheyne parted company with many physicians in his
emphasis on diet. He stated his purpose at the outset: "The chief Design
of these Sheets is to recommend to my Fellow Creatures that plain *Diet*
which is most agreeable to the Purity and Simplicity of uncorrupted
Nature, and unconquer'd *Reason.*"[146] Plain diet would return the corrupt
body to an Adamic purity, a purity that was peculiarly English. He
recommended the *"Diet* and *Manner of Living* of the middling Rank," a
yeoman's diet of plain local food and fermented (not distilled) drink,
nothing foreign or exotic. Refined down to its essentials of milk, vegetables, and seeds, this motherly diet would restore the abused body to
childlike health.[147] While the "Pop-gun Artillery" of coffee, tea, chocolate, and snuff could not damage health, cramming down luxurious food
certainly would. Foreign methods of cooking, "the ingenious mixing and
compounding of *Sauces* and foreign *Spices* and Provocatives" compelled
overeating.[148]

A debilitating, luxurious diet in turn "must necessarily beget an Inep-
titude for Exercise," and too much leisure depressed the spirits. When, as
in Bath, *"Assemblies, Musick Meetings, Plays, Cards* and *Dice* are the only Amusements," a lax habit of body necessarily followed, resulting in further
demands for luxury such as coaches with springs and *"Chairmen* [who]
wriggle and swim along." Equally damaging, and equally symptomatic of
English success, was the sedentary, intellectual life; English superiority in
the sciences had unforeseen consequences. The *"Great Wits"* who led intellectual life were also "Men of *Taste"* who indulged freely in the fruits of
civilization.[149]

Cheyne defended his views with citation of the classics as well as of Arbuthnot and Freind. He claimed he was neither enthusiast nor leveler but a true advocate of moderation. Far from enjoining his readers to "turn *Monks* [and] run into Desarts [*sic*]," his strictest diet, he said, was only for the most desperate cases. He did not quackishly presume to prescribe a single diet for every patient to follow. By means of the true natural philosophy, he had rescued nervous disorders from the throes of "Witchcraft, Enchantment, Sorcery and Possession" and established the true grounds of remedy. The only ones who might not benefit, he said, were "the *Voluptuous* and *Unthinking*," those who valued life only for pleasure, and those too stupid to care."[50] Mankind, he wrote, is commonly divided into "*Quick Thinkers, Slow Thinkers,* and *No Thinkers,*" and the doctor only concerned himself with the first category.[51]

Roy Porter has described *The English Malady* as a highly secularized work, noting that, with our knowledge of Cheyne's own mystical religion, his "silence is almost deafening." Certainly religion overtly intrudes very little into his text, and Porter rightly asserts that "no discussion of souls in crisis appears."[52] Cheyne himself characterized fasting and abstinence as "not more a *religious* than it ought to be reckon'd a *medical* Institution."[53] I suggest, however, that a pervasive sense of sin underlies Cheyne's discussion, culminating in his autobiography. As Wesley was beginning to recognize—inspired by Cheyne's *Essay of Health and Long Life*—discipline of the body was an essential counterpart to discipline of the soul. "Luxury and Laziness," said Cheyne, caused most nervous problems; if these acted upon the body, they were ultimately the result of bad behavior. Cheyne's patients had the free will to choose the way they lived, to choose to sin or not. They could choose to be Flavia or Miranda, Beau Nash or Lady Betty. Bad choices resulted in the cases described in the last third of his book.

Cheyne included case histories for several reasons. Particularly among his fellow Bath practitioners, they demonstrated the skill of the author and the rank of his patients, although Cheyne disdained this motive. He hoped to redefine the English malady as a legitimate disease, distinct from "a lower Degree of *Lunacy*" or mere whimsy. The vapours were "as much a bodily Distemper . . . as the *Small-Pox* or a *Fever*," and therefore as susceptible to medical intervention. But this "medicalization" would empower the patient as much as the doctor: while the doctor would prescribe the medicines, only the patient could affect the necessary changes in lifestyle. Cheyne wished to "illustrate and confirm the several Steps of the preceding Doctrine, and to direct the *Valetudinarian*, in the less obvious and uncommon Symptoms."[154] His case histories are narratives of both illness and disease, giving the points of view of both patient and healer, and in great detail. Cheyne's case histories partake of a genre Thomas Laqueur has termed "the humanitarian narrative," characterized by realistic detail, a focus on the body as the sympathetic link between reader and text, and the implicit possibility of amelioration. Other examples of this genre include the autopsy report and the novel. One purpose of these narratives, according to Laqueur, was to elicit sympathy for the suffering body; like Cheyne himself, the reader would experience the suffering of his patients. Yet unlike the Puritan perception of illness as something to be endured, Cheyne's narratives also offered the prospect of recovery.[155]

Cheyne classified his cases into three categories. The least serious disorders were "chiefly confin'd to the *alimentary Tube*" and could be cured by dietary adjustment and evacuations. The second class of illness was more serious, extending to the "juices" and organs, and required a stricter diet and stronger medicines. The third category was of "almost incurable" cases when the body was almost irreparably damaged. Here only the strongest medicines and the strictest diet of vegetables and milk would do.[156] Yet the goal of this diet was not slenderness: Cheyne's patients were often thin or even emaciated before his therapy, while after they are "hale," "brawn," "hearty," and most of all, "chearful."

The first category of illnesses ranged from headaches to "low spirits" and "Hysterick fits." Four out the six cases in this section were women, all described as hysteric to some degree. Cheyne's prescriptions differed little: after an initial purging regimen that included drinking Bath water, along with strengthening medicines such as bitters and steel, the main cure was a moderate regimen. This was by no means extreme: "the plainest, lightest and most simple *Animal Foods*, at noon only, and a little of the best *French Wines*" was a typical prescription.[157] The usual exercise recommended was horseback riding. Obviously, this was a diet for those who could afford to diet.

The second set of cases also numbered six, only one of which was female. They suffered from *"Lowness* and *Oppression,"* accompanied by various degrees of *"Nervous, Hypochondriacal,* and *Convulsive Fits* and *Paroxysms."* They had run the gamut of physicians and cures, coming finally to Cheyne in desperation. Here too, the head was directly connected with the stomach, and these nervous cases were relieved by various purging medicines. A lasting cure, however, was only accomplished by a change of regimen, in these cases more drastic than in the first set. Here Cheyne allowed meat (and only young white meat) on alternate days only; on the other days only milk and vegetables were allowed. Yet this regime too was hardly extreme: he allowed a gouty patient a pint a day of "some generous, soft, balsamick Wine (as *Sack, Canary,* or *Palm*)." As he pointed out, lovers of fine food could "bear a *Maigre* day more easily, when they know they shall have a *Gaudy* one the next."[158]

The final set of six cases was evenly divided between men and women. Not all of these seemed strictly to be nervous cases: a gentlewoman from Oxfordshire had a tumor in her breast, and a gentleman of Wales appeared to be crippled by arthritis. But the seriousness of their disorders led the patients to Cheyne as a last resort. In these cases, only the strictest diet would do: milk and vegetables. The recoveries wrought by these means were nothing short of miraculous, though far from instantaneous, taking as long as two years. Cheyne followed these cases with a further defense of his vegetable diet. He then appended two additional cases: the curious case of Colonel Townshend, and the more conventional case of Doctor Cranstoun. Colonel Townshend, who could will himself into a near-death state, left Cheyne baffled but was explained by the Edinburgh physician William Porterfield as an example of the intimate connection between the soul and the body, an explanation Cheyne later endorsed.[159]

The spectacle of Cheyne's fine gentlemen and ladies of eminent worth being afflicted with "bilious vomiting," "hysterick paroxysms," flatulence, convulsions, and "a fix'd *Melancholy, Terror,* and *Dread,*" "crucified" with pain, led to the conclusion that earthly wealth and eminence was no pre-servative from suffering.[160] But one could choose to alter one's behavior and save one's life. In his case histories, his voice and conversational therapy clearly emerge: the vivid description of symptoms, the doctor's own doubts and hesitations, the moral digressions, and the conversational tone are quite unlike the more schematic case histories of his Bath colleagues. In his use of self-motivation and persuasion, Cheyne anticipated the moral treatment of the end of the eighteenth century.[61] Cheyne's case histories crescendoed in intensity, reaching a peak with the doctor's own case. For forty agonizing pages, the reader could trace his pilgrim's progress from luxury, obesity, and depression to health and cheerfulness. In this context, the spiritual dimensions of Cheyne's case and its cure take on added significance as the conclusion of a work only seemingly secular, whose subtext was one of repentence and forgiveness.

Yet Cheyne was no typical evangelical, berating the sinful masses with fire and brimstone. As always, he attempted to find a *via media* between the extremes of atheism and enthusiasm. But Cheyne's response continued to hold a significant spiritual component. His popularity indicated that the ruling classes were perhaps not quite as confident in either secularization or the smoothed-out Anglicanism of Tillotson's church as we might think. They felt guilty, and Cheyne, as much priest as physician, afforded them absolution.

7

THE GREAT MUSE

The English Malady reached a sixth edition within two years, as well as a pirated Dublin edition. Cheyne's earlier writings, from the *New Theory of Fevers* onward, were also reprinted every few years in the 1730s, indicating his continued popularity among the "middling Gentry" he judged to form his audience.[1] The new and popular *Gentleman's Magazine* published a laudatory poem about the doctor in 1733, comparing him to Sydenham as a "great wondr'ous Genius." Highly favorable summaries of his ideas appeared in that magazine in 1735 and 1738, both reprinted from the religiously oriented *Weekly Miscellany*; the 1735 piece included a lengthy excerpt from his autobiography.[2] Mary Chandler's 1734 *Description of Bath* condemned the "Fatal Effects of LUXURY and EASE"; "'Tis to thy Rules, O TEMPERANCE! we owe/All Pleasures which from *Health* and *Strength* can flow." Matthew Green advocated "the plainest food/To mend viscidity of blood" in his 1737 poem "The Spleen."[3]

The English Malady also reestablished its author's status as a Newtonian, for in 1735 Bryan Robinson asked him to intervene in his controversy with Thomas Morgan. Although in *The English Malady* Cheyne had criticized some of Robinson's ideas, the Dublin physician expressed only admiration for him in the second edition of his *Treatise of the Animal Oeconomy*, published in 1734, appending a section on the effects of age, weather, and exercise on "Animal Fibres."[4]

Morgan (d. 1743) had published in 1725 his *Philosophical Principles of Medicine*, which Robert Schofield has described as a "journeyman's version of Pitcairne or James Keill." Morgan criticized Cheyne for apparently abandoning his iatromechanical principles: "the Mathematicks and Mechanism can signify nothing, when a Man has once raised an Indolent implicit

Reputation, and Experience has taught him an easier way of getting Money."[5] Morgan appended some "Remarks on Dr Robinson's Treatise of the Animal Oeconomy" to his 1735 *Mechanical Practice of Physick*, which criticized Robinson's account of fluid dynamics as inaccurate and indicative of a poor understanding of Newtonian theory. He also claimed to refute the "Beleineian hypothesis of animal secretion and muscular motion."[6] Robinson replied to Morgan in a *Letter to Dr. Cheyne* published in 1735, also included in the third edition of Robinson's book (1738), in which he asked Cheyne to determine who was the better Newtonian. No reply by Cheyne is extant, but Morgan issued in 1738 his own *Letter to Dr. Cheyne*, which ended the controversy for the time.[7] Both authors addressed Cheyne in highly flattering terms.

During Cheyne's last decade of life, from 1733 to 1743, he was at last happy, wealthy, and successful. During his recovery in 1728, the duke of Chandos wrote to him, "If your Spirits were thereupon for the time retired into a heap together I hope & make no question but that your usual Vigour of Mind will soon dissipate them, and make them flow regularly through the great Muse they animate."[8] Cheyne wrote Richardson that if he followed his advice, the printer would reach "a moderate, Active, gay Temper and Habit and write Books without End, as I have done, and grow as rich as a Jew and settle all your Family to your Heart's Content."[9] Since regaining his health in the late 1720s, he told Richardson, he had tripled his income.[10] Apart from his contributions to the Bath hospital, his newfound wealth allowed him to subscribe to several books, including Philip Miller's 1731 *Gardener's Dictionary* and John Quinton's 1733 treatise on Bath.[11] He occupied a comfortable house in Monmouth Street, a new street just outside the old west gate, not far from the new and fashionable Queen Square, constructed in 1728. Cheyne's house was among the most expensive in the neighborhood, comparing favorably to the nearby dwellings of his fellow physicians Richard Frewin and William Oliver the younger.[12]

Cheyne sent his fourteen-year-old son John off to Oxford in 1731, accompanied by the doctor's half-brother William, both to prepare for careers in the Church of England.[13] They attended St. Mary Hall, whose

principal, Dr. William King (1685–1763), was a noted Jacobite and friend
of Ramsay. King, along with William Cheyne, had acted as amanuenses
for Nathaniel Hooke when he translated the *Travels of Cyrus* at Cheyne's
house.[14] Like his older half-brother, William Cheyne had spent time as a
tutor. The doctor later sought the patronage of the countess of
Huntingdon in securing William a clerical post; he wrote, "I can get
small livings enough for him, but I think it were losing him to place him
but in some creditable situation, where he might labour for life."[15] With
or without the assistance of the countess, William gained a living in
Weston, not far from Bath, while John Cheyne died in 1768 as vicar of
Brigstock, near Northampton.[16]

Of the doctor's two daughters, the elder, Frances, married William
Stewart, an advocate and king's remembrancer, on 30 April 1741 at St.
Paul's Cathedral. The remembrancer was a royal officer responsible for
collecting debts (such as first fruits and tenths) due the sovereign. It
could be quite a lucrative post; in the *Drapier's Letters* Swift noted that the
first remembrancer made the princely sum of two thousand pounds per
annum.[17] The Stewarts resided in London, while Cheyne's favorite, Peggy,
remained at home in Bath with her parents. Peggy Cheyne inherited her
father's interests and intellect, and later advised Richardson on Clarissa
much as her father had advised him on Pamela. She was of uncertain
health. Richardson described her in 1746 as "a young Lady of Taste and
Reading," and Cheyne often referred to her as Richardson's favorite.[18]

Cheyne's patients included the earl and countess of Huntingdon, the
earl of Chesterfield, Lord Hervey, Lord Bateman, Lord Barclay, the earl
of Essex, and the earl of Bath as well as such lesser folk as "Mr and Mrs
Thomson of Yorkshire."[19] He regularly got one of his government friends
to frank his letters. In 1738 Cheyne traveled to Burford to attend his and
Pitcairne's old friend George Baillie of Jerviswood on his deathbed.[20]
George Lyttelton wrote with approbation of Cheyne to his friend
Alexander Pope in 1736: "Immortal Doctor Cheyney bids me tell you
that he shall live at least Two Centuries by being a Real and practical
Philosopher, while such Gluttonous Pretenders to Philosophy as You,
Dr Swift and My Lord Bolingbroke die of Eating and Drinking at

Fourscore."[21] Although Oliver was his usual physician at Bath, Pope consulted Cheyne in the 1730s and was an ardent admirer. Chronically in
poor health, Pope followed a Cheynean regimen of little wine, few suppers,
and much mineral water.[22] He recommended the doctor to others, writing
of him, "there lives not an Honester Man, nor a Truer Philosopher."[23] He
often asked his Bath friend Ralph Allen to convey his "Religious Respects"
to Cheyne, describing him in 1739 as "yet so very a child in true Simplicity
of Heart," comparing him to Don Quixote.[24]

While Cheyne consorted with the rich and powerful, his more intimate circle continued to be heavily biased toward religion. He named
John Heylyn one of the executors of his will and referred to William
Law as "the greatest best Man, and the most solid and deep of this
Island." Law regularly sent Cheyne copies of his books.[25] Upon the death
in 1740 of Cheyne's friend Archibald Hutcheson, his widow, Elizabeth,
joined Hester Gibbon at Law's Northamptonshire house to lead a life of
charity.[26] Also part of Cheyne's circle were Law's disciple John Byrom and
the London surgeon John Freke. Byrom and his brother visited Cheyne in
1738. Cheyne wrote Byrom a long letter in December 1741 about the
French mystic writer the marquis de Marsay (1688–1753) and offered him
a copy of his own *Natural Method.* He wrote again about Marsay in August
1742.[27] Byrom's friend, the physician David Hartley (1705–57), moved to
Bath in 1742 and became Cheyne's friend as well.[28] Samuel Richardson
was another member of what Cheyne referred to as "the Brethren."[29]
They shared mystical literature and opposed "meer Rationalists" on
every front. Cheyne's brother-in-law, the goldsmith George Middleton,
his daughter Frances Stewart, and John Heylyn acted as his London
contacts, at times lending books.[30] In the Bristol area, two physicians—
Cheyne's other brother-in-law John Middleton and his translator John
Robertson—were also part of this circle. Robertson edited Ramsay's
posthumous *Philosophical Principles of Natural and Revealed Religion,* published in
1748–49, and issued a new edition of James Garden's *Comparative Theology* in
1756. However, Robertson became a follower of the anti-Newtonian John
Hutchinson, whose doctrines Cheyne explicitly repudiated.[31] Wesley read
Ramsay's book "with great attention" in 1753 and wrote a long letter to
Robertson about it.[32]

The last decade of Cheyne's life is ironically both the least eventful in terms of dramatic change and the best documented. Some thirty of Cheyne's letters to the countess of Huntingdon survive, written between about 1730 and 1739. Eighty-two letters to Samuel Richardson, written between 1733 and 1743, are also extant. Both these collections were published in the 1940s by Charles F. Mullett. Lady Huntingdon and Richardson were both patients, but Cheyne's bedside manner varied considerably between them. In addition, amanuensis copies of fourteen letters from the duke of Chandos to Cheyne written in the late 1720s and early 1730s survive.

Cheyne's letters to Lady Huntingdon are serious and respectful, befitting the rank of the addressee. He recognized that she had other physicians with other opinions and expended much ink in persuading her of the merits of his therapy, citing other noble patients he had cured. Unlike the doctor-patient relationship today, Cheyne was a supplicant for the patronage of the countess, and he was not above obsequiousness. Yet he was also chatty and loquacious, assuring the countess that he valued her as an individual as well as a patient. He promoted himself to Lord Huntingdon, sending a copy of *The English Malady* as it came off the press, and later dedicating his *Essay on Regimen* (1740) to him, although they had never met.[33] Cheyne occasionally ran errands for Lady Huntingdon, as in 1736 when his wife ordered some shoes for her. In 1734 he recommended a tutor for the young Huntingdon daughters. He was rewarded in turn by gifts, of a whole deer on one occasion, a "fine cane" on another.[34] Similarly, Cheyne acted as the duke of Chandos's agent in Bath, seeking real estate for purchase, checking on the duke's tenants, and in one case even collecting rent.[35] These acts underscore the ambivalent relationship between the eighteenth-century physician and his noble patients, to whom he was both caregiver and client.

Lady Huntingdon first visited Bath and met Cheyne in 1732. She was twenty-four, three years married, and had already given birth to three sons.[36] While her husband was wealthy, she had been brought up in rural Ireland in comparative poverty; her dowry was small and because of family lawsuits it was not actually paid until 1810. Lady Betty and her half-sisters arranged the match between the young earl and "Lady Liney,"

but by all accounts it was a love match and a happy marriage. Correspondence between the earl and his lady on her many visits to Bath was
frequent and affectionate.[37]

Lady Huntingdon did not have fits like Catherine Walpole, but she
too suffered from "lowness of spirits" and abdominal pains, complicated
by "heats." Cheyne described Lady Huntingdon's case as a "distracting,
sinking nervous complaint" while acknowledging that her symptoms,
while in part hereditary, were largely due to her almost continuous state
of pregnancy, for she gave birth in 1729, 1730, 1731, 1732, 1735, 1737, and
1739.[38] He also detected evidence of bladder stones, that curse of the
upper classes. Cheyne wrote in 1735, "I greatly hope the worst is over with
your ladyship if you do not breed again, for had it not been for that you
must have been well ere now."[39] The maidenly difficulties of Catherine
Walpole, particularly lack of appetite and of menstruation, were not
evident.

Cheyne diagnosed Lady Huntingdon's ailment as an "acrid, hot humour
of the juices."[40] He prescribed the usual bleeding, vomiting, and purging;
bleeding would lessen the heat of inflammation, while vomiting and
especially purging would rid the body of the noxious humor. He supplemented this with a "cool regimen" of a "cool and scanty diet," consisting
mainly of milk and vegetables and liberal use of mineral water. During
her pregnancies, he prescribed abstinence from alcohol and only the
mildest of purgatives, avoiding the stronger combinations of mercury
and antimony. As we have seen, Cheyne lavishly praised the countess for
following his regime, apparently in the face of considerable criticism
from her friends and family. A low diet, however, had long been prescribed
in pregnancy.[41]

But too often Lady Huntingdon ignored the doctor's advice, for he
repeated his instructions again and again. She asked Cheyne to give his
opinion of her case to another doctor; each physician, however, had his
own pet remedies, and the countess apparently took them all, a model of
Mandeville's "over-physicked" patient. Similarly, the duchess of Chandos
alternately ignored Cheyne's advice and sought it, comparing his advice
to that of Freind and Arbuthnot.[42] Lady Huntingdon's relatives also
prescribed remedies; Lady Betty sent a recipe for "snail-watter" in 1731,

noting that "Phisicians will seldome approve what they don't recomend [*sic*]."[43] Lady Huntingdon also diagnosed herself: she wrote her husband in 1735, "I was so much out of order . . . I was forced to take a puke last night."[44] The duchess of Chandos also took "a gentle Pewk" to relieve the "Swimming and giddyness in her head."[45] Cheyne exasperatedly told Lady Huntingdon in 1734, "you must give over all medicines. I fear you have suffered by taking so many without a full notion of your case." The countess was further at fault for neglecting to detail all of her symptoms to her physicians, because of her natural "modesty and reservedness."[46]

"Modesty and reservedness" aside, the countess was a strong-willed and at times imperious woman. She disliked Bath, which she thought "stupid," and she disliked being away from her family on her trips to the spa. It is a measure of the severity of her symptoms that she nonetheless continued to travel to Bath as well as to Bristol, Buxton, and Scarborough for treatment and to consult Dr. Cheyne and follow his advice, however half-heartedly. Meanwhile she had herself begun to administer medical care to her "poor Neighbours" at home in Leicestershire.[47] Her sisters-in-law, the Ladies Elizabeth, Margaret, Ann, and Frances Hastings, also followed the doctor's prescriptions, though their ailments were often vague. Lady Betty wrote Lady Huntingdon, "My sister Ann has taken several things and thinks she is something better but I fear not much, tis not easy even to gess [*sic*] whether she is sick or well. I can't say she has follow'd Dr Cheney's prescription any farther than drinking a pint of whey in a morning which she thinks agrees with her."[48] Lady Ann's main problem was that "she eats & drinks as she use'd to do."[49]

By the mid-1730s the religious concerns Cheyne had long shared with Lady Betty now extended to other members of the family. Lady Huntingdon had revealed a puritanical streak in the early 1730s; on the affair of Miss Vane and the prince of Wales, she wrote to her husband, "I am quite out of patience with the wickedness of them all, for I believe no age ever came up to it."[50] Lady Huntingdon possessed copies of some of Cheyne's favorite mystical texts, including works of Guyon and Bishop Fénelon. She corresponded with William Law and was friendly with John Byrom, who through her met Cheyne.[51] It is not clear, however, whether Cheyne specifically prescribed religious texts as part of his therapy.

Cheyne and Lady Betty already knew John Wesley, and Lady Betty had supported the missionary efforts in Georgia of the Wesleys and George Whitefield in the mid-1730s.[52] David Shuttleton has argued that Whitefield's conversion in 1735 was directly inspired by his reading of Cheyne's works.[53]

By 1738 Lady Margaret Hastings (1700–1768) had become deeply involved with the Methodists, particularly with Benjamin Ingham (1712–72), recently returned from Georgia and a member of the Holy Club. They married in 1741. The Hastings sisters, like the Wesleys and William Law, also read the works of the German pietists known as the Moravians in the mid-1730s, whose emphasis on conversion and evangelism greatly influenced the Methodist movement. Lady Betty's fortitude during the long and painful illness (probably breast cancer) that caused her death at the end of 1739 undoubtedly influenced her family's conversion, which began in July 1739. While Lady Huntingdon and her husband at first inclined toward the Moravians, after Lady Betty's death, and with the influence of Lady Margaret and Ingham, they turned toward Wesley and the Methodists. By 1743 Lady Huntingdon was inviting Wesley to preach before the colliers at the Huntingdon's mine near Oakthorpe in Leicestershire.[54]

John and Charles Wesley and Benjamin Ingham had journeyed to the new American colony of Georgia in 1735, returning early in 1738. Upon his return, John Wesley consulted Cheyne about his health. While he had followed Cheyne's regimen during his Holy Club days, he indulged in wine and "Animal food" during his stay in America. Cheyne urged him to return to his old abstemiousness, which he did, later crediting his good health to Cheyne's plan.[55] Like Cheyne, the crisis in his health was also a crisis in his soul, and Wesley had to experience a conversion to resolve this, which occurred in May 1738. Soon after, Wesley founded a congregation that met at Fetter Lane in London.

The conversion of the Hastings family horrified many of their acquaintances. Lady Mary Wortley Montagu reported, "Lady Margaret Hastings has disposed of herself to a poor wandering Methodist," and the duchess of Buckingham wrote Lady Huntingdon in 1743,

I thank your ladyship for the information concerning the Methodist preachers. Their doctrines are most repulsive and strongly tinctured with impertinence and disrespect toward their superiors, in perpetually endeavouring to level all ranks and do away with all distinctions. It is monstrous to be told that you have a heart as sinful as the common wretches that crawl the earth. This is highly offensive and insulting, and I cannot but wonder that your ladyship should relish any sentiments so much at variance with high rank and good breeding.[56]

Her conversion markedly changed the tone of Lady Huntingdon's relationship with Dr. Cheyne. She shared a "most friendly" New Year's Eve dinner with the doctor and his wife in 1741. The countess told her husband, "[we] spent our evening in most pious and religious conversation, a thing hard to be found here. . . . He is I think more in favour than ever with me, though much out of fashion here."[57] A few days later Cheyne visited her, "and has been talking like an old apostle. He really has the most refined notions of the true spiritual religion I almost ever met with. The people of the Bath says [*sic*] I have made him a Methodist, but indeed I receive much light and comfort from his conversation."[58]

Did Cheyne become a Methodist? Despite his sympathy with many Methodist doctrines, particularly the notion of conversion, Cheyne was disturbed by the "enthusiastic" tendencies of Wesley and his followers. He wrote to the son of Lady Betty's friend Bishop Thomas Wilson in 1740, "even the Methodists, though novices, indiscreet and precipitate, may be sent to move the waters," hardly a ringing endorsement.[59] Cheyne continued to believe that the quietist mystics he had discovered in 1705 offered the surest guidance to salvation, the surest middle way between enthusiasm and deism. At the same time, Wesley grew to reject the mysticism of Law and others, which he had found so inspiring a decade earlier. He dismissed Law's Behmenist *Grounds and Reasons of Christian Regeneration*, published in 1739, as "philosophical, speculative, precarious; Behmenish, void, and vain"; a few years later he found Boehme's own work to be "sublime nonsense," and he resolved to "drop Quietists and Mystics altogether."[60] While Wesley and Cheyne thus parted ways on doctrine, Wesley nonetheless continued to admire and employ Cheyne's ideas on regimen. Lady Huntingdon also continued to correspond with Law.[61]

Cheyne also wrote of religion to Samuel Richardson, his patient, his printer, and eventually, his friend and a member of "the Brethren." Cheyne's letters from Bath to Richardson in London are chatty, informal, and highly opinionated; with his autobiography, they are the most revealing documents we possess of Cheyne's character. Cheyne is in turn impish, peevish, and pious, dispensing literary and medical advice with equal lavishness. Despite his age and years of success, he also remained at times a bumbling, tactless bumpkin. A nonstop talker, he overflowed with enthusiasm, indignation, or whatever emotion seized him; quick to anger, but quick to forgive, and ever ready with an aphorism or quip. Small wonder that Cheyne asked Richardson to destroy these very revealing documents: "Be sure you destroy all my Letters when perused, for though I value little wh[a]t the present or future World of this State, thinks of me, yet for my Family's Sake I would not be counted a mere Trifler, as these long Nothing-Letters, merely to amuse you, would show me."[62]

Their friendship began as a business transaction, for Richardson, perhaps recommended by his brother-in-law James Leake, printed Cheyne's books from *The English Malady* onward. Mullett has well described the business side of authorship.[63] But this relationship soon blossomed into friendship; by the end of 1734, Richardson was sending Cheyne apples, oysters, and copies of religious works and his *Weekly Miscellany*, while Cheyne gave Richardson medical advice.[64] Cheyne refused payment for this advice, but accepted favors: a "catechism" printed in 1738, a "handsomely bound" collection of Law's works in 1742.[65]

Cheyne was well familiar with Richardson's symptoms, which included lack of appetite and "lowness of spirits," and for the next decade the doctor and the printer negotiated both printing contracts and regimens. Cheyne prescribed his old favorites, mild purges along with cinchona bark and mineral water, for Richardson's ongoing symptoms. But at times of crisis he added stronger purgatives and emetics, all the while advising moderation in diet, exercise, and diversion. A recommendation from 1738 is typical:

I hope your Case is more Hypochondriacal than Apoplectic. I am for losing a
little Blood once in 2 or 3 Months, taking a Vomit some Days after, drinking
only Valerian Small Beer and Valerian Tea—the more the better of either—living
on Half a Chicken in Quantity of any fresh tender Meat (any Things else to fill
Chinks you please), and drinking only half a Pint of Wine with Water and
Small Beer a Day, useing all the House or Abroad Exercise you can, keeping
good Hours, and never applying [i.e., working] long at a Time, and for Drugs
only these Pills,

following with a prescription for a purging pill made of mercury and
ecphractic, another purging drug. Valerian was diuretic.[66]
    Richardson was "a staunch Epicure" and hated to exercise.[67] He tended
to overwork, especially at the end of the decade, when he wrote *Pamela*
while still working as a printer. Cheyne urged him to relax, eat and drink
less, and exercise. Like most of the doctor's patients, Richardson followed
this advice only intermittently, even though the doctor tried to tailor his
regimen to suit Richardson's tastes. Vomits were beneficial not only for
evacuation but also for the exercise they afforded.[68] Cheyne advised
Richardson to exercise upon the "chamber-horse" if he would not go out-
doors; he himself rode "an Hour every Morning" on it and found "great
Benefit" by it.[69] The chamber horse was a long board supported on each
end, with a chair in the middle that bounced up and down. Carol
Houlihan Flynn presents "The image of a plump Richardson, that senti-
mental Traveler of the imagination, jogging cautiously back and forth in a
motion designed to get precisely nowhere" as a symbol of the times, when
both early novelists such as Richardson and "writers against the spleen"
such as Cheyne "were searching for ways to come to terms with a mor-
tality becoming all too pressing in a secularized world."[70] As in his own
case, Cheyne tended both to Richardson's body and to his spirit.
    Richardson's symptoms ebbed and flowed, causing him considerable
distress and depression. He consulted other doctors, who prescribed
"nauseous and loathsome" drugs and such quackish devices as a "sweating
Machine for the Head."[71] "Get rid of Doctors and all the quacking Trade
as soon as you can. I find few of them that understands [*sic*] your Case,"
Cheyne wrote to Richardson in 1742, adding "I have tried all their

Medicines in my own Bacon, which is more instructing than any Thing can be known in anothers."[72] Cheyne again appealed to his patient not only as a physician but as a "sadly experienced" fellow sufferer. Richardson's preoccupation with his health categorizes him as a hypochondriac in the modern sense, and Cheyne's characterization of him as "a true genuine Hyppo" carried with it both meanings of the term.[73]

Most of all, Cheyne tried to divert Richardson's mind with a "hobby-horse" corresponding to the "chamber-horse" for his body.[74] He recommended games such as the popular quadrille and picquet, or reading "interesting Stories, Novels or Plays." Cheyne counted his own letters as diversions, although they contained mainly his instructions for Richardson interspersed with comments on theology and religion.[75] Theology and devotional works had calmed Cheyne's mind in his own crisis, and he firmly believed that they would also soothe the wounded spirits of his patients. He urged Richardson to compile a "Catalogue of Books for the Devout, the Tender, Valetudinarian, and Nervous" that would include devotional works but also "the most entertaining books of History Natural and Political," travel accounts, "Allegorical Histories, Adventures, and Novels that are Religious, Interesting, and Probable," poetry, and "Choice Plays, if any such, that recommend Virtue and Good Manners." J. Paul Hunter's characterization of most contemporary writing as religious in subject matter and didactic in intent well describes Cheyne's proposed catalogue.[76]

Yet the doctor recognized that to capture the public's attention, books could not be merely didactic, however uplifting their content. They needed also to entertain and, by the use of empirical, concrete examples, to engage the reader's sympathy in vicarious experience. The case histories in *The English Malady* had served these purposes, and the French novels Cheyne loved were full of incident, if at times indifferently didactic. Richardson's *Pamela; or, Virtue Rewarded*, which he began in 1739 and published in 1740, fulfilled many of Cheyne's criteria. The doctor noted that his catalogue "would come in very aptly with the Design of Pamela and might perhaps be called a Catalogue of her Library. . . . Such a Catalogue for England would be as useful as Bedlam is, and perhaps more so."[77]

Richardson's epistolary novel about the virtuous Pamela, who found love and upward mobility while retaining her virginity, was intended, the author declared in his preface, "to inculcate *religion* and *morality* in so easy and agreeable a manner, as shall render them equally *delightful* and *profitable* to the *younger* class of readers, as well as worthy of the attention of persons of *maturer* years and understandings."[78] The twentieth-century critic Ian Watt more succinctly claimed it held "the combined attractions of a sermon and a strip tease."[79] Modest and virtuous, Pamela was a model of Christian womanhood, rejecting the finery offered by Mr. B. in exchange for her virtue, and willing to live on a "poor pittance."[80] The fits she suffered when her chastity was threatened testified to her sensitive nature, as Cheyne had explained in *The English Malady*. Although she was merely a servant girl, this upper-class sensibility indicated that she was a suitable mate for Mr. B. Robert Erickson has argued that in the scenes of attempted rape, Pamela's fits in addition served to throw off her tormentors in the same way in which, by Cheyne's definition, hysteric fits "worked off . . . the offending Matter" in the body.[81]

Cheyne delighted in *Pamela*, "which entertained me and all mine." "It is really finely wrought up, and delicately imagined in a great many Incidents, and I never thought you Master of so much Wit and Gallantry as are couched in it," Cheyne told Richardson in a typically left-handed compliment.[82] Pope, he reported, "had read Pamela with great Approbation and Pleasure, and wanted a Night's Rest in finishing it, and says it will do more good than a great many of the new Sermons." Cheyne offered to introduce the two writers to each other.[83]

Pamela created an immediate sensation. Critics praised its anonymous author for the novel's morality and realism.[84] Six editions appeared by the end of 1741, as well as a number of parodies and imitations, including Henry Fielding's *Shamela*, which presented the heroine as a conniving tart. Richardson hastened to add a final two volumes, which described Pamela's life after her marriage to Mr. B. He asked several of his friends for advice, including Cheyne, who sent him a list of comments in August 1741. Cheyne advised Richardson to cut down on the scenes of "Fondling and Gallantry . . . clasping, kissing, stroking, hugging" as "not becoming the Character of Wisdom, Piety, and Conjugal Chastity." Pamela, he added, should convert her husband, "for Religion and Seriousness is more the Character of the Women than the Man"; and for this purpose, she should be acquainted with "the best, purest and strongest Writers in Morality and Christianity," offering to compile such a library for verisimilitude's sake. He also urged Richardson to provide more "interesting Incidents," noting that Richardson had begun the work with the "least interesting Parts." "A broken Leg, a disjointed Limb, a dangerous Fever. . . . The Death of a favourite Child, a sudden Conflagration," would provide opportunity for Christian behavior in the characters while gaining the reader's attention.[85]

Richardson defended his work in his reply. Display of "matrimonial Tenderness," he said, was necessary to "catch young and airy Minds," for he was conscious of criticisms that he had made Pamela "too much of a Methodist."[86] He did not respond to Cheyne's other comments, but in a letter to another friend who had also complained about the lack of incident in the new volumes, Richardson replied:

An excellent Physician was so good as to give me a Plan to break Legs and Arms and to fire Mansion Houses to create Distresses; But my Business and view was to aim at Instruction. . . . I hate so much the French Marvellous and all unnatural Machinery, and have so often been disgusted with that sort of Management . . . that I am contented to give up my Profit, if I can but Instruct.[87]

Richardson sent Cheyne copies of the volumes upon publication at the end of 1741; the doctor thought "the Moral extreemly good," but added that some unnamed "Critics" continued to complain about the lack of incident. With these friends and critics it is not surprising that Richardson continued to suffer from anxiety; a friend described him to Cheyne as "full puffed, short necked, and Head and Face bursting with Blood."[88] With characteristic tactlessness Cheyne asked Richardson to send him a copy of Fielding's *Joseph Andrews* "by the very first Coach," even though he feared correctly that it was written "in Ridicule of your Pamela." Upon reading it, Cheyne reported that "Fielding's wretched Performance . . . will entertain none but Porters or Watermen."[89]

Cheyne directed his own writings at a more elevated clientele, despite his comment to Thomas Wilson that "the highest and greatest . . . be extremely ignorant, corrupted, and vicious," and that the only hope for redemption lay among "the middling sort."[90] He wrote two books and several shorter pieces in this decade. These works revealed no new insights but reiterated the ideas expressed in the *Essay of Health and Long Life* and *The English Malady* to a waiting and appreciative audience.

Cheyne's obituary of his patient George Baillie of Jerviswood (1664–1738) appeared in the *Gentleman's Magazine* in 1738; Cheyne had asked Richardson to print in addition several copies "in a handsome legible Character" on "a Half Sheet of Imperial Paper" to be distributed in London, Oxford, Bath, and Scotland and sent to the editors of the *Weekly Miscellany* and *London Journal*.[91] Baillie was the scion of a noted Presbyterian family. His father had been implicated in the Rye House Plot and executed, whereupon George fled to Holland and entered the service of William of Orange. George Baillie had been a longtime Whig member of Parliament, not particularly noted for his piety. Cheyne mentioned this history only obliquely; the elder Baillie lost his life to "the Necessity of the Times," forcing the son by circumstance into the Orange camp. The doctor instead lauded Baillie as a model of the Christian gentleman. He claimed that Baillie had spent the last twelve years of his life in "constant Prayer, and uninterrupted Contemplation," having "passed through several States of Purification and Trial." Cheyne's purpose in the eulogy was to condemn "the present Degeneracy and Lapse of Human Nature, the present deep Corruption of the Age and this Nation."[92] He forcibly expressed the "new morality" of *Pamela,* and this dark view of contemporary humanity strongly colored his last works.

Astonished to be nearing seventy, Cheyne rushed to codify his legacy. He intended the *Essay on Regimen* and *The Natural Method* to be complementary works summarizing his theory and practice; the *Essay on Regimen,* he told Lady Huntingdon, contained "the substance and principles of all I know, or have learned by study or experience."[93] No longer fearing criticism, Cheyne freely expressed himself in both works, revealing the profound interconnections between his natural philosophy and his religion. Both books combined old and new wisdom, reaching back to his early sources of inspiration and gleaning new ideas from contemporary texts in both religion and natural philosophy.

The history of the composition of these works is tangled. As Cheyne's correspondence with Richardson suggests, he completed the *Essay on Regimen* with particular difficulty, continually revising and adding to it, knowing that this was his last chance to get it right. Cheyne had seemingly completed this book by the autumn of 1737, when he asked Richardson and Lord Bateman for their opinions of it. Yet in August 1739 Cheyne wrote, "I have been forced to make many Alterations and Additions [that] I must have another Revise," even though the book was already being printed.[94] The first essay was apparently inserted at the last minute before publication in 1740, since it is separately paginated. In 1738 Cheyne referred to his *Philosophical Amusements in Three Dissertations* (the final version of the *Essay on Regimen* contained six essays), and had apparently already composed *The Natural Method* as a companion volume, although it was not published until 1742. Early in 1739 both Lord Chesterfield and Pope's friend George Lyttleton read the *Essay* in manuscript; Chesterfield described its author as "sublimely mad."[95] Cheyne spent much effort negotiating with publishers and badgering Richardson about the quality of his printing: "I must beg your Pardon for the many Emendations and Corrections. . . . The Subject is abstracted, obscure and difficult; and if it be incorrectly printed, it will be unintelligible and intirely spoil the Sale." His longtime publisher George Strahan would not accept Cheyne's terms, and the doctor finally went with Charles Rivington instead.[96]

Cheyne correctly judged the difficulty of the *Essay on Regimen*, for it was not only abstract but also even more rambling in style than his earlier works, consuming much italic type. It was not intended for popular consumption, he wrote Lady Huntingdon, but for "learned and philosophical men"; therefore he dedicated it to her husband, fearing "impropriety" if he addressed it to her.[97] His dedication, dated 15 August 1739, delicately toed the line of the patron-client relationship. Lord Huntingdon was "a true friend to Christianity in general, [and] to the Church in particular." Several members of the earl's family, he added, had benefited from his care; and he added for good measure a laudatory sentence about Lady Betty.[98]

Despite his excuses to Lady Huntingdon, Cheyne intended his "Discourses" for a wide audience of his *Fellow-sufferers*," serving, like the works in his projected catalogue, as "suitable *Entertainments* and *Amusements*" for the valetudinarian. The juxtaposition of natural philosophy and religion was not inconsistent but essential; that Cheyne turned from salvation to the formation of salt crystals on the same page simply illustrated the essential unity of heaven and earth.[99] As Hélène Metzger has noted, Cheyne's goal was not merely to add to knowledge but to lead to action, to change lives.[100]

The doctor was not concerned with proof, for the truth of what he spoke was assumed. He would display "the *final Causes*, the *moral Consequences*," to disclose "the true *Reason* of the present *Darkness*, both in *Providence* and *Revelation*," which he defined as "the Difficulty of Recovering this *Purity* of *Heart* and *Life*." One key to this disclosure was the method of analogy, defined as "in *Things* only, what *Proportion* is in *Numbers*," a moral algebra capable of solving any problem in "*Nature, Providence, or Revelation*." True happiness consisted in following a middling way of life in diet, occupation, and manners, cultivating an "innocent, benevolent" character rather than the rancorous acrimony of the "*malicious, critical, spurious Free-thinker*."[101] Cheyne alternated straightforward exegesis of natural philosophy and matter theory with mystical excursions and revealed the full range of his sources, from Newton to Garden, Bourignon and Guyon, Wesley to Law.

Cheyne began with the conduct of daily life. In the title essay he reiterated the reasons for his "regimen of Diet." The most "pernicious Error in *Physic*," he expostulated, was that medicines were at all effective. Heredity and diet were the greatest determinants of constitution, that "*hydraulic Machin*." The solids of the body were fixed at birth; the fluids or "juices," on the other hand, were under the domain of medicine and could be changed, particularly by diet. The goal was to retain lively fluidity and fend off congealing death. Cheyne expounded on his favorite topics of water drinking, a vegetable diet, and the evils of alcohol, concluding with thirty-seven aphorisms.[102]

The first of the five "philosophical conjectures" that composed the rest of the volume summarized Cheyne's mature theory of matter, life, and creation. This theory centered on the continuum between matter and spirit, explained by the method of analogy presented in the 1715 *Philosophical Principles*. The original or *"primitive Animal Body"* at the Creation was composed of pure elements, "harmoniously combined, and elegantly ranged," but this had since the fall of Adam decomposed into "our present patch'd gross Bodies," in the same way that the earth was only the "putrified Carcase" of the original planet. These original pure elements were closer to spirit than to matter, and therefore the descent of the body toward matter and toward imperfection and disease was inextricably linked to the decline of faith and the spirit. As the body became more material, the earth became "really and literally a Prison or Gaol," from which only death provided relief. This, to Cheyne, proved the "perpetual *Analogy* running through all the works of God, *Natural, Moral,* and *Spiritual.*" By the use of analogy, Cheyne skirted around a claim that matter was in fact condensed spirit, a notion implicit in his narrative; in good Newtonian fashion, he declared we could know only appearances, while God's causes and methods remained hidden. The doctor admitted that some might find his description to be *"an imaginary and enthusiastical Romance."*[103]

Cheyne's second essay returned to his familiar dietary exhortations. Animal food, he said, following Arbuthnot's chemical analysis, contained more salt and oil and therefore its fibers were more strongly attractive, more "tenacious and glewy," and less healthy. God may indeed have sent us animal food "to punish, admonish, and correct us, by bodily Distempers."[104] Certainly the present deficiencies of the ruling classes, so *"Stunted"* in comparison to ancient Britons, were solely attributable to "the free and frequent Use of strong and *spirituous Liquors,* and rich and high Foods, with foreign *Cookery* . . . and living in great Towns, and using only Coaches and Chairs, and sedentary Employments and Diversions."[105] According to *Genesis,* prelapsarian humans were vegetarians; a 1747 vegetable cookbook was titled *Adam's Luxury, and Eve's Cookery.*[106] Eating animal food was therefore another sign of human descent since the fall. Moreover, animal foods increased passions and therefore led to vice; a vegetable diet was not only healthy but virtuous, a means of returning to a prelapsarian state of grace. Despite his gloomy view of the present state of humanity, hope remained; medicine and regimen could, to some extent, undo the effects of the fall. Repairing the body could help repair the spirit. Spiritual reform was in process, and humankind acted to "throw off this present *Load of Corruption, Deteriority,* and *Lapse,*" as in a fever crisis, to emerge purified. Even animals, Cheyne believed, were in the process of a "progressive Purification" that would lead to their membership in the kingdom of God "in some Degree or Order," and "produce at last *pure Love* and *naked Faith.*"[107] This "progressive purification" took place not in some millennial future but as he wrote. Following Boehme and Law, Cheyne believed heaven on earth was not only possible but underway.[108]

In his next essay Cheyne explained Newtonian matter theory in the form of propositions with medical corollaries, a summary of the *Philosophical Principles* of twenty-five years earlier. This short essay prefaced a lengthy discourse on "Spiritual Nature, the Human Spirit in Particular," which contained much of what Wesley might have called "Behmenish nonsense." Here Cheyne revealed just how far he had traveled from mainstream Anglicanism in his lifelong spiritual journey. He began by defining the willed acts of thinking, including perception, choice, and memory, as "rational spirits." All such finite spirits were merely emanations from the one divine spirit, "so that all *Spirits* are, in their own Natures, diminutive or infinitely small *Deities,* and necessarily . . . must partake of his . . . *Divine Nature.*" The properties of mind necessarily followed from God by the principle of analogy; intelligent creatures were "analogous *Infinitesimals* of the Deity."[109] Hélène Metzger rightly identified this view as Neoplatonic, but Cheyne's sources were not only Newton, as she believed, for Cheyne had imbibed Platonism since he first heard Scougal's lectures at Aberdeen half a century earlier. Now he returned to his earliest sources of inspiration. Ramsay's *Travels of Cyrus* had explicitly drawn upon the work of Ralph Cudworth, the Cambridge Platonist.[110]

Cheyne contrasted passive, inert matter to self-active, penetrable spirit, claiming that Newton, Huygens, Leibniz, and Fatio de Duillier all agreed that the cause of gravity was an infinitely rarefied substance that Cheyne defined as spirit. Both in religion and in natural philosophy the doctor found principles that would unify all sects. However, Cheyne went on to defend the doctrine of the Trinity against heresies that denied the tripartite character of God and therefore, to Cheyne, debased divine nature."[111] His defense included an elaborate network of threes in nature and faith.

His final essay on analogy began with propositions and corollaries on method but moved on once more from gravity to the analogous principle of reunion with God. The physical principle of repulsion also had its moral analogy, which Cheyne extended far beyond what Newton might have accepted. Moral repulsion away from God was the "Essence of *Misery* and *Hell*," and the resulting "*Unhappiness* and *Tortures*" of intelligent beings was "like the *Chill* and *Cold* in the *Comets*, while in the Parts of their *Orbit* most distant from the *Sun*." Indeed, Cheyne argued, it was more than possible that the planets were literally "the more tolerable *Jails*, *Prisons* and *Dungeons* of the several *Orders* and *Degrees* of *lapsed, probationary, sentient* and *intelligent* Beings."[112] While this was an old idea, Cheyne had most likely learned it from the *Témoignage d'un enfant de la verité & droiture de voyes de l'esprit* of the Huguenot refugee Charles Hector Saint-Georges de Marsay (1688–1753).[113] Cheyne praised Marsay in a letter to John Byrom in 1742: "I think him infinitely more plain, simple, universal, luminous, and unctuous than any I ever met with." Jean Orcibal has described Marsay's work as an Enlightenment adaptation of Bourignon, which replaces hell with "a process of gradual purification in the stars." Yet Cheyne was not entirely certain of Marsay's "new scriptural manifestations and discoveries about the states and glory of the invisible world and the future purification of lapsed intelligences, human and angelical," and his account, while similar, is more hellish than the "luminous" Marsay's.[114]

The volume ended not with this last essay but with a further forty pages of "Miscellaneous Observations on, and Explications of, the Preceding Discourses." Answering charges of enthusiasm, Cheyne readily admitted that he preferred enthusiasm to infidelity: "both *Enthusiasm* and *Infidelity*, I think, equally imply a wrong Head, some *nervous* Disorder, and want of *common Sense*; but both *Excesses* and *Defects* strongly evidence, that there is a just *Medium* wherein *true* Virtue and sole *Right* consist: And still of the *two* Evils, *Infidelity* and *Tepidity* is infinitly the worst. . . . *Pure Love* and *naked Faith* only," he concluded, were the keys to salvation."[115]

In the *Essay on Regimen* Cheyne revealed his innermost thoughts on the relationship between medicine, natural philosophy, and salvation; it was,

he said, "the best, most useful, and solid Work I ever composed." He
anxiously awaited its reception among London "Criticks and Connois-
seurs."[116] To his great disappointment, his message was poorly received.
Fielding criticized Cheyne's prolix style in his periodical the *Champion* in
1739–40.[117] Cheyne's "barbarous treatment" of the English tongue was
satirized in a 1740 pamphlet entitled *The Tryal of Colley Cibber*, in which the
author, a "T. Johnson," "arraigned" Cheyne for the "Philosophical,
Physical, and Theological Heresies" in the *Essay on Regimen*. Ironically
echoing Oliphant's description forty years earlier of Cheyne's "barbarous
perplext stile," "Johnson" wrote, "The M.D.&c. hath so mangled and
mauled it, that when I came to examine the Body, as it lay in Sheets in a
Bookseller's Shop, I found it an expiring heavy Lump, without the least
Appearance of Sense."[118]

In fact most copies of the book remained in sheets in Charles Rivington's shop, for the *Essay on Regimen* was the least successful of Cheyne's
mature works, and he was forced to buy back the unsold copies from
Rivington for eighty pounds. Characteristically, he blamed this failure
not on the difficulty of the text but on the rapaciousness of the booksellers, complaining that Leake had ordered three thousand copies
printed, far too many (though an indication of Cheyne's popularity).
Leake had added insult to injury by including Cheyne's book among the
titles he loaned by subscription through his Bath lending library, which,
as Cheyne noted, "will quite ruin it's [*sic*] Sale here."[119]

Meanwhile, Cheyne turned to the practical, writing "two Sheets" on
spas for Richardson's new edition of Daniel Defoe's *Tour thro' the Whole
Island of Great Britain*, published in 1742.[120] He is identified in the text only
as "a very eminent Physician," offering learned analyses of the waters of
Bath, Tunbridge, Cheltenham, and Bristol. Not surprisingly, Bath waters
received the highest approbation. In a lengthy chemical analysis, Cheyne
attributed their heat to a mixture of sulfur and iron, which resulted in a
"hot, milky, soft, salutiferous Beverage . . . far beyond any hot mineral
Waters for its Delicacy, and supportable, tho' comfortable Heat."
Although Bath water was "beneficial in almost all chronical Distempers,"
it needed to be joined to the proper regimen for the greatest efficacy: "if
a light Regimen, due Exercise, and good Hours, be joined with them,

they would truly work Wonders: but by the Neglect of these, their Efficacy is often lost, and their Credit brought into Question."[121]

Despite dark threats never to publish again after the failure of the *Essay on Regimen*, Cheyne was soon negotiating with Strahan for his next book, *The Natural Method*. Strahan agreed to pay off the debt to Rivington in exchange for the unsold sheets of the *Essay on Regimen*, and Cheyne finally agreed to £205 for both books, plus fifty free copies of the *Natural Method*. Cheyne was as usual anxious about the book, asking Richardson for his opinion on the text even as he printed it.[122]

The Natural Method of Cureing the Diseases of the Body, and the Disorders of the Mind Depending on the Body, published in 1742, comprised Cheyne's "last Labours in Medicin," as he wrote Chesterfield in his dedication. In it he summarized his therapeutic and preventive advice in the most general and comprehensible terms. Attentive readers, he noted, would find reminders of his earlier works. He would not include theory, already contained in the *Essay on Regimen*, and advice on particular symptoms and ailments remained the physician's duty, although much of the book was devoted to particular diseases and remedies. Individual experience, he added, was the patient's best guide. He summarized his therapeutic guidelines in four steps: evacuations; attenuating and unclogging medicines; astringents and strengtheners of the solids; and always diet, air, and exercise.[123] Cheyne envisaged his audience as those "whose Sufferings have soured the *false Pleasures* resulting from *sensual Appetites*, and who are at length willing to renounce *Luxury*, in order to lessen *Misery*." His regimen would not only lengthen life but "soften the *Terrors of Death*" by conducing to virtue.[124]

Despite his claim to eschew theory, the first part of the *Natural Method* reiterated the basics of Cheyne's physics and physiology, though in a more readable form than the *Essay on Regimen*. He discussed the structure of the nerves and their action, arguing once more that the nerves were put in motion by an immaterial spirit and not by a mythical nervous fluid. The structure of the nerves, however, was not well understood; we could only reason from its effects. Cheyne reiterated that "unnatural appetites" and other signs of nervous disorder signified not an imperfect God but the failure of our own free will.[125]

For the remainder of the book Cheyne elaborated on this favorite theme: "How it may be in other *Countries* and *Religions*, I will not say, but among us good *freethinking Protestants* of *England*, *Abstinence*, *Temperance* and *Moderation*, (at least in Eating) are so far from being thought a *Virtue*, or their Contrary a *Vice*, that it would seem, not eating the fattest and most delicious, and to the *Top*, were the only *Vice* and Disease known among us."[126] All chronic illness was a result of "Mal-regimen," he flatly declared. Dietary therapists argue similarly today, but for different reasons. According to Cheyne, inorganic salts, such as those contained in highly seasoned food, were responsible for contagion. Madness was caused by an obstruction of the nerves, occasioned by excess; the "*Christian Philosophy*," however, was a sovereign cure for such ailments. Excess particularly affected the "children of God," those natural governors of intellect and sensitivity, those who came to Bath seeking Cheyne's help. They must forgo sensual pleasures altogether. The "children of Men," the naturally governed, those of manual rather than mental occupations, were of more material composition and could indulge in material excess for a longer time without damage, though ultimately they too would pay a price.[127]

In the last section Cheyne had the final word against his critics, detailing a long list of particular medicines and cures for diseases from hypochondria to dropsy. He discussed his favorite medicinal therapies: bleeding, vomits ("in Diseases what Bombs are in besieging *Forts*"), and mercury.[128] Yet the *Natural Method* was not merely a rehash of familiar themes. Returning to his earliest influences to find new wisdom, he harked back to that "women's doctor" David Hamilton and addressed a section specifically to women.

In the first part of the *Natural Method* he had detailed his ideas on preformation first given in the 1705 *Philosophical Principles* and repeated in the *Essay on Regimen*. The spermatozooist or animalculist version of that theory claimed that the generative principle was contained in the sperm.[129] Cheyne believed that the sexes formed a continuum rather than a dichotomy, and he had previously only minimally distinguished between male and female ailments; hypochondria and hysteria were to him almost identical.[130] His long association with Lady Huntingdon, however, as well as his reconsideration of generation, led him also to reconsider female illnesses as specific to the sex. By his spermatozooist view, the male contribution to generation far outweighed that of the female, who contributed only nourishment to the embryo preformed in the male seed. But the importance of diet to Cheyne's general scheme meant that the female role in generation was nonetheless critical. The decline of "great and opulent Families" in Britain owed at least as much to difficult pregnancies and births as to the diseases of adults, and both causes could be placed at the door of luxury. The increase in difficult births, which made "*Man-Midwifery* so necessary and profitable a profession," was directly attributable to bad regimen. Being weaker in body, in part from the stresses of childbirth, women were naturally more susceptible to the effects of bad living and "their Sufferings not being so intense as Men's, and their being more used to Sickness they are rarely brought into the greatest Abstinence."[131] Moreover, the doctor complained to Richardson, women were also more susceptible to the blandishments of luxury. The combination was disastrous. Lady Huntingdon suffered continuous malaise throughout her many pregnancies and lost at least one child shortly after birth. Others fared far worse.[132]

Cheyne had attempted to resolve Lady Huntingdon's symptoms with regimen, but management of pregnancy could not in itself solve the deeper problem. Catherine Walpole and her sisterhood had taught Cheyne that the vapors and related symptoms began long before marriage. Contrary to popular wisdom, as well as experts including Astruc and Mandeville, Cheyne emphatically argued that "greensickness" and other such ills were not to be cured by marriage and childbirth. If anything, childbearing would exacerbate existing symptoms; he told Lady Huntingdon that her symptoms would be relieved only if she stopped having children. Ideally, she should have followed the proper regimen from an early age. Had Cheyne contemplated the case of Catherine Walpole twenty years on, he would have concluded that she died because he had been called in too late. A proper regimen would prevent symptoms from appearing in the first place.[133]

Cheyne advised women to take control of their bodies by maintaining their own health. This is far from the stereotypical image of the male doctor as exploiter of women. Cheyne saw his role as a guide and advisor

to his patients, male and female, who had in the end to make their own
decisions about health and sickness, salvation and damnation. He was a
prophet, not a god.

As Cheyne predicted, the *Natural Method* "was a more popular and
consequently a better Bookseller's Book" than the *Essay on Regimen*, and it
reached a third edition within the year and a fifth edition and a French
translation within a decade.[134] Practical advice, which Cheyne dispar-
agingly referred to as "more to the Vulgar Taste and Capacity" than the
theory of the *Essay on Regimen*, continued to be eagerly sought, and the
Natural Method boosted sales of the *Essay on Regimen* as well. Even
doctors liked it. Cheyne bragged to Richardson: "I have already high
Compliments from them and 3 Bishops."[135] Wesley called it "one of the
most ingenious books which I ever saw. But what epicure will ever regard
it? for 'the man talks against good eating and drinking'!"[136] That epicure
Chesterfield wrote to Cheyne, "I read with great pleasure your book. . . .
The physical part is extremely good, and the metaphysical part may be so
too, for what I know; and I believe it is; for, as I look upon all metaphysics to be guess-work of imagination, I know no imagination likelier
to hit upon the right than yours; and I will take your guess against any
other metaphysician's whatsoever."[137]

Cheyne lived for another year after the publication of the *Natural
Method*. He considered a revised edition of that book but planned no new
books other than the "Catalogue" he discussed with Richardson. He also
sponsored the translation into English of a French work he referred to in
fractured Franglais as "L'essence de le extract de la religion chretiene,"
but the translation was unsatisfactory and was never published.[138] Continuing his medical practice in Bath, he dispensed epistolary advice to
Richardson and no doubt to others with his usual prolixity. He read Law,
whose *Appeal to All That Doubt, or Disbelieve the Truth of the Gospel* he pronounced
"admirable and unanswerable," adding, "I wish all the Methodists might
get it by Heart." He also reread Boehme, sent to him by Richardson, as
well as popular novels and travel accounts.[139] His own health, carefully
monitored, continued "tolerably well," somewhat to his surprise, and he
enjoyed the companionship of his wife, "Pegg," and daughter Peggy. He
had reached seventy and more, outliving his contemporaries Arbuthnot,

Cockburn, Freind, and the Keill brothers. Now he prepared himself for a good death, the final proof of his theories.

The end came on 13 April 1743. Only a few weeks earlier he had warned Richardson about the "Spring Fermentation," which generally led to a "plunge."[140] Peggy Cheyne described to Richardson the doctor's own illness, which began with flulike symptoms in early April and quickly progressed. By the time Cheyne called his physicians—his Bath colleague David Hartley and his brother-in-law John Middleton—the end was near. He had already spoken to his family "of his Death as of a natural Consequence," and when it came, "his Death was easy, and his Senses remained to the last."[141] Here was the ideal of the good death, a gentle transition in the company of loved ones. Hartley later approvingly described the scene to Wesley: "He seemed quite loose from all below, till, without any struggle, either of body or mind, he calmly gave up his soul to God."[142] Cheyne was buried in the church at Weston, where his brother was vicar.

A contemporary obituary described Cheyne as "that learned Physician, sound Christian, deep Scholar, and warm Friend . . . those that best knew him most loved him." The *Gentleman's Magazine* compared him as a physician to Hippocrates and Sydenham, noting that "he might be mistaken in some Parts . . . but it plainly appears that he writ from the full Conviction of his Heart." The author recommended Cheyne's autobiography, part of which had been reprinted in the magazine a few years earlier. A number of panegyric poems on Cheyne appeared in the *London Weekly*. A Latin ode commended Cheyne's spirit to the Milky Way, an appropriate abode for one of his dietary predilections. A female patient bemoaned the loss of his serene smile in purple phrases, while a more sober poet praised his "unaffected Modesty, Sound Judgment, Manly Sense."[143] A month after Cheyne's death, John Byrom remembered the doctor with William Law, who recalled Cheyne's influence on him.[144]

In material terms, Cheyne left his family well provided for. He had written his will in 1738 and revised it a few weeks before he died to acknowledge the marriage of his daughter Frances. He left each of his daughters three thousand pounds, and his wife received the house in Monmouth Street, five hundred pounds, and an income of one hundred pounds a year. He left various legacies of one hundred or two hundred pounds to his sister, brother, and nephew as well as to a favorite servant, and paid for the apprenticeship of the son of another servant. The remainder of the estate was to be managed by the executors for Cheyne's son John until he reached the age of twenty-five. The executors, William Stewart, John Heylyn, William Cheyne, and George Middleton, were given two thousand pounds for administering the estate.[145] Margaret Cheyne, probably with her daughter Peggy, continued to live on Monmouth Street until her death in 1752. She was buried next to her husband.[146]

In the last decade of his life, Cheyne had achieved his goal of perfection of the life as well as of the work. He had successfully resolved the tensions and conflicts of his life, finding a middle way that balanced mind and body, matter and spirit, profession and family. He had few enemies and many friends. He ended his life a happy man.

CONCLUSION:
CHEYNE IN HIS TIME
AND OURS

Like his life, the doctor's intellectual legacy was paradoxical. Although he viewed his work as a unity, few shared his vision. His medical theories, the center of his enterprise, were soon outmoded. By 1784 *Biographia Britannica* stated that his "metaphysical notions . . . may . . . be thought fanciful and ill-grounded."[1] But his broader philosophy, as well as his views on religion and regimen, were widely disseminated and cited throughout the eighteenth century. Cheyne's emphasis on personal well-being fits well with the general shift toward moral philosophy exemplified in the work of Francis Hutcheson from the 1720s onward, in which worldly happiness is legitimated and sentiment is exalted. Yet in Cheyne's own moral outlook, worldly pleasure was ultimately to be rejected.

The new value of sentiment and sensibility was, of course, especially expressed in the novel. The popularity of Cheyne's doctrines among the literati has been well documented by David Shuttleton.[2] As John Mullan has stated, "In novels, the articulacy of sentiment is produced via a special kind of inward attention: a concern with feeling as articulated by the body. . . . Here sensibility is both private and public, and here, transcending the influences of speech, the novelist finds an eloquence which promises the true communication of feelings."[3] J. Paul Hunter's emphasis on the didacticism of the early novel also describes Cheyne's aims.[4] Cheyne's greatest achievement in terms of its impact on his time and ours was his definition of the sensitive character and the interaction between the body and the soul. While he was not the first to write on the "English malady," his work was, in the words of Roy Porter, "a remarkable ideological coup" that codified "the hyp" as the disease of the elite, the by-product (and not a wholly undesirable one) of English success.[5]

Literary scholars have exhaustively detailed the impact of "nerves" on the eighteenth-century British character.[6] Samuel Richardson's second novel, *Clarissa*, published in seven volumes in 1747–48, provides one example of how Cheyne's concept of sensibility was translated into the language of popular culture and the novel. The nervous crises of Pamela, Richardson's earlier heroine, occurred at critical moments in the novel, providing both a means of propelling the plot and evidence of her moral character. However, Pamela was essentially a woman of robust nerves, more yeoman than gentlewoman; she was, after all, a servant. In Clarissa, on the other hand, Richardson created a character of unambiguous sensitivity and, by extension, morality; the conflict between Clarissa and Lovelace is, unlike that of Pamela and Mr. B., clearly a struggle between good and evil. Pamela ends by marrying Mr. B., but Clarissa dies.

Raymond Stephanson and John Mullan, among others, have discussed the uses of Cheyne's ideas by Richardson.[7] Stephanson in particular has argued that eighteenth-century readers of *Clarissa*, familiar with Cheyne's ideas, would readily recognize Clarissa's physical decline as a necessary consequence of the psychological trauma of her rape by Lovelace. Mind and body, Cheyne had argued, were so intimately related that excessive feeling inevitably expressed itself in bodily ills. The sensitivity that made Clarissa such a highly moral and refined character also meant that her reaction to the events of the novel would be extreme. Stephanson argues that Lovelace himself comes to recognize that Clarissa's delicacy is in fact a desirable trait, one he needs to emulate; as a "man of feeling" himself, Richardson did not limit sensitivity to the female sex.[8]

At the same time, as Cheyne had always argued, the concept of sensibility fit into a larger framework of sin and redemption, and Richardson's novel epitomized Cheyne's model of moral entertainment. As Jina Politi has pointed out, *Clarissa* outlines a struggle between spirit and corrupt matter, in which the heroine's death indicates the triumph of the spirit.[9] Clarissa's case can also be seen an example of anorexia, a too-zealous following of the saintly models whose works Cheyne shared with Richardson. The poet Mary Chandler (1687–1744), author of the popular *Description of Bath* (1734), was said to have died of "extreme sensibility," exacerbated by her excessive devotion to an ascetic diet.[10]

Cheyne's ideas permeated the works of his friends. Andrew Michael Ramsay's posthumous *Philosophical Principles of Natural and Revealed Religion*, published by John Robertson in 1748, had more in common with Cheyne's ideas than merely the title. Although Ramsay's theology traveled even farther from the mainstream than Cheyne's, the two men shared views on the preexistence of souls, the importance of free will, and the present fallen state of humankind. Their Scottish backgrounds also bequeathed to them a passionate belief in toleration and in the evils of sectarianism.[11]

David Hartley's *Observations on Man* a year later also bore signs of Cheyne's influence. Hartley was close to Cheyne during his last years and acted as his physician. His work, printed by Richardson and sold by Leake, has been remembered since for its concept of the association of ideas. Hartley's physiology of "vibrations" in the nerves that caused association owed much to Cheyne's explanations of nervous activity.[12] However, Hartley's second volume, which contained "observations on the duty and expectations of mankind," has been less regarded; indeed, some commentators have had difficulty fitting this volume together with the "enlightened" naturalism of the first half.[13] The natural theology of this volume showed the influence both of Cheyne and of their mutual friend William Law. Hartley followed his discussion of God's attributes with a chapter on "the rule of life" that advised, with these mentors, that "sensible pleasure" could not be the guideline for life and that its pursuit needed to be regulated by "Benevolence, Piety, and the Moral Sense." He went on to give rules for diet and other daily activities.[14]

It is more difficult to trace a direct influence of Cheyne on physiological thinking. While strict mechanism had been largely rejected as an explanation of physiological phenomena by the mid-eighteenth century, no single system replaced it. As we have seen, the works of Nicholas and Bryan Robinson, Thomas Morgan, and Cheyne himself in the 1730s each offered differing "Newtonian" explanations for phenomena. Cheyne's contemporary Richard Mead rewrote his early works in the 1740s and early 1750s, exchanging the particles in motion of earlier Newtonian matter theory for the later Newtonian orthodoxy of ethers.

However, Cheyne's ideas on sensibility and mind-body interaction found special relevance to his fellow Scots centered at the Edinburgh

Medical School. In a well-known article, Christopher Lawrence has discussed the "preoccupation with the nervous system" that he found characteristic of Scottish medicine in the eighteenth century. Lawrence emphasizes
the culture of "improvement" (in opposition to the barbarism of the
Highlands) as an important component of this intellectual development.
Yet he does not mention any intellectual forebears; Robert Whytt, noted
as the first to emphasize the nervous system in Edinburgh medicine,
appears sui generis. But Cheyne was well known in Scotland—his election
to the Edinburgh College of Physicians in 1724 acknowledged his fame—
and Whytt's ideas bear more than a passing resemblance to his. Moreover,
in the context of building what Lawrence calls "a specifically *Scottish*
cultural identity," the work of Scots such as Cheyne and Pitcairne, as well
as Whytt's Edinburgh predecessor William Porterfield, takes on added
significance.[15]

    We have seen how Porterfield used Cheyne's case of Colonel Townshend
in the *English Malady* as evidence of the action of will in sustaining vital
functions.[16] John Wright has shown how Whytt built on and transformed
Porterfield's ideas about will and nervous function into his famous
concept of the "sentient principle," centered on the nerves. Roger French
has described this as an "immaterial principle intermediate between the
incoming disturbance of the nerves and the consequent outgoing, execu-
tive disturbance . . . compromised between the old mechanical theories
and the older animist ideas."[17] This resembles Cheyne's "active, self-motive,
self-determining Principle," analogous to gravity, described in the *Essay of
Health and Long Life* and subsequently elaborated upon. To both, feeling
becomes the central motivation for human action, and external environ-
mental influences such as diet and exercise determine the health of the
nervous system and therefore of both mind and body. Although Whytt
did not name Cheyne, their ideas are too similar to be merely coincidental.[18]

    Cheyne's notions of regimen were continually reread and rewritten
over the course of the eighteenth century. Some works, such as Bernard
Lynch's *Guide to Health* (1744), James Mackenzie's *History of Health* (1758),
and the numerous works of the Bath physician James Makittrick Adair
(1728–1802) attempted to update Cheyne's ideas for new generations of
elite patients. Others translated the concept of regimen for different

audiences, demonstrating that the gap between popular and elite medicine remained easily bridged. A few months after the doctor's death appeared a sixty-page pamphlet, *Dr. Cheyne's Account of Himself and of His Writings*, "faithfully extracted" from his works. It included extracts from his autobiography as well as his most pithy aphorisms and immediately went into a second edition.[19] In the next year appeared a poetic version, John Armstrong's *The Art of Preserving Health*.[20] John Wesley's *Primitive Physick*, first published in 1747, was a popular handbook of medicine designed for the use of literate working people; priced at one shilling, it was readily affordable. In the *Essay of Health and Long Life* Cheyne had emulated the seventeenth-century handbook tradition for a more upscale audience. Wesley reversed the process, appropriating the doctor's ideas for popular consumption. Wesley had already embraced Cheyne's dietary dicta, and these would prove to be central to the Methodist experience, for the body required discipline so that the spirit could fully unfold.[21]

Like Cheyne, Wesley viewed medicine as a means of repairing some of the damage wrought by the fall of Adam, when the original incorruptible body had become subject to pain and sickness. Wesley viewed his work as a return to an earlier, simpler empirical medicine that had since been complicated and corrupted by theory and science. He named the unlikely trio of Sydenham, Thomas Dover (known for his "powders"), and Cheyne as examples of a return to "primitive" medicine; Cheyne, he added, would have "countenanced the modern practice" less had he not feared to offend his colleagues.[22]

Although *Primitive Physick* was essentially a recipe book, with remedies for some three hundred diseases, Wesley also told his readers to "observe all the time the greatest exactness in your regimen or manner of living," including such favorite Cheynean advice as plain food, water drinking, exercise, and early bedtimes. To enforce his admonitions, Wesley added a list of "plain easy rules, briefly transcribed from Dr. Cheyne." These were comments from the *Essay of Health and Long Life* and *The Natural Method* presented in the form of aphorisms.[23]

Wesley's book was fabulously popular, with at least twenty editions during its author's lifetime.[24] Equally popular was William Buchan's *Domestic Medicine*, first published in 1769 and continually reprinted until

1913.[25] Buchan's intended audience, who paid six shillings in comparison to Wesley's one, occupied the social stratum between Wesley's literate workers and Cheyne's fashionable elite, comprising those upwardly mobile members of the "middling ranks" who aspired to Bath if they did not attain it. Buchan borrowed freely from Cheyne and other popular authors such as S. A. Tissot, whose *Avis au peuple sur la santé* appeared in 1761. Like Cheyne, Buchan castigated luxury as the origin of many ills and advocated the lifestyle of the yeoman as the best guarantor of health. In addition, the argument from design pervaded *Domestic Medicine*. However, important differences between Buchan's work and Cheyne's indicate the changes both in their audiences and in the state of medicine that had taken place in the half-century since the *Essay of Health and Long Life*. Buchan's work followed the *Natural Method* rather than the *Essay* in emphasizing specific diseases (though not specific remedies) rather than the "non-naturals," and his discussion of disease was in the language of infection rather than humors. Charles Rosenberg has emphasized in addition the secularism of Buchan's text, which takes a "cool and instrumental" stance toward religion in comparison to Cheyne's passionate engagement.[26]

Cheyne was a man of the Enlightenment, and not merely by the date of his birth. But his was not the Enlightenment of Voltaire and "écrasez l'infame," of relentless secularization. It was, however, the Enlightenment of sensibility and sociability, of the emergence of the "public sphere" and the reevaluation of women's roles, of Newtonian science and Edinburgh medicine. Cheyne's role in all of these intersecting areas must lead us to reappraise and complicate our concept of "Enlightenment" and how it is relevant to the United States in the late twentieth century, when many of our own ills and confusions are traced back to that age whose label seems increasingly ironic.

Cheyne speaks above all to our obsession with the body, the middle term in the triad of food, flesh, and spirit. As one who equated thinness with virtue, he seems a progenitor of our weight-conscious culture, the first of a long line of dietary reformers from Sylvester Graham to W. K. Kellogg to Nathan Pritikin. As Susan Bordo has noted, the idea of the body as a deceptive prison of the soul is an old one in Western philosophy.[27] As she points out, the body/spirit duality is frequently a gendered distinction, and this too is borne out in Cheyne's valuation of the feminine virtues of sensibility and sensitivity. To him, the feminine was obviously the more spiritual while at the same time the masculine was more intellectual; to both, therefore, the body is the enemy to be conquered, the animal lurking within. Although Cheyne did not discuss sex, it too is a ravenous appetite to be restrained.[28]

Yet, despite his admiration for anorexic medieval saints, Cheyne did not follow their route, nor did he recommend it. His long struggle to be thin was a struggle with his own sinful self, but he did not aspire to sainthood, only to the good life, that most enlightened of goals. While neither the doctor nor his audience was presumably of sufficient sanctity to survive a truly ascetic diet for long, Cheyne's passion for moderation was deeply felt. Religious and political extremism held no appeal; only the middle way promised a true equilibrium. In our present age of extremes, this emphasis on moderation is, I suggest, both timely and highly relevant.

NOTES

Introduction

1. Guerrini, "Newtonian Matter Theory, Chemistry, and Medicine, 1690–1713"; "James Keill, George Cheyne, and Newtonian Physiology, 1690–1740"; "The Tory Newtonians: Gregory, Pitcairne, and Their Circle"; "Archibald Pitcairne and Newtonian Medicine"; "Isaac Newton, George Cheyne, and the 'Principia Medicinae'"; "John Keill's *De operationum chymicarum ratione mechanica*"; "'A Club of Little Villains': Rhetoric, Professional Identity, and Medical Pamphlet Wars"; "Ether Madness: Newtonianism, Religion, and Insanity"; "Chemistry Teaching at Oxford and Cambridge, circa 1700."

2. De Maria, *Samuel Johnson*, 113; unfortunately this book appeared too late for me to incorporate its discussion of Cheyne.

3. *Gentleman's Magazine*, 1743, quoted in *Dr Cheyne's Account of Himself*, 34.

4. On the medical marketplace, see Cook, *Decline of Old Medical Regime*; Porter, *Health for Sale*.

5. Clark, *English Society*, esp. 216–324; on science and religion, see Brooke, *Science and Religion*. However, one needs to distinguish between religion and the established church.

6. Porter, *Mind-forg'd Manacles*; MacDonald, *Mystical Bedlam*; Scull, *The Most Solitary of Afflictions*.

7. Greenhill, *Life of George Cheyne, M.D.*

8. *Dictionary of National Biography*, s.v. "Cheyne, George."

9. *Biographia Britannica*, 2nd. ed., s.v. "Cheyne, George."

10. Brown, *Mechanical Philosophy and the "Animal Oeconomy."*

11. Viets, "George Cheyne"; King, "George Cheyne, Mirror of Eighteenth Century"; McCrae, "George Cheyne"; Siddall, "George Cheyne, M.D."; Riddell, "George Cheyne."

12. Porter, *Mind-forg'd Manacles*.

13. Henderson, *Mystics of the North-east*; Rousseau, "Mysticism and Millenarianism." It will become clear in the following chapters that I do not agree with Rousseau's interpretation of Cheyne.

14. Shuttleton, "My Own Crazy Carcase." Despite its title, this is not a full biography of Cheyne. I did not obtain a copy of this work until after the present book was completed, but I have tried to note significant aspects of Shuttleton's arguments.

15. Child, "Discourse and Practice"; Kramnick, "Cheyne and the Eighteenth-Century Body." I regret that B. J. Gibbons's *Gender in Mystical and Occult Thought* (Cambridge: Cambridge University Press, 1996) did not come to my attention until after this book was completed.

16. Stone, "Revival of Narrative," 10.

17. A good summary of these arguments is found in Harlan, "Intellectual History and the Return of Literature," 581–609, and the subsequent responses in that issue of the *American Historical Review*.

18. By using the term context I recognize that I place myself in a certain intellectual camp. See Spiegel, "History and Post-Modernism, IV"; Appleby, "One Good Turn Deserves Another"; LaCapra, "Rethinking Intellectual History."

19. A similar approach is described in more detail in Spiegel, "History and Post-Modernism." Rousseau emphasizes the interdisciplinary nature of Cheyne as a topic in "Mysticism and Millenarianism."

20. For an example of this approach, see Shapin and Schaffer, *Leviathan and the Air-Pump*.

21. Kleinman, *Patients and Healers*; Kleinman, *The Illness Narratives*.

22. Bynum, *Holy Feast and Holy Fast*.

23. On Bourignon, see especially van der Does, *Antoinette Bourignon*; on Guyon, see Balsama, "Madame Guyon, Heterodox"; Gondal, *Madame Guyon*.

24. On changing views of the female, see Mullan, "Hypochondria and Hysteria: Sensibility and the Physicians"; Castle, "The Female Thermometer"; Schiebinger, *The Mind Has No Sex?*; Laqueur, *Making Sex*; Moscucci, *The Science of Woman*; Tomaselli, "Reflections"; Tuana, *The Less Noble Sex*. On women and religion see among others Davis, "City Women and Religious Change"; Mack, *Visionary Women*. I explore this issue in greater detail in "The Hungry Soul," forthcoming.

25. MacDonald, *Mystical Bedlam*, 230; Scull, *The Most Solitary of Afflictions*.

26. Porter, *Mind-forg'd Manacles*.

27. See also Porter and Porter, *In Sickness and in Health*; Porter and Porter, *Patient's Progress*.

Chapter 1. A Soul in Crisis

1. Schwartz, *French Prophets*, 37–50; on Mason, see Hill, "John Mason"; on van Helmont, Coudert, "Forgotten Ways of Knowing," 83–99; on Lead, DNB s.v. "Leade, Jane." See also Rousseau, "Mysticism and Millenarianism," 87–89; Force, *William Whiston, Honest Newtonian*, ch. 4; Thomas, *Religion and the Decline of Magic*, 168–72; Hill, "Sir Isaac Newton and His Society," 268–71.

2. Walsh, "Origins of the Evangelical Revival," 140; see also Bennett, "King William III and the Episcopate," 104–31; and Holmes, "Science, Reason, and Religion in the Age of Newton," 164–71.

3. Ward, *The London Spy*, 10–12 and passim; Mandeville, *The Fable of the Bees*, 64. This first portion of *The Fable of the Bees*—"The Grumbling Hive"—first appeared in 1705.

4. Rupp, *Religion in England*, 72–76, 214–17, 295–98; Sykes, *Church and State*, ch. 1, pp. 1–40; Redwood, *Reason, Ridicule, and Religion*, 18–21; Jacob, *The Newtonians and the English Revolution*, 97–99; Holmes, "Science, Reason, and Religion in the Age of Newton"; Curtis and Speck, "The Societies for the Reformation of Manners."

5. Cheyne, *The English Malady*, 325; for his Edinburgh years, see chapter 2 below; Cheyne does not discuss these in his autobiography. For a fuller discussion of this work, see Guerrini, "Case History as Spiritual Autobiography." See also Barker-Benfield, *The Culture of Sensibility*, 6–15.

6. Mandeville, *Hypochondriack and Hysterick Diseases*, 40–41.

7. Cheyne, *English Malady*, 326; Cheyne later wrote to Samuel Richardson, "I never wrote a Book in my Life but I had a Fit of Illness after": Cheyne to Richardson, 7 July 1741, in Mullett, ed. *The Letters of Doctor George Cheyne to Samuel Richardson*, 69, hereafter cited as *Letters to Richardson*. See also Rousseau, "Mysticism and Millenarianism," 83. On his book, see chapter 3 below.

8. Cheyne, *English Malady*, 327; David Gregory may have been referring to Cheyne when he commented in the autumn of 1704 "He has been lately very ill, & is low in his circumstances": Hiscock, *David Gregory, Isaac Newton, and Their Circle*, 20, memorandum for 24 October 1704.

9. Cheyne, *English Malady*, 327.

10. Jackson, *Melancholia and Depression*, 139, 284.

11. Cheyne to Richardson, July 1742, *Letters to Richardson*, 104.

12. Jackson, *Melancholia and Depression*, 274–310; Porter, *Mind-forg'd Manacles*, 49–54; Veith, *Hysteria: The History of a Disease*; Fischer-Homberger, "Hypochondriasis"; Mullan, "Hypochondria and Hysteria"; Rousseau, "A Strange Pathology," 151–57.

13. Quoted in Jackson, *Melancholia and Depression*, 284.

14. Purcell, *Vapours, or Hysterick Fits*, 7–8, quoted in Porter, *Mind-forg'd Manacles*, 50–51.

15. Mandeville, *Hypochondriack and Hysterick Diseases*, 162.

16. Kleinman, *Distress and Disease*, 143–79.

17. See ch. 5 below.

18. Mandeville, *Hypochondriack and Hysterick Diseases*, 270.

19. The historiography of hysteria is immense. A good summary of medical opinion is Veith, *Hysteria*; a good introduction to recent scholarship is Gilman et al., *Hysteria beyond Freud*; Rousseau's discussion of Sydenham in the same volume is especially relevant, 138–45. See also Micale, "Hysteria and Its Historiography," 223–62, 319–51.

20. Astruc, *Diseases Incident to Women*, 287; on Hoffmann, see Jackson, *Melancholia and Depression*, 285.

21. Quoted in Jackson, *Melancholia and Depression*, 284.

22. Cheyne, *English Malady*, 327–28; Hiscock, *Gregory*, 23, memorandum dated 5 January 1705.

23. See Guerrini, "Case History as Spiritual Autobiography."

24. On "self-fashioning," see Greenblatt, *Renaissance Self-Fashioning*; Nussbaum, *Autobiographical Subject*. On Cornaro, see Flynn, *Body in Swift and Defoe*, 47–48.

25. Cheyne, *English Malady*, 327. Pitcairne had attributed melancholia to a sluggish circulation: *Elements of Physick*, 192–93, 288; see Jackson, "Melancholia in the Eighteenth Century," 300–301. Illness as a prelude to conversion in this period is noted by Schwartz, *French Prophets*, 217–19.

26. Cheyne, *English Malady*, 328.

27. Walton, *William Law*, xvii–xix.

28. Flynn, *Body in Swift and Defoe*, 7.

29. Cheyne, *English Malady*, 330–34.

30. See MacDonald, "Narrative, Identity, and Emotion," 59–61. On Cheyne's religious melancholy, see below and also Guerrini, "Newtonianism, Religion, and Insanity."

31. Flynn, *Body in Swift and Defoe*, 21.

32. Porter, "Medicine and Religion."

33. *John Craige's "Mathematical Principles of Christian Theology."* To cite Craig as a representative of millenarian beliefs, as do both Schwartz and Rousseau, is therefore somewhat misleading.

34. Cheyne, *English Malady*, 328. In my 1989 article "Isaac Newton, George Cheyne, and the *Principia medicinae*" I implied that Cheyne's "retirement" was to Bath; as I shall argue

below, I now believe that he did not go to Bath until 1706. In terms of contemporary therapy, the discharge effected by a seton would have relieved symptoms caused by excess fluid elsewhere in the body.

35. Daniel Defoe, *Conjugal Lewdness* (1727), quoted in Flynn, *Body in Swift and Defoe*, 45.

36. Cheyne, *English Malady*, 329–30.

37. Cheyne, *English Malady*, 330–31. The best description of the latitudinarian strain of thought remains Jacob, *Newtonians*.

38. Cheyne, *English Malady*, 331–32; Clarke, *Demonstration of the Being and Attributes of God* (1705), cited in Emerson, "Latitudinarianism and the English Deists," 27.

39. Burton, *Anatomy of Melancholy*, quoted in Jackson, *Melancholia*, 332–33. See also Rosen, "Enthusiasm," 412; MacDonald, *Mystical Bedlam*, 223–24; Porter, *Mind-forg'd Manacles*, 76–81.

40. Cheyne, *Essay of Health and Long Life*, 157.

41. Cheyne, *English Malady*, 331.

42. Ibid.

43. *DNB*, s.v. "Garden, George"; Hunter, *Royal Society and Its Fellows*, 58; see below, ch. 2.

44. "A Discourse Concerning the Modern Theory of Generation, by Dr. George Garden of Aberdeen," 474–83; Cheyne, *Philosophical Principles of Natural Religion*, 2:24–29. Garden's paper is discussed in Gasking, *Investigations into Generation*, 29–30.

45. Roger Emerson has pointed out to me that there was no standardized service anywhere in Scotland in 1704, and that a Presbyterian service in Aberdeen may simply have been one at which the reigning monarch—Queen Anne in 1704, a far more accept-able monarch than King Billy—was prayed for.

46. Henderson, *Mystics of the North-east*, 24, 33–34; Tayler and Tayler, *Jacobites*, 226–27; *DNB*, s.v. "Garden, George." James Garden did not acknowledge his deprivation and later sued for reinstatement, claiming to be covered by an act of oblivion.

47. See Henderson, *Mystics of the North-east*, and below. The Gardens' views were specifically condemned by the Church of Scotland from 1700 to 1736 and explicitly refuted during that period by professors of divinity in the Scottish universities.

48. For the following account, I have relied particularly upon Mullan, *Episcopacy in Scotland*; Henderson, *Burning Bush*; Buckroyd, *Church and State*; Snow, *Patrick Forbes*.

49. Many Scottish Episcopalians accepted the Calvinist notion of bishops as super-vising clerics rather than as heirs of the apostolic succession. By 1689, however, political polarization led Scots Episcopalians increasingly to adopt the more extreme divine-right views of the English nonjurors.

50. Garden acknowledged this succession with his biography of Forbes, still the main source for his life. This was published with Garden's edition of the works of Forbes's son John in 1703. The main modern source for Forbes's life is Snow, *Patrick Forbes.*

50. Editions of Thomas à Kempis were published in Scotland in 1678 and 1687.

51. G. D. Henderson, "The Aberdeen Doctors," in *Burning Bush,* 75–93.

52. See Henderson, *Mystics of the North-east,* 11–12; Selwyn, *John Forbes,* introduction; *Opera Johannis Forbesii;* according to Henderson, mss. of Forbes's *Spiritual Exercises* exist in Edinburgh and Aberdeen.

53. G. D. Henderson, "Henry Scougall," in *The Burning Bush,* 94–104; *DNB,* s.v. "Scougal, Henry."

54. *DNB,* s.v. "Scougal, Patrick." Patrick Scougal was uncle to John Cockburn, antagonist of George Garden (see below), and granduncle to the natural philosophers James and John Keill; see Guerrini, "Tory Newtonians," 305–6.

55. *The Works of Robert Leighton;* Stewart, *Life and Letters of Leighton; DNB,* s.v. "Leighton, Robert, 1611–1684"; the *DNB* author describes Leighton's "Rules and Instructions for a Holy Life" as "an ideal which perhaps tends too much towards mysticism and abstraction from the world."

56. Orcibal, "John Wesley and Continental Spirituality," 83–84.

57. On Leighton's mysticism see especially Stewart, *Life and Letters of Leighton,* 267–82.

58. [Scougal], *Life of God,* preface (not paginated). On Burnet's opinions see Buckroyd, *Church and State in Scotland.*

59. Scougal, *Life of God,* 3–5.

60. Henderson, *Burning Bush,* 99–101; on Scougal's course see also Shepherd, "Arts Curriculum at Aberdeen," 148, and chapter 2 below. On Scougal and Leighton, see also Emerson, "Science and Moral Philosophy," 11–16.

61. Leighton, *Works,* sermon 14, p. 417.

62. On Poiret, see Henderson, *Mystics of the North-east,* and sources for Bourignon listed below. Poiret began his career as a Cartesian and turned to mysticism after an illness. He wrote several theological works on Bourignon and later on Jeanne Guyon.

63. Bourignon and Poiret, *Antoinette Bourignon.* The most complete biographical source for Bourignon's life is van der Does, *Antoinette Bourignon,* which includes a very full bibliography of Bourignon's works. See also *Nouvelle biographie française,* s.v. "Bourignon" (which describes her as "*laid*" [ugly] and castigates her refusal to marry); Macewen, *Antoinette Bourignon, Quietist;* Reinach, *Cultes, mythes et religions,* 426–58; Irwin, "von

Schurman and Bourignon"; and especially de Baar, "Prophecy, Femininity, and Spiritual Leadership."

64. [Garden], *Apology for M. Antonia Bourignon*, 61.

65. Van der Does, *Bourignon*, 185; Irwin, "von Schurman and Bourignon," 303; on Jansenism see Sedgwick, *Jansenism in Seventeenth-Century France*, esp. ch. 8, pp. 193–207.

66. Bourignon, *Renovation*, 98–132 and passim.

67. Bourignon, *Renovation*, 29, 112; Irwin, "von Schurman and Bourignon," 306.

68. Bourignon, *Renovation*, 11.

69. Ibid., 27; italicized in text.

70. Ibid., 59.

71. Poiret's catalogue is reproduced in Walton, *William Law*, 129–87; Bynum, *Holy Feast and Holy Fast*. See also Curran, *Grace before Meals*, and ch. 5 below.

72. Macewen, *Bourignon*, 29; Bourignon, *Light of the World*, preface, xiv–xv.

73. On the Quaker definition, see Nussbaum, *Autobiographical Subject*, 165–67.

74. Bynum, *Jesus as Mother*.

75. Bourignon, *Renovation*, 59, 67. De Baar, "Prophecy, Femininity, and Spiritual Leadership," has noted that Bourignon's disguise was for practical reasons and was soon penetrated; but it also has a certain doctrinal resonance.

76. Castelli, "Pieties of the Body," 43–45.

77. For works, see van der Does, *Bourignon*, ch. 1, and Macewen, *Bourignon*, 6–11; for criticisms see van der Does, 49–52, and Macewen, 6–16.

78. Cockburn, *Bourignianism Detected*, preface, unpaginated. Bourignon had been accused of Quakerism in her lifetime, a charge she vigorously refuted on the grounds of her disagreement with the Quaker lifestyle. See *DNB*, s.v. "Cockburn, John, D.D. (1652–1729)."

79. Bourignon, *Light of the World*, preface, xiv–xv; Cockburn, *Bourignianism Detected*, 35, 40–41.

80. Quoted in Macewen, *Bourignon*, 10. For White, see Tayler and Tayler, *Jacobites*, 245. White was deposed from his parish in Maryculter in 1717.

81. Garden, *Apology*, 73, 77; J. Garden, *Comparative Theology*, 40.

82. Cheyne, *English Malady*, 331; cf. Garden, *Comparative Theology*, 37–38: "so the other means of Salvation that I have already named [having to do with renunciation of the body] do spring from a higher and far more Noble Principle than our Nature."

83. Scougal, *Life of God*, 16–18.

84. Cheyne, *English Malady*, 330–31.

85. McGee, "Conversion and Imitation," 35–36.

86. Henderson, *Mystics of the North-east*, passim. Pitsligo is discussed on pp. 44–46. Shuttleton, "My Own Crazy Carcase," details this circle exhaustively, but I remain unconvinced by his argument that Cheyne played a dominant role.

87. Shuttleton, "My Own Crazy Carcase," 62.

88. Henderson, *Mystics of the North-east*, 56–61, relates most of the scanty information available about Keith, whose letters to Lord Deskford are published in this volume. James Keith's father, John, replaced George Garden as minister at Old Machar in Aberdeen in 1684 when Garden moved to Saint Nicholas. See also Smith, *English-speaking Students*, 131 (he identifies the "Jacobus Kiets" of the Leiden records as James Keill, an identity Henderson disputes); Munk, *Roll*, vol. 2, s.v. "Keith, James."

89. Henderson, *Mystics of the North-east*, 59 and passim. Rousseau, "Mysticism and Millenarianism," states that correspondence of both Cheyne and Garden formerly existed at the Seafield residence at Cullen House (which he calls Culladen House). Henderson, who published the Cullen House correspondence between Keith and Deskford in *Mystics of the North-east*, does not mention any other letters; the Seafield Muniments at SRO (GD 248) do not, as far as I have ascertained, contain any Cheyne or Garden letters. However, Cullen House burned down in 1985, and any on-site archives were lost.

90. Henderson, *Mystics of the North-East*, 59; Keith's correspondence with Ockley is in British Library, Add. MSS 15, 911.

91. Cheyne to Ramsay, 29 November 1708, National Library of Scotland, Fettercairn MSS. Cheyne's letters to Ramsay will be discussed below.

92. Cheyne, *English Malady*, 334–44.

93. Henderson, *Mystics of the North-east*, 160 (Keith to Deskford, 5 July 1718); Keith added, "But I believe he must alter his mind," but Cheyne apparently stuck to his resolve, not returning to London until 1725 (see ch. 6). Cheyne, *English Malady*, 339. On Cheyne's medical practice, see ch. 5.

Chapter 2. The Education of a Newtonian

1. Cheyne, *English Malady*, 325. The spelling and pronunciation of Cheyne's name varies. Aberdonians inform me that the proper pronunciation is "Sheen," but spellings include Chein, Cheyn, Cheyney; the man signed himself most often Cheyne, and I have adopted the English pronunciation of "Cheyney."

2. Porter, *English Society*, 208–9; Flinn, *European Demographic System*, 16–17.

3. Smout, *History of the Scottish People*, 143–45.

4. Little has been written on the important topic of medical patronage. See Holmes, *Augustan England*, 166–235, and references in ch. 3, below.

5. Pitcairne to Sloane, 29 September 1701, in Johnston, ed., *Best of Our Owne: Letters of Archibald Pitcairne*, #16, p. 37 (hereafter cited as Pitcairne, *Corres.* #16:37).

6. Useful biographical accounts include: Shuttleton, "My Own Crazy Carcase"; Viets, "George Cheyne"; Bulloch, "Cheyne." Viets argues for a later date of birth based on baptismal records, but Bulloch notes that Cheyne was described as seventy-two when he died in 1743. Shuttleton argues for 1672 as the probable date of birth.

7. This account is drawn largely from Bulloch, "Cheyne," 394–96; Cheyne was also a kinsman of Charles Maitland, the inoculator (1668–1748). See Burnett, *Family of Burnett*, 133–40. Sir Thomas Burnet, M.D. (1638–1704), should not be confused with the half-dozen of his contemporaries bearing the same name, notably Thomas Burnet, D.D. (?1635–1715), author of the *Sacred Theory of the Earth* (1680), and Thomas Burnet, ejected regent at the University of Edinburgh in 1690. On kinship in the seventeenth century, see Cressy, "Kinship," and Stone, *Family, Sex and Marriage*, 123–42.

8. *List of Pollable Persons in the Shire of Aberdeen*, 2:222; Bulloch, "Cheyne," 395.

9. See below, ch. 3. Pitcairne, his patron, was the son of a minor laird and Edinburgh magistrate; John Arbuthnot, Richard Mead, and John Freind were all sons of clergymen; James Keill's father was a writer to the signet in Edinburgh, a position somewhat equivalent to a solicitor in England; William Cockburn was the younger son of a Scots baronet. For more detail, see Guerrini, "The Tory Newtonians." In that article I stated that the father of John and James Keill was a draper; in fact their mother, Sarah Cockburn, inherited the draper's business from her father. See *Roll of Edinburgh Burgesses*, 295.

10. Cheyne, *English Malady*, 330; Anderson, *Fasti maris*. 2:263; Rosner, *Medical Education*, 27–28.

11. Shepherd, "Arts Curriculum at Aberdeen," 149–51; the earliest notebook she examined dated to 1688. See also her "Philosophy and Science."

12. Shepherd, "Arts Curriculum at Aberdeen," 147–48; Henderson, "Henry Scougall," 99–100. Although Scougal died in 1678, Shepherd notes that his lectures continued to be delivered well into the 1690s, and lecture notes passed freely between King's and Marischal.

13. Anderson, *Fasti maris*. 2:39. His brother Alexander, who became a regent two years later, was a noted Jacobite.

14. Pitcairne to Colin Campbell, 1 October 1703, National Library of Scotland, MS 3440, f.20r (copy) in Pitcairne, *Corres.*, #18:38.

15. *Fasti aberdonenses*, 441. Bower resigned his post in 1717.

16. Ouston, "Patronage of Learning"; Emerson, "Sir Robert Sibbald"; Lenman, "Physicians and Politics," 74–79; Clive, "Scottish Renaissance"; Christie, "Scottish Scientific Community."

17. On the vast topic of science as culture, see Schaffer, "Natural Philosophy"; more recently, see Rossi, *Dark Abyss of Time*; Jacob, *Scientific Revolution*; Stewart, *Rise of Public Science*; Golinski, *Science as Public Culture*; Biagioli, *Galileo Courtier*; Markley, *Fallen Languages*; and a number of articles by Steven Shapin, particularly "Natural Philosophy and Politics" and "Problematic Identity." See also the suggestive essays in Hunt, *New Cultural History*.

18. Sibbald, *Memoirs*, 75–76; Ritchie, *Early Days*, 54–56; Grant, *Edinburgh* 1:217–19; see also Lenman, "Physicians and Politics," 75–77; *DNB*, s.v. "Sibbald, Robert"; and especially Emerson, "Sir Robert Sibbald," 43–46.

19. Biographical accounts of Pitcairne include Webster, *Dr Archibald Pitcairne*; *Biog. Brit.*, 1st ed., 5:3359–66; *DSB* 11:1–3; *DNB*, s.v. "Pitcairne, Archibald"; Ritchie, *Early Days*, 159–89; *Edin. Cat.*, 100.

20. The chief biographical source for David Gregory is Eagles, "Gregory"; See also Stewart, *Academic Gregories*; *Biog. Brit.* 4:2365–72; *DNB*, s.v. "Gregory, David"; *DSB* 5:520–22, 524–30; Anderson, *Univ. and King's*, 37; Anderson, *Fasti maris*. 2:219; Lawrence and Molland, "Gregory's Inaugural Lecture," 143–44. I have not seen Lawrence's Ph.D. thesis, "The Gregory Family: A Biographical and Bibliographical Study" (Aberdeen University, 1971). David Gregorie later adopted the Anglicized spelling of "Gregory" for his family name, and I shall use this spelling.

21. Eagles, "Gregory," 17–18; Bower, *Edinburgh* 1:306–7, 2:82; *Graduates of Edinburgh University*, 123. See also Stewart, *Gregories*, 53; Lawrence and Molland, "Gregory's Inaugural Lecture," 144.

22. Gregory to Newton, 9 June 1684, *Correspondence of Isaac Newton* 2:396 (hereafter cited as Newton, *Corres.*).

23. Pitcairne, *Assembly*, introduction, 12, citing Robert Chambers, *Domestic Annals of Scotland* (Edinburgh, 1861). Consultation in coffeehouses, if not in taverns, was commonplace in the early eighteenth century.

24. Wodrow, *Analecta* 2:255.

25. Pitcairne, *Corres.*, #11:25–32. Other mentions of drinking include #15, 21, 30, 54; Gregory to Arthur Charlett, 17 September 1692, Bodleian Library, Ballard MS. 24, f. 30.

26. Ferguson, *Scotland's Relations with England*, 178; on drink in general in the eighteenth century, see Porter, *English Society*, 33–34, 235; Porter, "Alcoholism in Georgian Britain."

27. Wodrow, *Analecta* 2:255, 3:520–22; MacPike, *Edmond Halley*, 265, citing an anecdote among the Rawlinson MSS in the Bodleian Library; Eagles, "Gregory," 35–45.

28. Robert Baillie, quoted in Smout, *History of the Scottish People*, 174.

29. Ferguson, *Scotland's Relations with England*, 146–50; Riley, *King William*, 1–10; Lenman, "Scottish Episcopal Clergy."

30. Riley, *King William*, 4; Lenman, "Scottish Episcopal Clergy," 39.

31. Stewart, *Gregories*, 55–58; Lenman, "Scottish Episcopal Clergy," 39–41; Lenman, *Jacobite Risings*, 25.

32. Pitcairne's 1689 Latin epitaph for Dundee, the hero of Killiecrankie, was translated by John Dryden and is printed, with extensive commentary, in Dryden, *Works* 11:113–15.

33. Pitcairne, *Assembly*, 83. The play was first published anonymously in 1722, but earlier manuscript copies exist: see Scottish Record Office, Episcopal Church of Scotland MSS, Jolly Kist CH12/16, #25, "The Assemblie" with the date 6 March 1696 written on the back.

34. Eagles, "Gregory," 41.

35. Pitcairne, *Assembly*, 65; Schaffer, "Glorious Revolution and Medicine," 173.

36. Lenman, *Jacobite Risings*, 23–27.

37. Pitcairne, *Assembly*, 84. On Pitcairne's politics, see also Cunningham, "Sydenham versus Newton," 90–91; Lenman, "Physicians and Politics," 78–79; Schaffer, "Glorious Revolution and Medicine," 172–77.

38. Cheyne, *Philosophical Principles* (1705), dedication. For Roxburghe, see *DNB*, s.v. "Ker, John"; Riley, *Union*, passim. John Ker was born between 1678 and 1680: see *Scots Peerage*, s.v. "Roxburghe," and ch. 3 below.

39. Viets, "Cheyne," 439, claims Burnet's influence, adding that Cheyne would have been resident at Floors Castle. Rousseau, "Mysticism and Millenarianism," 86–88, claims the influence of Garden and the existence of "Roxburgh House."

40. Shuttleton, "My Own Crazy Carcase," 40, speculates that Cheyne may have met the Ker brothers in Edinburgh through Pitcairne. This is certainly possible, but undocumented.

41. Yester papers, National Library of Scotland, MSS 7011–22. Most of the letters are dated from 1688 to 1695; Tweeddale, Lady Roxburghe's father, died in 1697.

42. Countess of Roxburghe to Marquis of Tweeddale: NLS, MS 7011, ff. 228 (7 October 1689), 242 (6 November 1689), 250 (19 November 1689), 257 (17 December 1689); MS 7012, ff. 1 (2 January 1690), 185 (14 October 1690), 191 (21 October 1690), 221 (29 November [1690]), 234 (30 December 1690); MS 7013, f. 3 (10 January 1691). James Gray is first mentioned in MS 7017, f. 100 (29 October 1694).

43. Smith, *English-speaking Students*, 113.

44. Lindeboom, "Pitcairne," 280–82; Cunningham, "Sydenham versus Newton," 90; Webster, *Pitcairne*, 17, 20; Christie, "Scottish Scientific Community," 124; see also Shirlaw, "Pitcairn and Newton."

45. Pitcairne to Gray, 23 September 1694, Pitcairne, *Corres.*, #3:18–19.

46. Cunningham, "Sydenham versus Newton," is the best account of the fever dispute up to 1695, and I have based my account largely upon his. See also Howie, "Sir Archibald Stevenson."

47. Cunningham, "Sydenham versus Newton," 82–83, 84–87; Pitcairne, *Curatione febrium*; Pitcairne, *Works*, 188–207.

48. Cunningham, "Sydenham versus Newton," 84. See also Schaffer, "Glorious Revolution and Medicine"; Cook, *Decline of Medical Regime*; Cook, "Sir John Colbatch."

49. Brown, "Animal Oeconomy," 120–21 and ch. 3; Frank, *Harvey*, ch. 11; Guerrini, "Ethics of Animal Experimentation."

50. Brown, "Acceptance of Iatromechanism"; on fever as the model for disease, see Risse, *Hospital Life*, 180–82.

51. Dewhurst, *Sydenham*, 60–63; Bates, "Sydenham and 'Method.'"

52. Howie, "Stevenson," 271–73.

53. Pitcairne, *Apollo staticus*, preface, n.p. See Stigler, "Apollo Mathematicus."

54. Howie, "Stevenson," 273–74; Craig, *Royal College of Edinburgh*, 410–17; the College declared an amnesty in 1703. For a list of the pamphlets up to 1695, see Cunningham, "Sydenham versus Newton," appendix; this list is continued to 1702 in Guerrini, "Club of Little Villains," at appendix, 238–40.

55. Smith, *English-speaking Students*, 173; Sedgwick, *House of Commons* 2:306–7; Howie, "Stevenson," 273–74; Craig, *History of the Royal College*, 408–12. Gregory mentions his marriage to Elizabeth Oliphant in a letter to Arthur Charlett, 26 September 1695, Bodleian Library, MS Ballard 24, f. 38; see Eagles, "Gregory," 59, who notes that "the Oliphants were generally a Jacobite family."

56. Oliphant, *Usefulness in Vomiting in Fevers*, preface. The death of Oliphant's patient is mentioned in C[hamberlen], *Vomits in Fevers*. For a more detailed account of the following, see Guerrini, "Club of Little Villains."

57. *Answer to the Pretended Refutation of Dr. Olyphant's Defence*. The National Library of Medicine catalog attributes this pamphlet to Oliphant, but this is certainly incorrect. For Johnston, see Smith, *English-speaking Students*, 129.

58. Charles Oliphant to William Bennet of Grubet, 11 December 1702, Ogilvy MSS, Scottish Record Office, GD 205/34/4.

59. *Privy Council of Scotland*, 178, 699; Foster, *Members of Parliament, Scotland*, 349 (he says Wallace was MP for Kintore, Elgin); *Register of the Society of Writers to Her Majesty's Signet*, 330 (states Wallace was MP for Burgh of Aberdeen); *Register of Marriages for the Parish of Edinburgh*, s.v. "Wallace, Hew."

60. Wallace was a heritor for Corstorphine, the Edinburgh district that included Ingliston.

61. [Oliphant], *Short Answer to Two Lybels Lately Published against D.O*, 4.

62. Cheyne, *Health and Long Life*, preface, vii.

63. Cheyne, *English Malady*, 325, 352.

64. Pitcairne to Gray, 27 November 1700, Pitcairne, *Corres.*, #13:34. Rousseau, "Mysticism and Millenarianism," 86n, claims that the *New Theory* was first written as a Latin dissertation, but I have found no evidence of this, although Pitcairne referred to it as "De febribus."

65. Pitcairne to Gregory, 20 February 1701, Pitcairne, *Corres.*, #14:35; Pitcairne to Gray, 27 February 1701, ibid., #15:36; although Pitcairne told Gray not to mention to Gregory that the copies of Cheyne's book had been sent to Strahan (since Gregory was brother-in-law and friend to Charles Oliphant), Pitcairne had in fact already told Gregory this. For Strahan, see Plomer, *Dictionary of Printers and Booksellers*, 282, and chs. 6 and 7 below. His address, the Golden Ball in Cornhill, was occasionally used as a mailing address by Gray; Pitcairne, *Corres.*, 36n.

66. Oliphant to Bennet, 11 December 1702, Ogilvy MSS, Scottish Record Office, GD 205/34/4. Other holders of Aberdeen M.D.s included William Cockburn and James Keill; see Guerrini, "The Tory Newtonians." On Arbuthnot, see ch. 3 below.

67. Anderson, *Univ.and King's*, 124.

68. Foucault, *Order of Things*, 56–57. On Newton's theology, see Force and Popkin, *Essays on Newton's Theology*, and further references below.

69. Gregory kept a medical notebook: British Library, Add. MS. 29, 243. "Praxeos Pitcarnianae specimina," University Library Edinburgh, Gregory MS. Dc.I.62, includes medical notes by both Gregory and Pitcairne. Gregory appears to have practiced medicine in Oxford and corresponded with Pitcairne about his cases: see Pitcairne, *Corres.*

70. On the English style of natural philosophy, see Shapin and Schaffer, *Leviathan and the Air-Pump*; Shapiro, *Probability and Certainty*, 72–73; Hunter, *Science and Society*; Webster, *Great Instauration*.

71. King [Shepherd], "Science and Philosophy." In a lengthy commentary on the Scots universities addressed to Newton, Gregory claimed that "the general contrivance of the universities in Scotland is the same with that of these in France": Gregory to Newton, 8 August 1691, Newton, *Corres.* 3:157–63, at 157.

72. Mead, *Influence*, 43–44 (referring to a case history from Pitcairne in which he stated that he was lodging with Gregory in 1687); Gregory to Newton, 2 September 1687, Newton, *Corres.* 2:484; Westfall, *Never at Rest*, 468–70. For the composition of the *Notae*, see Eagles, "Gregory," 26–34; the original is among the Gregory MSS at the Royal Society, and contemporary MS copies exist in Oxford, Edinburgh and Aberdeen; see also Wightman, "Gregory's Commentary."

73. Borelli, *De motu animalium* 2:53–54: "cum naturae operationes sint faciles, simplices et juxta leges mechanicis, quae sunt leges necessitatis." See Descartes, *Regulae ad directionem ingenii*, in *Oeuvres*. For a detailed account of the following, see Guerrini, "Varieties of Mechanical Medicine."

74. Markley, "Representing Order"; Markley, *Fallen Languages*, ch. 5; Guerrini, "The Tory Newtonians."

75. Pitcairne, *Works*, 135–63. All subsequent quotations from Pitcairne's works are from this translation, somewhat modified for clarity. I have compared it to the Latin: Pitcairne, *Elementa medicinae*. See King, *Philosophy of Medicine*, 109–18.

76. Pitcairne, *Works*, 135–36.

77. Westfall, *Never at Rest*, 504.

78. Lindeboom, "Pitcairne's Leyden Interlude," 278; Westfall, *Never at Rest*, 527–28; "De natura acidorum," Newton, *Corres.* 3:205–14. Pitcairne's visit and the transmission of his manuscript to Gregory is described in n. 1, 212–13. Gregory's copy is among the Gregory MSS at the Royal Society.

79. See Heimann and McGuire, "Newtonian Forces and Lockean Powers"; Schofield, "Evolutionary Taxonomy"; Shapin, "Of Gods and Kings"; Markley, *Fallen Languages*.

80. I explored this topic in my Ph.D. dissertation, "Newtonian Matter Theory."

81. Westfall, *Never at Rest*, 469–550, especially 524–29; Dobbs, *Newton's Alchemy*, 217–21.

82. Newton, "De natura acidorum," 205–6 (English), 209–10 (Latin); Dobbs, *Newton's Alchemy*, 217–21.

83. Newton, "De natura acidorum," 206–9, 210–12.

84. Gregory, Memorandum, Royal Society, Gregory MS 247, f. 80. The page is undated, but I do not know of another time Gregory was required to "emitt Theses." The works he refers to are Thomas Wharton, *Adenographia* (1656); William Cole, *De secretione*

animali cogitata (1674); François Bayle's *De usu lactis*, the third of his *Dissertationes medicae tres* (1670); the works of Thomas Willis; and Daniel Sennert, *Institutiones medicinae* (1611).

85. Gregory, "Tres lectiones cursoriae," University Library Aberdeen, MS 2206/8 ff. 1–48, at ff. 1–2. See Eagles, "Gregory," 156–62; Schaffer, "Glorious Revolution and Medicine," 174–75.

86. Pitcairne, *Works*, 11–12, 13. Cf. King, *Philosophy of Medicine*, 113–14. He prefers a weaker translation of *vires* as "phenomena" or "data" to contrast with the Galenic *causae* or essences.

87. Pitcairne, *Works*, 17.

88. Newton, *Philosophiae Naturalis Principia Mathematica* (hereafter cited as Newton, *Principia*) 2:552n: "Corpus omne in alterius cujuscunque generis corpus transformare posse, & qualitatum gradus omnes intermedios successive induere"; this passage was omitted in subsequent editions of the *Principia*. Newton, "De natura acidorum," 207, 211. See also McGuire, "Transmutation and Immutability."

89. Pitcairne, *Works*, 19; Schaffer, "Glorious Revolution and Medicine," 275; Brown, "Animal Oeconomy," 220–21.

90. Lindeboom, "Pitcairne's Leyden Interlude," 280–82.

91. Smith, *English-speaking Students*, 115–16. Three of the four respondents were Scots: George Hepburn twice and James Johnston. See Cunningham, "Sydenham versus Newton," 89; Schofield, *Mechanism and Materialism*, 49–50.

92. Pitcairne, *Works*, 43–44; Newton, *Principia* 2:550: "Causas rerum naturalium non plures admitti debere, quam quae & vera sint & earum Phaenomenis explicandis sufficiunt. Natura est enim simplex & rerum causis superfluis non luxuriat." In later editions, this appeared in slightly different form as "Regula I" of the "Regulae Philosophandi."

93. Pitcairne, *Works*, 56–57.

94. On mathematical knowledge, see Funkenstein, *Theology and the Scientific Imagination*, 32–35, 315–17; on the certainty of Newtonian science, Bechler, "Newtonian Historiography," 2–6 and passim.

95. Craig, *John Craige's "Mathematical Principles,"* Introduction, xvii.

96. Lindeboom, "Pitcairne," 279–80. On the lectures' publication, see Pitcairne, *Philosophical and Mathematical Elements of Physick*, preface, xi–xii. I have found three sets of manuscript student notes, dating from 1692 to 1713: George Hepburn, Leiden, 1693, Wellcome Institute for the History of Medicine, MS 3915; John Fullerton, 1713–14, Wellcome Institute, MS 2451; Josiah Holmes, 1712, University of British Columbia, Vancouver (not

seen). The notes I have seen correspond closely to the published lectures. Cf. Brown, "Animal Oeconomy," 233–34, who refers to these as the "Edinburgh lectures," dating them after Pitcairne's return from Leiden.

97. Pitcairne, *Elements*, 3–6.

98. Ibid., 8, 10–11, 20–21, 25.

99. Ibid., 30; Cunningham, "Sydenham versus Newton," 91; Harvey, *Circulation of the Blood*, 3. See also Hill, "Harvey and the Idea of Monarchy"; White, "Harvey and the Primacy of the Blood"; Straka, "Final Phase of Divine Right Theory in England."

100. Pitcairne, *Works*, 164–67.

101. Newton to Richard Bentley, 17 January 1692/3, Newton, *Corres.* 3:240.

102. Pitcairne to Robert Grey, 24–25 October 1694, Pitcairne, *Corres.*, #4:19–20; in a note dated 16 October 1695, Pitcairne asked Gregory "To endeavour to get Newton's papers about the mythologies; & Christian religion for me": Hiscock, *Gregory*, 3–4.

103. Newton, *Corres.* 3:338, 384; Westfall, "Newton's *Theologiae Gentilis Origines Philosophicae*"; see also Schaffer, "Glorious Revolution and Medicine," 176–77.

104. Westfall, "Newton's Theological Manuscripts"; Westfall, "Newton's *Theologiae Gentilis Origines Philosophicae*"; Westfall, *Never at Rest*, 344–56; Manuel, *Religion of Isaac Newton*; Manuel, *Isaac Newton, Historian*; Gregory's memoranda from his 1694 visit are reproduced in Newton, *Corres.*, 3; McGuire and Rattansi, "Newton and the 'Pipes of Pan'"; McGuire, "Force, Active Principles, and Newton's Invisible Realm."

105. Pitcairne, *Works*, 8–10, 12, 19. Cf. Schaffer, "Glorious Revolution and Medicine," 176–77.

106. Kuhn, "Mathematical versus Experimental Traditions."

107. Foucault, *Order of Things*, 55–57; Schaffer, "Natural Philosophy," 72–91; Cunningham, "How the Principia Got Its Name." See also Cantor, "Eighteenth-Century Problem"; Barbara Shapiro, "History and Natural History"; B. Shapiro, *Probability and Certainty*; Miller, "Valley of Darkness."

108. On the relationship between theology and natural philosophy, see especially Westfall, *Science and Religion*; Funkenstein, *Theology and the Scientific Imagination*. On the role of religion in society, see Holmes, "Religion and Party"; more generally, Geertz, "Religion as Cultural System" and "Ethos, World View, and Analysis." (See ch. 4 for further discussion.)

109. Westfall, "Newton's Theological Manuscripts"; Shapiro, "History and Natural History"; Funkenstein, *Theology and the Scientific Imagination*, 327–45; see also Force, *William Whiston*; Force and Popkin, *Essays on Newton's Theology*.

110. Holmes, "Religion and Party," 194–202.

111. Craig calculated that at least 1,454 years must pass before the Second Coming: Craig, *John Craige's Mathematical Principles*, 70.

Chapter 3. The Pursuit of Fame

1. Defoe, *Tour* (1971), 577; on London's growth, see George, *London Life*, 63–65; Stone, "Residential Development." On London's importance, see Wrigley, "Model of London's Importance," 44–45; Porter, *English Society*, 55–56; George, *London Life*, 109–41; Fisher, "Development of London."

2. Brown, *Amusements*, quoted in Varey, *Space*, 137.

3. Dickson, *Financial Revolution*, 3–14, 46–57; Wilson, *England's Apprenticeship*, part 2, passim, esp. 160–63, 206–25; Earle, *Making of the Middle Class*, 17–18; Defoe, *Tour* (1971), 306–7.

4. See Holmes, *British Politics in the Age of Anne*.

5. Lady Roxburghe's letters to Tweeddale are among the Yester MSS, National Library of Scotland, Edinburgh.

6. Ward, *London Spy*.

7. Cited in Earle, *Making of the Middle Class*, 18.

8. Wrigley, "Simple Model," 53–55; Earle, *Making of the Middle Class*, ch. 1–2, pp. 3–81; his phrase "petty capitalist" appears on p. 4.

9. McKendrick, "Consumer Revolution"; Brewer, "Commercialization and Politics."

10. See Stewart, "Public Lectures and Private Patronage"; Stewart, "Selling of Newton"; Stewart, *Rise of Public Science*.

11. [Macmichael], *Gold-Headed Cane*, 22; Earle, *Making of the Middle Class*, 72–73.

12. Clive, "Social Background of the Scottish Renaissance," 35–36; Ferguson, *Scotland's Relations with England*, 178; Clark, *Later Stuarts*, 281–85.

13. Smout, *History of the Scottish People*, 240; Stott, "Incorporation of Surgeons."

14. See Guerrini, "Tory Newtonians."

15. On the changing role of the college in the seventeenth century, see Cook, *Decline of the Old Medical Regime*; Cook, "Rose Case Reconsidered."

16. Cook, *Decline of Old Medical Regime*, 72–73, 77, 217–20.

17. Cook, *Decline of Old Medical Regime*, ch. 4, pp. 133–82; Brown, "Acceptance of Iatro-mechanism in England."

18. See Wear, "Medical Practice," 296–97; Trail, "Sydenham's Impact."

19. See Guerrini, "Newtonian Matter Theory," 122–28; Coleman, "Mechanical Philosophy and Hypothetical Physiology," 322–32; Zuckerman, "Dr. Richard Mead," and below.

20. Hamilton, *Diary*, introduction; on the displacement of midwives by physicians, see Donnison, *Midwives and Medical Men*.

21. Hamilton, *Diary*, 3, xxvi; Radcliffe quoted in Gregg, *Queen Anne*, 106.

22. The main biographical source for Arbuthnot remains Aitken, *Arbuthnot*. See also Beattie, *John Arbuthnot*; Steensma, *Dr. John Arbuthnot*; and Leslie Stephens's excellent article in *DNB*. Hans Freudenthal's article in *DSB* 1:208–9 completely ignores his medical career.

23. Arbuthnot to Charlett, 6 June 1696, quoted in Aitken, *Arbuthnot*, 17–18.

24. George Hamilton to Charlett, 14 September 1696, quoted in ibid., 19.

25. Pitcairne to [Alexander Monro, Provost of Old College, St. Andrews], 1 August 1696, in Pitcairne, *Corres.*, #7:22–23. The recipient is not identified by Johnston but is identified in the manuscript, National Library of Scotland, Delvine papers, MS 1393, f. 219.

26. Beattie, *Arbuthnot*, 208; on Woodward's work see Rudwick, *Meaning of Fossils*, 82–87.

27. This essay has also been attributed, equally plausibly, to John Keill and to Martin Strong.

28. Aitken, *Arbuthnot*, 24–26; For Gregory's plans see Gregory to Arthur Charlett, 11 August 1700, Bodleian Library, MS Ballard 24, f. 39.

29. Wanley to Charlett, 24 June 1698, quoted in Aitken, *Arbuthnot*, 24. Henry Aldrich, dean of Christ Church, was a powerful Oxford figure. Thomas Smith, a former Oxford don ejected for nonjuring in 1690, had been active in the Oxford Philosophical Society.

30. For biographical details, see Guerrini, "Tory Newtonians," 303–4; Cockburn, *Profluvia ventris*, preface, not paginated.

31. Harris, *Diseases of Infants*, dedication. A "Mr. Cockburne," possibly a relative of William Cockburn, acted as companion to the earl of Roxburghe on his European tour in 1695–96 (during the course of which he died): Countess of Roxburghe to Marquess of Tweeddale, 4 October 1695, Yester Papers, National Library of Scotland, MS 7019, f. 79r.

32. Cook, "Practical Medicine," 21.

33. Harris, *Diseases of Infants*, preface (not paginated), 5–6, 34–36; Harris believed that excessive acid caused most diseases in infants and cited Hippocrates to this effect; see Lonie, "Hippocrates the Iatromechanist." For a different interpretation see Cook, "Practical Medicine," 21–22.

34. Cockburn, *Sea Diseases*, 55–57, 73. This edition does not differ substantially from the first. See Brown, *Animal Oeconomy*, 242; Guerrini, "Newtonian Matter Theory," 104–5.

35. Cook, "Practical Medicine," 22–25; Keevil, *Medicine and the Navy* 2:286–92; *DNB*, s.v. "Cockburn, William"; Munk, *Roll* 1:507–9.

36. *DNB*, s.v. "Cockburn, William." See Cook, *Decline of Old Medical Regime*, 237–39; Brown, *Animal Oeconomy*, 239–49; Cook, "Practical Medicine," 24–25.

37. Frank, "Physician as Virtuoso"; Brown, *Animal Oeconomy*, 247–49.

38. Schaffer, "Natural Philosophy," 55–62, 72–75; Elias, "Scientific Hierarchies," 56–57; Mousnier, *Social Hierarchies*; on the definition of profession, see Freidson, *Professional Powers*; Freidson, *Profession of Medicine*.

39. Hunter, *Royal Society*, 25.

40. Elias, *Court Society*; Elias, "Scientific Hierarchies"; Mousnier, *Social Hierarchies*; Brewer, "Commercialization and Politics," 197–200; Stone, "Social Mobility"; on the social origins of Royal Society members see Hunter, *Royal Society*, 5–11; Hunter, *Establishing the New Science*; Mulligan and Mulligan, "Reconstructing Restoration Science." McClellan, *Science Reorganized*, unfortunately says little about this aspect of scientific societies.

41. Hunter, *Royal Society*, 6–8, rightly points out how London-centered Society membership was.

42. Espinasse, "Decline and Fall of Restoration Science"; Heilbron, *Royal Society*, 9–11; Westfall, *Never at Rest*, 627–29. See also Miller, "Into the Valley of Darkness."

43. Mulligan and Mulligan, "Reconstructing Restoration Science"; see also Hunter, "Problems and Pitfalls in Institutional History."

44. Hunter, *Royal Society*, 44–47; Heilbron, *Royal Society*, 12.

45. Quoted from the Council Minutes in Hunter, *Royal Society*, 46. See Westfall, *Never at Rest*, 627; Heilbron, *Royal Society*, 12–13.

46. Miller, "Valley of Darkness," 157–58; Shapin, "House of Experiment," 401; see also Hunter, *Science and Society*, ch. 2; Shapin and Schaffer, *Leviathan and the Air-Pump*; Dear, "Rhetoric and Authority."

47. Holmes and Speck, *Divided Society*, 66–68; an attempt to reimpose censorship in 1698 was thrown out of the House of Commons amid arguments for free speech. For some of the implications of this for medicine, see Guerrini, "Club of Little Villains."

48. Whiston, *Life of Dr. Samuel Clarke*, 5, referring to when he met Clarke in 1697.

49. Westfall, *Never at Rest*, 498–501, 560.

50. *Spectator* 1:88 (no. 21, 24 March 1711).

51. [Woodward], *Art of Getting into Practice in Physick*, 10.

52. "Proposals for the Advancement of the Royal Society," Royal Society MS DM 5.12, quoted in Hall, *Promoting Experimental Learning*, 20; this manuscript has been attributed to Robert Hooke, which would date it to ca. 1702: Hunter and Wood, "Towards Solomon's House," 62–63, 95–96.

53. Mandeville, *Hypochondriack and Hysterick Diseases*, 39–40.

54. Cheyne, *Acute and Slow Continu'd Fevers*, 3d ed., preface, not paginated. This edition is identical to the 1702 edition, although it claims to be a revision. For the role of this work in the fever dispute, see Guerrini, "A Club of Little Villains."

55. Cheyne, *New Theory*, preface.

56. Harris, *Lexicon Technicum*, vol. 1 (1704), cited in *OED*, s.v. "postulate."

57. On this distinction see Wear, "Continuity and Union."

58. Cheyne, *New Theory*, 37–47.

59. Ibid., 40–41, 42–44, 46, 61–64.

60. Ibid., 47–53.

61. Ibid., 103–5.

62. Ibid., 70–72.

63. Ibid., 124–29; for a critique of Pitcairne's (and Cheyne's) method of reasoning, see King, *Philosophy of Medicine*, 114–18.

64. Cheyne, *English Malady*, 325.

65. Roxburghe Papers, National Records Administration (Scotland), vol. 1100, bundle 1082. I am very grateful to Tristram Clarke of the Scottish Record Office for obtaining transcripts for me of the relevant items from this private collection. John and William Ker were born between about 1677 (their elder brother was born around 1676, since he was nineteen at his death in 1695) and 1682, when their father died. I have approximated John's date of birth at 1678 and William's at 1680. See *Scots Peerage*.

66. Pitcairne, *Corres.*, #21, 23, 24, 55; other correspondence is in the Ogilvy MSS, SRO. On Roxburghe as parton see below.

67. Their relationship is speculative. Pitcairne knew them both: see Pitcairne to William Jameson (the Roxburghe steward), 27 May 1705, SRO, Ogilvy MS GD205, 34/4/12; he sends greetings to Mr Gray, along with "talk in ye taverne yesternight."

68. [William Ker] to William Bennet of Grubet, n.d., Ogilvy MS GD 205/31/1/15, Scottish Record Office. The author has been identified by the cataloguer as Roxburghe, but from the context (including a reference to "Lord John"), Will Ker seems a more likely author.

69. See Guerrini, "Club of Little Villains," for a tentative chronology and a more detailed account of the following. Although Oliphant wrote his replies in the third person, there is no reason to doubt his authorship; he claims authorship of the *Short Answer to Two Lybels* in his December 1702 letter to Bennet. Johnston had been a student of Pitcairne in

Edinburgh and respondent to one of Pitcairne's *exercitio gratia* dissertations; see ch. 1 above, and Smith, *English-speaking Students*, 130.

70. [Oliphant], *Refutation of the Short Answer to the Examination of Dr. Pitcairn's Dissertations*, 14, 19.

71. See Guerrini, "Tory Newtonians"; Thackray, "Business of Experimental Philosophy."

72. *Biographia Britannica* (1757), s.v. "Gregory, David"; Gregory, *Astronomiae physicae et geometricae elementa*.

73. On Keill's lectures, see Guerrini and Shackelford, "John Keill's *De operationum*."

74. See *DNB*, s.v. "Lister, Martin"; *DSB* 8:415–17. Letters from Pitcairne to Lister are among the Lister MSS in the Bodleian Library, Oxford. (MS Lister 3, 36).

75. [Martin Lister], "A Letter from Dr Martin Lister, F.R.S. to Dr Tancred Robinson, F.R.S. concerning pouder'd Blues passing the lacteal Veins, &c," *Philosophical Transactions* 22 (1701): 819–20. Lister's letter was dated 2 May 1701; the issue of the *Transactions* bore the cover date of March–April 1701 but was in fact several months behind that date.

76. Ibid.; the passages to which he refers are Cheyne, *New Theory*, 78–79, 44.

77. Frank, *Harvey and the Oxford Physiologists*, ch. 11; Guerrini, "Ethics of Animal Experimentation." On sites of experiment see Shapin, "House of Experiment."

78. Brown, *Animal Oeconomy*, 253–55; *DNB*, s.v. "Lister"; Jeffrey Carr in *DSB* 8:417 calls Lister's last work, *Dissertatio de humoribus* (1709), "extremely speculative, containing little observation or experiment," and describes Lister as "unsympathetic" to iatromathematics.

79. Rousseau, "Mysticism and Millenarianism," 95–100; Viets, "George Cheyne," 443–44; Bowles, "Physical, Human, and Divine Attraction." The publication history of the *New Theory* is tangled; see bibliography. The 1722 edition, called the third, advertised extensive revisions on the title page but noted on a page before the preface that the author "being very much engaged" had not in fact revised the text. The 1722 text is identical to the second, 1702 edition.

80. Cheyne, *New Theory*, 1–3. For further analysis of the concept of gentlemanliness in this context, see Guerrini, "Club of Little Villains."

81. Brown, *Animal Oeconomy*, 246–47; these bridges were, he says, gradually rebuilt after 1703. See also Cook, *Decline of the Old Medical Regime*, 215, 251.

82. Cheyne, *New Theory*, 7; he seems never to have read deeply in ancient philosophy and unlike many of his contemporaries does not often cite ancient precedents.

83. Cheyne, *New Theory*, 7–8; see Stevenson, "New Diseases."

84. Cheyne, *New Theory*, 21–7.

85. Ibid., 23–25.

86. Ibid., 32–35.

87. See Guerrini, "Club of Little Villains," for detail.

88. Oliphant, *Refutation of the Short Answer*, 14–16.

89. Cheyne, *Essay*, 36.

90. Cheyne, *Remarks*, preface, n.p. Cheyne's use of "ingenious" here may mean simply "intelligent" or even "honest" rather than "clever": see *OED*, s.v. "ingenious."

91. Cheyne, *Remarks*, 2. Cf. the discussion of the Boyle lectures in Jacob, *Newtonians*.

92. Cheyne, *Remarks*, 4–9, 13, 19.

93. Cook, *Decline of Old Medical Regime*, "Conclusion," 254–63.

94. Cheyne, *Remarks*, 4. On the medical marketplace, see also Porter, *Health for Sale*, ch. 2.

95. For biographical sources, see above, n. 19. Mead practiced out of the house of his father, Matthew, one of the best-known dissenting ministers in London. The elder Mead had been implicated in the Rye House Plot in 1683. Stepney was a center of dissent.

96. Mead, *Mechanical Account of Poisons*, preface, not paginated.

97. The author of the article on Mead in *Biog. Brit.* 5 (1750): 3080, n. G notes that Mead's "talents lay neither to mathematicks nor mathematical philosophy."

99. Mead, *Mechanical Account*, 13–14.

99. Ibid., 13; Newton, "De natura acidorum," *Corres.*, 3:203–9.

100. Mead, *Mechanical Account*, 65–66.

101. Morland, "Dr. Mead's *Mechanical Account of Poisons*." Also in this issue was a letter from Joseph Morland to Mead on secretion and an abstract by Mead of a letter from Bonomo to Redi on mites.

102. On Newton's "young men" see Manuel, *Portrait*, ch. 13. Gregory's dislike of Cheyne was no doubt based at least in part on the latter's rivalry with the Keills.

103. William Cockburn to Hans Sloane, 8 March 1702/3, BL Sloane MS 4039 f. 94.

104. Craig, "Specimen methodi generalis," 1346. The Latin reads, "a te promota sit in Libro tuo, quem D. Archibaldo Pitcarnio Patriae nostrae & saeculi, hujus Ornamento inscripsisti."

105. Hiscock, *Gregory*, 13–14; Westfall, *Never at Rest*, 514–18, 638–39. The most complete account of the following is in Hall, *Philosophers at War*, 130–39.

106. Gregory's copy of *Fluxionem methodus inversa* is in the library of Christ Church, Oxford. Cheyne's letter to Gregory is pasted to the inside front cover: Cheyne to Gregory, 20 January 1702[/3?], reprinted in Hiscock, *Gregory*, appendix, 43–44.

107. Westfall, *Never at Rest*, 639.

108. Hall, *Philosophers at War*, 135.

109. Pitcairne to Colin Campbell, 1 October 1703, Pitcairne, *Corres.*, #18:39.

110. Hall, *Philosophers at War*, 132–34, 139; letter in Hiscock; this incident is also discussed in Shuttleton, "My Own Crazy Carcase," 28–30.

111. Pitcairne to Colin Campbell, 1 October 1703, Pitcairne, *Corres.*, #18:38–39; Thackray, "Business of Experimental Philosophy," 155–59.

112. Hall, *Philosophers at War*, 131.

113. Cheyne to Sloane, 28 May 1703, BL Sloane MSS 4039, f. 135; Hiscock, *Gregory*, 15 (1 March 1703/4). I do not know if Cheyne's request was a common one; he considered it his privilege as FRS.

114. De Moivre, *Animadversiones*, preface, not paginated.

115. Isaac Newton, *Opticks* (4th ed., 1730; rpt. New York: Dover, 1952), cxxii; Westfall, *Never at Rest*, 639.

116. Hiscock, *Gregory*, 17.

117. Cheyne, *Rudimentorum methodi*, 2; "Praefatio" (not paginated). My translation. The title on the first page of text may be translated "Response to de Moivre's Skirmishes" ("Responsio ad velitationes Ab. De Moivre"); Cheyne demonstrated the elegance of his own style by preserving the military metaphor throughout his text.

118. Cheyne, *Health and Long Life*, iv–v. He had similarly referred to "vain and airy fancies" in the preface to his response to de Moivre: *Rudimentorum*, "Praefatio."

119. Westfall, *Never at Rest*, 639.

Chapter 4. Philosophical Principles

1. David Gregory, Memorandum, Christ Church, Oxford, Gregory MS 346, f. 101: "Dr Cheyn librum scribit de existentia Dei ost[end]enda de Operibus ejus. Edidit, 10 Febr 1703/4, Addenda et Adnotanda (verius Emendanda) ad Fluxionum Librum." See Bentley, *Eight Boyle Lectures*, originally published 1692–93; Clarke, *Demonstration*.

2. Rousseau, "Mysticism and Millenarianism," 86, 90. Rousseau argues that "the Newtonians disapproved" of Cheyne's writings (without specifying who "the Newtonians" were) and that this disapproval "eliminated Cheyne from consideration as a future Boyle lecturer." Since Cheyne was not a clergyman, he was never in any case eligible to be a Boyle lecturer.

3. Craig, *John Craige's Mathematical Principles*, 83.

4. Cheyne, *Philosophical Principles* (1705), preface (not paginated); Hiscock, *David Gregory*, 24–25 (27 March 1705). Gregory's copy survives at Christ Church, Oxford. His

list of errata was included in the published copies. Both Theodore Brown (*DSB* 3:244) and Geoffrey Bowles ("Physical, Human and Divine Attraction," 477, n. 17) have misread Gregory's comment on this. They believe he referred to the *Fluxionem*, but from the context and the date the work is obviously the *Philosophical Principles*, as Hiscock pointed out.

5. Bentley, *Confutation of Atheism*, parts 1–3 (1692), in *Eight Boyle Lectures*.

6. Flynn, *Body in Swift and Defoe*, 15, 21.

7. Cheyne, *Philosophical Principles* (1705), dedication.

8. On this point see Shuttleton, "My Own Crazy Carcase," 42–43.

9. Cheyne, *Philosophical Principles* (1705), dedication. Cf. Viets, "George Cheyne," 439, who dated these "discourses" to 1690 (see ch. 2 above)—a dating repeated by most subsequent authors, including myself: Guerrini, "Newton, Cheyne, and the 'Principia medicinae,'" in *Medical Revolution*, 234. The quoted passage is from Hiscock, *Gregory*, 21.

10. Cheyne, *Philosophical Principles* (1705), dedication. The *Oracles of Reason* referred to the deist Charles Blount.

11. Cheyne, *English Malady*, 224–25.

12. Cheyne, *Philosophical Principles* (1705), part 1, pp. 6, 47 (parts 1, 2–3, and 4 are paginated separately). Newton distinguished between laws of creation and laws of nature in a letter to Thomas Burnet (of *Sacred Theory* fame), January 1680/81, Newton, *Corres.* 2:331. On Newton's post-1700 views of gravity, see Dobbs, *Janus Faces*. The relevant Boyle lectures are: Bentley, *Confutation of Atheism*, part 2 (1693) and part 3 (1693), both reprinted in *Eight Boyle Lectures*; Clarke, *Demonstration*. On Clarke, see Stewart, "Clarke, Newtonianism, and Factions." See also Metzger, *Attraction universelle*, especially part 3.

13. Cheyne, *Philosophical Principles* (1705) 1:91, 100–104.

14. See McGuire, "Atoms and the 'Analogy of Nature,'" especially 35–36. McGuire suggests that Cheyne only developed these ideas on analogy in the 1715 edition of the *Philosophical Principles*.

15. Cheyne, *Philosophical Principles* (1705) 1:110–17; cf. Newton, *Principia* 1:329 (book 1, prop. 90).

16. Cheyne, *Philosophical Principles* (1705) 1:3, 46–53, 60–80, 2:19. Cf Bentley, *Confutation*, part 1 (1692), the sixth Boyle lecture, in *Eight Boyle Lectures*. See Schaffer, "Newtonian Cosmology," 185–90.

17. Cheyne, *Philosophical Principles* (1705) 1:95–97.

18. Ibid., part 2, p. 50 and passim.

19. Schwartz, *French Prophets*, 235; Schaffer, "Halley's Atheism"; Kubrin, "Newton."

20. Cheyne, *Philosophical Principles* (1705) 2:98. Cf. Thackray, "Matter in a Nut-shell."

21. Cheyne, *Philosophical Principles* (1705) 2:40–70. This argument had earlier been made by Sir Matthew Hale in his *Primitive Origination of Mankind* (1667; see Rossi, *Dark Abyss of Time*, 32–33), and may be of even earlier provenance; see also Tuveson, *Millennium and Utopia*, 126–28.

22. Clarke, *Being and Attributes*, quoted in Tuveson, *Millennium and Utopia*, 127–28; Jacob, *Newtonians*, 190–200.

23. Cheyne, *Philosophical Principles* (1705) 2:22–23, 28–29. Bowles, "Place of Newtonian Explanation," 224, n. 1.

24. Cheyne, *Philosophical Principles* (1705) 3:74–76, 208–10. John Toland's *Letter to Serena*, a book such as Cheyne described, had appeared in 1704.

25. Shuttleton, "My Own Crazy Carcase," 36–38. Royal Society, MS 82, f.14v, dated Ash Wednesday 1713/14. This commentary will be further discussed below.

26. See Arber, "Analogy"; Hesse, *Forces and Fields*; Ritterbush, *Overtures to Biology*; Bono, "Science, Discourse, and Literature."

27. On this topic, see particularly McGuire, "Atoms and the 'Analogy of Nature.'" On the *Philosophical Principles*, see also Metzger, *Attraction universelle*, 140–53; her discussion mostly concerns the 1715 edition, for which see below. See also Bowles, "Physical, Human, and Divine Attraction," 481–82; Rousseau, "Mysticism and Millenarianism," 90–92. For Pitcairne, see above, ch. 2.

28. Hiscock, *Gregory*, 23, 25. Pitcairne told Colin Campbell in April 1705 that Cheyne's *Philosophical Principles* was "daylie expected" (Pitcairne to Campbell, 2 April 1705, Pitcairne, *Corres.*, #22:41); Gregory received the errata page, showing corrections he had suggested, on 15 May, and the book was in print by early June.

29. Campbell papers, Edinburgh University Library.

30. Westfall, *Never at Rest*, 639n, citing Royal Society, Journal Book (Copy) 10, 107. Gregory's comment appeared in Hiscock, *Gregory*, 25, memorandum dated ?3 June 1705.

31. Jonathan Barry, "Piety and the Patient," 167–68 and n. Cheyne's will in the PRO (727/193) lists his children. John was not yet twenty-five when Cheyne wrote his will in 1738; Foster, *Alumni Oxon.*, lists John Cheyne as fourteen when he matriculated in 1731. For Patrick Middleton, see *DNB*; he died in Bristol. On George Middleton see Anderson, *Univ. and King's*, 27; Henderson, *Mystics of the North-east*, 26 and passim. Schwartz, *French Prophets*, 157, 301, confuses George Middleton with his son or nephew Thomas Middleton, a follower of the French Prophets. Cheyne frequently mentioned his brothers-in-law in his correspondence with Richardson: see *Letters to Richardson*, passim.

32. Henderson, *Mystics of the North-east*, passim; 129 n. 10 refers to a group of books Cheyne received around 1710, including works of Poiret and Garden's *Apology for M. A. Bourignon*.

33. Cheyne to Ramsay, 5 June 1708, National Library of Scotland, Fettercairn MSS.

34. Ibid., Schwartz, *French Prophets*, 157, quoting National Library of Scotland, MS/493/73 [*sic*], letter of 21 May 1709 (recipient not named).

35. Henderson, *Mystics of the North-east*, 199–208 (James Cuninghame to George Garden, n.d. [ca. November 1709]); on *Fides et ratio collatae*, see Hobhouse, *Selected Mystical Writings*, appendix 1, pp. 381–83. Poiret published the anonymous *Fides et ratio* in 1708; an English translation appeared in 1713.

36. Cheyne to Ramsay, 1 June 1709, National Library of Scotland, Fettercairn MSS.

37. See Schwartz, *French Prophets*, ch. 5 on the Prophets in Scotland.

38. Bourignon, *Warning against the Quakers*, xix–xxi. Many of Bourignon's English-speaking critics such as Cockburn quickly equated her ideas with Quakerism, but Bourignon had rejected Quakerism as merely another sect. See above and Macewen, *Bourignon*, 78–79.

39. Ramsay to ?, 12 November 1709, NLS MS 493/73, cited in Schwartz, *French Prophets*, 156. Interestingly, Cuninghame is one of the two exceptions Ramsay cites to this phenomenon. Schwartz lists both Ramsay and Keith as followers of the prophets, which is certainly incorrect: Schwartz, *French Prophets*, 298, 310; cf. Henderson, *Mystics of the North-east*, 197.

40. Holmes, *Trial of Doctor Sacheverell*; on the riots, see Holmes, "Sacheverell Riots."

41. Holmes, *Trial of Doctor Sacheverell*, 62–69; Sacheverell, *Perils of False Brethren*, 9–10, quoted by Holmes, *Trial*, 65.

42. She figures prominently in the Keith-Deskford correspondence: Henderson, *Mystics of the North-east*, 38–39 and passim.

43. A very full bibliography is included in Gondal, *Madame Guyon*; see also Henderson, *Mystics of the North-East*, passim; Balsama, "Madame Guyon, Heterodox"; Mallet-Joris, *Jeanne Guyon*; and the suggestive essay in Kristeva, *Tales of Love*, 297–317. A useful summary of Guyon's views is found in *New Catholic Encyclopedia* 6:869–71.

44. No letters directed to Cheyne survive. However, at the very least he was aware of the group through Keith, who mentions Cheyne frequently in his letters to Deskford.

45. George Cheyne, *Philosophical Principles of Religion, Natural and Revealed* (1715), part 2, preface (not paginated); this work will hereafter be referred to as *Philosophical Principles* (1715). On this dating, see Bowles, "Physical, Human, and Divine Attraction," 478.

46. Royal Society MS 82, ff. 11–14, dated "Ash Wednesday, 1713/14." Bowles, "Physical, Human, and Divine Attraction," 478, surmises that the date 23 September 1713

at the end of the 1715 edition is the date of completion for the whole work, but Cheyne cites several works published in 1713, making this dating more problematic. For Taylor, see *DNB, DSB*. He was apparently not related to the Dr. Taylor of Croydon who so influenced Cheyne's dietary reforms.

47. Cheyne, *Philosophical Principles* (1705) 1:13; Royal Society MS 82, f. 11r; on the "steady state" see Schaffer, "Newtonian Cosmology and the Steady State."

48. Cheyne, *Philosophical Principles* (1705) 2:42–43; Taylor, RS MS 82, ff. 12v–13r. On the arguments against deism, see Schaffer, "Newtonian Cosmology and the Steady State." I am grateful to Dr. Schaffer for providing me with a draft chapter of this thesis (not included in the final copy) in which he discusses the particular case of Taylor and Cheyne.

49. Cheyne, *Philosophical Principles* (1715), preface to part 1, not paginated. On the second edition of the *Principia*, see Westfall, *Never at Rest*, 748–50. See Stewart, *Rise of Public Science*, 71–73.

50. Holmes, *Trial of Doctor Sacheverell*, 269–70; Henderson, *Mystics of the North-east*, 63–64 and passim; Tayler and Tayler, *Jacobites; DNB*, s.v. "Garden, George."

51. Cheyne, *Philosophical Principles* (1715) 1:2, 46.

52. Leighton, *Works*, 563–64; see Emerson, "Science and Moral Philosophy," 11–12.

53. Cheyne, *Philosophical Principles* (1715) 1:42.

54. See Westfall, *Never at Rest*, 303–8; McGuire, "Neoplatonism and Active Principles."

55. Cheyne, *Philosophical Principles* (1715) 1:47.

56. Cheyne, *Philosophical Principles* (1715), preface to part 2.

57. Cheyne, *Philosophical Principles* (1715) 2:3, 39–40, 53; Newton, *Opticks*, query 28.

58. Cheyne, *Philosophical Principles* (1715) 2:61–66.

59. Ibid., 74–83. Newton's rejection of the Trinity was a well-kept secret; see Westfall, *Never at Rest*, 649–53. This undermines Rousseau's claim of Whiston's influence on Cheyne, since Whiston was a well-known Arian; see Rousseau, "Mysticism and Millenarianism."

60. Newton, *Principia*.

61. Bourignon, *Renovation*, 36.

Chapter 5. A Bath Physician and His Practice

1. Manuel, *Religion of Isaac Newton*, 35. Manuel does not cite any source for this assertion.

2. Cheyne, *Essay of Health and Long Life*, viii.

3. Wordsworth, *Scholae academicae*, 79, 129, 332–37; on Oxford, see Shuttleton, "My Own Crazy Carcase." 103.

4. Moore and Silverthorne, "Gershom Carmichael," 78–79; Emerson, "Science and Moral Philosophy," 19; Wood, "Science and the Pursuit of Virtue," 130.

5. Barfoot, "Hume," 153, 155, 159.

6. LeClerc, *Bibliothèque ancienne et moderne* 3:42–43; Vermij, *Secularisering*, 108, 114. On LeClerc, see Colie, *Light and Enlightenment*, 31–35 and passim; *Nieuw nederlandsch biografisch woordenboek*, 430–33; Vermij lists several other secondary works on LeClerc (in Dutch) in his bibliography.

7. See bibliography for editions. The Dutch translator was the philologist Lambert ten Kate (1674–1731). See Vermij, *Secularisering*, 108, 156; I have not been able to determine whether this translation is of the first or second edition. I have not located a copy of LeClerc's French translation. Hartsoeker's review appeared in *Bibliothèque ancienne et moderne* 8:303–50, 1717.

8. Leibniz to Cheyne, 25 September 1716, cited in Leibniz, *Briefwechsel*, 35, described by the editor as "Betr. die Streitigkeiten mit Newton u. Clarke." Cheyne had written to Leibniz in 1704 about the calculus.

9. Henderson, *Mystics of the North-east*, 104, n. 10; 141 (Cheyne leaves London for Bath 4 April 4 1717); 160 (5 July 1718).

10. Cheyne, *Essay of Health and Long Life*, preface; for his family, see ch. 4 above.

11. [Macmichael], *Gold-Headed Cane*, 39–40.

12. Mullan, *Sentiment and Sociability*, 2–4.

13. *Letters to Richardson*, introduction, 9, citing *Historical Manuscripts Commission, Portland MSS* 4:584; *Historical Manuscripts Commission, Downshire MSS* 1: part 2: 906–7.

14. Hamilton, *Diary*, xxiv–xxv, n. 48, refers to Hamilton's visit to Bath in 1715, citing undated letters to Sloane. Some of the letters to which Roberts refers date from 1720–21; see below.

15. Cheyne to Hugh Campbell, Earl of Loudoun, 11 May 1709, Huntington Library, MS LO 7882, published in *Letters to the Countess of Huntingdon*, 1–2.

16. Henderson, *Mystics of the North-East*, 193. For Cuninghame, see above, ch. 4.

17. Scott-Moncrief, *Household Book of Lady Grisell Baillie*, 31. Pitcairne was consulted several times in 1707: ibid., 16, 18. Cheyne later attended George Baillie on his deathbed: Cheyne to ?Grisell Baillie, Burford, 3 August 1738, Scottish Record Office, MS GD 158/2923; in his obituary for Baillie he mentions thirty years acquaintance (see below, ch. 7).

18. Cheyne to Harley, 4 August 1716, BL Add. MSS 4291, f. 241. For Harley's connection with the Keith-Garden circle, see Henderson, *Mystics of the North-east*, 93.

19. Mead was born in 1673, Arbuthnot in 1667, Freind in 1675. See above, ch. 3.

20. *DNB*, s.v. "Sloane, Hans"; Munk, *Roll*, 1. Sloane's medical practice has never, to my knowledge, been studied.

21. Hamilton, *Diary*, xxiii–xxiv.

22. On the development of Bath, see Mullett, *Public Baths and Health*; Chalklin, *Provincial Towns*; McIntyre, "Bath"; Corfield, *Impact of English Towns*; MacInnes, "Emergence of a Leisure Town"; Borsay, *Urban Renaissance*; Neale, "Bath: Ideology and Utopia"; Hembry, *English Spa*; Varey, *Space*, part 2 and passim.

23. Fiennes, *Journeys*, 44.

24. McIntyre, "Bath," 214.

25. Defoe, *Tour* (1971), 360.

26. Hamilton to Sloane, n.d.(but ca. 1715 from context), BL Sloane MS 4059, f. 100.

27. Borsay, *Urban Renaissance*; MacInnes, "Emergence of a Leisure Town." On increased wealth, see Weatherill, *Consumer Behaviour*.

28. Eaves and Kimpel, *Samuel Richardson*, 17, 74; Defoe, *Tour* (1742) 2:255.

29. Corfield, *Impact of English Towns*, 54–58; Neale, "Bath: Ideology and Utopia"; Varey, *Space*, ch. 4.

30. Wood, *Description of Bath*, 224–25.

31. On the development of the "season" see Corfield, *Impact*, 59–60; *A Step to the Bath, with a Character of the Place* (London, 1700), quoted in Neale, "Bath: Ideology and Utopia," 226. Mullett attributes this work to Ned Ward: *Public Baths and Health in England*, 20 and bibliography no. 42.

32. McIntyre, "Bath," 205–6. For a more balanced view of Nash's influence, see Varey, *Space*, 76–77; Gadd, *Georgian Summer*.

33. *A Step to the Bath*, cited in Neale, "Bath: Ideology and Utopia," 126.

34. Varey, *Space*, 76; Gadd, *Georgian Summer*, 78–80; Melville, *Bath under Beau Nash*; Barbeau, *Life and Letters at Bath*.

35. Defoe, *Tour* (1971), 360.

36. Wood, *Description of Bath*, 437–43. A good account of Bath's daily round, still intact nearly a century later, is in Jane Austen's *Northanger Abbey*.

37. Thomas Pitt to Robert Pitt, 5 February 1708/9, Historical Manuscripts Commission, *Manuscripts of J.B. Fortescue, Esq. preserved at Dropmore* 1:41 (hereafter referred to as *Grenville Papers*).

38. Scott-Moncrief, *Household Book of Lady Grisell Baillie*, 307–9; on wages, see Earle, *Making of the English Middle Class*, 73.

39. Peirce, *Bath Memoirs*, preface, not paginated.

40. Floyer and Baynard, *History of Cold-Bathing.*

41. Quinton, *Practical Observations in Physick,* 17.

42. Oliver, *Practical Dissertation on Bath Waters,* 33–36, 50–54; see also McIntyre, "Bath," 208; *DNB,* s.v. "Oliver, William (1659–1716)"; Munk, *Roll,* 1.

43. Webster, *Great Instauration,* 264–68.

44. Beier, *Sufferers and Healers,* 4–5.

45. Duden, *Woman beneath the Skin,* 25, citing Gianna Pomata, *Un tribunale dei malati: Il protomedicato bolognese* (Bologna, 1983).

46. Peirce, *Bath Memoirs,* preface.

47. Anstey, *New Bath Guide* (1766), in *Poetical Works of Christopher Anstey,* 19.

48. Smollett, *Humphry Clinker,* 65–66.

49. Garrison, "Medicine"; Lane, "The doctor scolds me"; Porter, "Laymen, Doctors and Medical Knowledge"; Porter, "Lay Medical Knowledge"; Porter and Porter, *Patient's Progress,* 189–207; Porter and Porter, *In Sickness and in Health,* 133–52. On fees, see Holmes, *Augustan England,* 223; Andrews, "A Respectable Mad-Doctor," 181.

50. Kleinman, *Patients and Healers,* 104–18.

51. Duden, *Woman beneath the Skin,* 26. See n. 45 above.

52. Jewson, "Medical Knowledge and the Patronage System"; Nicolson, "Metastatic Theory of Pathogenesis." Nicolson, however, dismisses the nuances of medical theories, which, as I have argued, could be as important as therapy in establishing the physician's persona to his patients.

53. Paster, *Body Embarrassed,* 17–19.

54. Kleinman, *Patients and Healers,* 34–42.

55. Klein, "Liberty, Manners, and Politeness." See also his "Politeness for Plebes: Some Social Identities in Early Eighteenth-Century England," paper presented at a Clark Library seminar, January 1991.

56. Borsay, *English Urban Renaissance;* Porter and Porter, *Patient's Progress.*

57. Rousseau, "Nerves, Spirits, and Fibers"; Barker-Benfield, *Culture of Sensibility;* on the literary discussion of sensibility, see (among a vast bibliography) Todd, *Sensibility.*

58. Mullan, *Sentiment and Sociability,* 201.

59. See King, *Medical World of the Eighteenth Century.*

60. Mandeville, *Hypochondriack and Hysterick Diseases,* xxi.

61. Holmes, *Augustan England,* 231–35.

62. James Keill to Hans Sloane, 14 May 17??, British Library, Sloane MSS 4078, f. 289; Keill to Sloane, 20 February 1710/11, Sloane MSS 4042, ff. 254–55. See Valadez and O'Malley, "James Keill of Northampton."

63. James Keill to Hans Sloane, 13 September (1711?), BL Sloane MSS 4078, f. 182; Keill to Sloane, n.d., Sloane MSS 4059, ff. 226, 228.

64. See her letters in the Hastings MSS, Huntington Library.

65. Duke of Chandos to Cheyne, 26 June 1728, Huntington Library, Stowe MSS 57 (Chandos Letterbooks), vol. 32, f. 18.

66. Scott-Moncrieff, *Household Book*, 15; Cheyne to Sloane, 14 November 1720, BL Sloane MS 4034, f. 330. Cheyne is obviously trying to justify his apparent neglect of this patient by laying the blame at her door.

67. Anstey, *New Bath Guide*, 21.

68. Beier, *Sufferers and Healers*, 4.

69. See Coleman, "Health and Hygiene."

70. Paster, *Body Embarrassed*, 16–19.

71. Smith, "Prescribing the Rules of Health," esp. 249–62; Riley, *Eighteenth-Century Campaign*.

72. Smollett, *Humphry Clinker*, 75.

73. Peirce, *Bath Memoirs*, book 1, ch. 6.

74. Defoe, *Tour* (1742), 257–58.

75. Ibid.; Peirce, *Bath Memoirs*, book 1, ch. 9. On the analysis of spa waters, see Coley, "Physicians, Chemists, and Analysis," and Hamlin, "Chemistry, Medicine, and Legitimization." On chlorosis, see especially Figlio, "Chlorosis and Chronic Disease"; Brumberg, *Fasting Girls*, 172–75.

76. Porter and Porter, *In Sickness and in Health*, 147; see also Fraser, "Stukeley and the Gout." A modern clinical description of the gout is Talbott, *Gout*.

77. I have not been able to identify Tennison. He may have been related to Archbishop of London Thomas Tenison, or to Richard Tennison, bishop of Meath.

78. Cheyne, *Gout*, 3.

79. Ibid., 7.

80. Sydenham, *Treatise on Gout* (1683), in *Works of Sydenham*, 130. For a survey of views on gout in this period, see Fraser, "Stukeley and the Gout."

81. Cheyne, *Gout*, 82–84.

82. Sydenham, *Gout*, 129; Hamilton, *Diary*, xxv–xvii.

83. Cheyne, *English Malady*, 342–43. Cheyne's ulcerated legs were a sign of impaired circulation, perhaps even congestive heart failure.

84. Quoted in *Letters to Richardson*, 7.

85. Cheyne described his yearly spring visitation of the gout in *English Malady*, 359.

86. Cheyne, *Gout*, 32–37; he cites query 31 of Newton's 1718 *Opticks* but does not mention "De natura acidorum."

87. Fraser, "Stukeley and the Gout," 166–67.

88. Cheyne, *Gout*, vi–vii, 42.

89. Ibid., 41, 96–98.

90. On providentialism, see Porter, "Medicine and Religion"; Guerrini, "Newtonian Medicine and Religion."

91. Rousseau, "Nerves, Spirits, and Fibres."

92. Quoted in Gregg, *Queen Anne*, 106.

93. Porter, *Mind-forg'd Manacles*, 57.

94. Speck, *Stability and Strife*, 196–200; for financial details, see Dickson, *Financial Revolution*.

95. On Hamilton's losses, see Hamilton, *Diary*, xxii and n; Roberts disputes the figure of eighty thousand pounds but admits he cannot refute it. Cheyne wrote Harley in 1720, "I most gratefully accept being a Subscriber in the next Subscription to the South Sea-Stock," 8 May 1720, BL Add. MSS 4291, f. 237r. I have not been able to learn how much Cheyne invested or lost. On Newton's losses, Westfall, *Never at Rest*, 861–62.

96. Keith to Deskford, 2 July 1720, 20 September 1720: Henderson, *Mystics of the Northeast*, 167, 169.

97. Jane Pitt to Hon. Mrs. Pitt, 2 October 1720, *Grenville Papers* 1: 65–66.

98. Cheyne to Sloane, 21 December 1720, BL Sloane MS 4034, f. 332.

99. Quoted in Rogers, "This Calamitous Year," 160. Rogers attributes this and other writings on the Bubble in *Applebee's Journal* to Daniel Defoe.

100. Rogers, "This Calamitous Year."

101. Mead, *Medical Precepts and Cautions* (1751), cited in Andrews, "A Respectable Mad-Doctor," 184.

102. Plumb, *Walpole*, ch. 8.

103. On Lord Montrath, see Cheyne to Sloane, 4 March 1719/20, BL Sloane MS 4034, f. 317; n.d., Sloane MS 4034, ff. 340–41. The patient Cheyne described as having "dos'd his life away" may have been Lord Montrath: Cheyne to Sloane, n.d., Sloane MS 4034, f. 344.

104. Cheyne to Sloane, 13 April 1720, BL Sloane MS 4034, ff. 325–26; 9 May 1720, Sloane MS 4045, f. 329; 11 July 1720, Sloane MS 4034, ff. 323–24. In the 1730s Pitcairne's Edinburgh protégé George Hepburn also treated the Walpole family (see Hepburn to Sloane, 22 June 1734, Sloane MS 4078, ff. 6–7); I have not found any connection between Hepburn and Cheyne.

105. See *Letters to the Countess of Huntingdon*, and ch. 7 below.

106. On anorexia, see Brumberg, *Fasting Girls*; Cohen, *Daughter's Dilemma*.

107. Cohen, *Daughter's Dilemma*, 24.

108. Tryon, *Monthly Observations*, 3.

109. Cheyne to Sloane, 21 December 1720, Sloane MS 4034, f. 332.

110. *Praxeos Pitcarnianae specimina*, University Library Edinburgh MS Dc.1.62, f. 4, dated 28 May 1704.

111. Cheyne to Sloane, 13 April 1720, BL Sloane MS 4034, ff. 325–26; 11 July 1720, Sloane MS 4034, ff. 323–24. Between Pitcairne and Cheyne lay an edition of the *Edinburgh Pharmacopoeia* that had eliminated some of the more exotic remedies.

112. Hamilton, *Diary*, 6; Freind, *Emmenologia*, 67 and passim; Duke of Chandos to Cheyne, 15 June 1728, Huntington Library, Stowe MSS 57 (Chandos Letterbooks), vol. 31, f. 334; Pitcairne, "Some Observations Concerning Womens Monthly Courses," (ca. 1704), in *Works*, 221–37; Crawford, "Menstruation," esp. 50–57; Schofield, *Mechanism and Materialism*, 52–53.

113. Bynum, *Holy Feast and Holy Fast*, 201–2, 214.

114. Paster, *Body Embarrassed*, 81; see also Crawford, "Menstruation," 70–72.

115. Cheyne to Sloane, 13 April 1720, Sloane 4034, ff. 325–26.

116. Freind, *Emmenologia*, 22.

117. Cheyne to Sloane, 11 July 1720, Sloane MS 4034 ff. 323–24; 9 May 1720, Sloane MS 4045 f. 329; 31 August 1720, Sloane MS 4034, f. 327.

118. Cheyne to Sloane, 11 July 1720, Sloane MS 4034, ff. 323–24.

119. Bennet Dyer to ?, Bath, 2 October 1736, Edinburgh University Library, MS Gen (Dyer) 130, #11.

120. Robert Walpole to Sloane, 26 August 1720, Sloane MS 4046, f. 6. Walpole refers to a letter from Cheyne to Sloane that Sloane then forwarded to him. I have not found this letter.

121. Cheyne to Sloane, 31 August 1720, Sloane MS 4034, f. 327.

122. Pitcairne, "A Dissertation upon the Circulation of the Blood in Born Animals and Embryons," in *Works*, 164–87, at 173. See Kramer, "Opium Rampant," Andrews, "A Respectable Mad-Doctor," 174–75. On Cheyne's use of opiates in therapy see ch. 6 below.

123. Cheyne to Sloane, 24 October 1720, Sloane MS 4034, f. 319.

124. Oliver, *Practical Dissertation on Bath Waters*, 25–26.

125. Cheyne to Sloane, 14 November 1720, Sloane MS 4034, f. 330.

126. Cheyne to Sloane, 30 November 1720, Sloane MS 4034, f. 334.

127. Cheyne to Sloane, 21 December 1720, Sloane MS 4034, f. 332.

128. Ibid.

129. Cheyne to Sloane, 23 January 1720/21, Sloane MS 4034, f. 336.

130. Cheyne to Sloane, 20 August 1721, Sloane MS 2034, f. 339.

131. Cheyne to Sloane, 19 September 1721, Sloane MS 4034 ff. 342–43.

132. Cheyne to Sloane, 30 July 1722, Sloane MS 4034 f. 346.

133. Borsay, "Cash and Conscience," 217; Andrew, *Philanthropy and Police*, 21.

134. On the history of the Bath hospital, see Wood, *Description of Bath*; Falconer, *Mineral Water Hospital, Bath*; Rolls, *Hospital of the Nation*; Borsay, "Cash and Conscience."

135. Committee Minute Book 1737–44, Royal National Hospital for Rheumatic Diseases, Bath, 51–52.

136. On eighteenth-century hospitals, see Foucault, *Birth of the Clinic*; Andrew, *Philanthropy and Police*, 53–54; Granshaw and Porter, *Hospital in History*; Wilson, "Politics of Medical Improvement."

137. Committee Minute Book, 1737–44, 52; Porter, "The Gift Relation," 150.

138. Perry, *Mary Astell*, 258–65, 238–42 (on the Chelsea school) and references. See also *DNB*, s.v. "Hastings, Lady Elizabeth." There are two biographies of Lady Betty, neither very satisfactory: Barnard, *Lady Elizabeth Hastings*; Medhurst, *Life and Work of Lady Elizabeth Hastings*.

139. See the letters of Lady Elizabeth Hastings, HA 4719–4760, Huntington Library. The earliest mention of "Dr Cheney" I have found is Lady Elizabeth Hastings to Selina, Countess of Huntingdon, 9 August [?1728], MS HA 1726. Internal evidence suggests that this letter may date from 1730 or after.

140. For Hoare, see Perry, *Mary Astell*, passim; *DNB*, s.v. "Hoare, Sir Richard" (father of Henry); on the Charitable Society, Wilson, "Politics of Medical Improvement," 15–24. The Hoare family continued to be prominent London philanthropists throughout the eighteenth century; see Andrew, *Philanthropy and Police*, passim. For Cockburn, see *DNB*, s.v. "Cockburn, Patrick"; he had been ejected from his curacy of a London church for refusing to take the required oaths on the accession of George I. He later published an edition, to which Cheyne subscribed, of the works of his kinsman Henry Scougal, including Garden's funeral sermon for Scougal. His wife, Catharine Trotter Cockburn, was a well-known playwright and philosopher.

141. Porter, "The Gift Relation," 151–54; Borsay, "Cash and Conscience," 219.

142. *DNB*, s.v. "Jekyll, Sir Joseph"; Holmes, *Trial of Doctor Sacheverell*, passim.

143. Borsay, "Cash and Conscience," 217 and passim.

144. Wood, *Description of Bath*, 274–83; Rolls, *Hospital of the Nation*, 12–13; Committee Minute Book, 1737–44, Royal National Hospital for Rheumatic Diseases, passim. Cheyne's patient Lord Montrath is listed on the committee in 1728.

145. Committee Minute Book, 1737–44, Royal National Hospital for Rheumatic Diseases, passim; Wood, *Description of Bath*, 274–304.

Chapter 6. The Passions of the Soul

1. Cheyne to Jekyll, 9 March 1724, Edinburgh University Library, MS La.II.303, Div. II.

2. Cheyne, *Health and Long Life*, preface, xi.

3. For editions, see bibliography. Extracts appeared in an Italian work in the 1850s. In comparison, Richard Mead's 1720 treatise on the plague reached its ninth edition in 1744.

4. Cheyne, *Health and Long Life*, preface, xvi. Robert Peirce had also referred to himself using the phrase "crazy Carkasse": Peirce, *Bath Memoirs*, preface, not paginated.

5. Flynn, *Body in Swift and Defoe*, 49–50.

6. Cheyne, *English Malady*, 344–45.

7. Cheyne, *Health and Long Life*, preface, i, vii.

8. Cheyne, *Acute and Slow Continu'd Fevers*.

9. See above, ch. 5.

10. Cheyne, *Health and Long Life*, 115. In addition to punch, a popular drink of the time was negus, a mixture of port, sugar, spices, and hot water named after its inventor, Colonel Negus (d. 1732).

11. Cheyne, *Health and Long Life*, 5–6; on Calvinist ideas, see Wear, "Puritan Perceptions of Illness." The Puritan divine William Perkins described the body as "God's workmanship" in *A Golden Chaine* (1612), quoted in Wear, 63.

12. Barnard, *Lady Elizabeth Hastings*, 26–27.

13. Cheyne, *Health and Long Life*, xviii–xix, 2.

14. Ibid., xviii–xix, 21–27, 29. See Turner, "Government of the Body," esp. 259–66; see also his *Body in Society*.

15. Woodward, *State of Physick*; Flynn, *Body in Swift and Defoe*, 45–46.

16. Cheyne to Richardson, 2 February 1742, in *Letters to Richardson*, 82. See Sekora, *Luxury*.

17. Cheyne, *Health and Long Life*, 84.

18. Ibid., 95, 98, 100–104; Flynn, "Running out of Matter," 158–59.

19. On Cornaro and Lessius, see *Letters to Richardson*, 14 and n.; Flynn, *Body in Swift and Defoe*, 47–48.

20. Cheyne, *Health and Long Life*, 4; Mandeville, *Hypochondriack and Hysterick Diseases*, 1–20; *Elizabeth Montagu, the Queen of the Blue Stockings: Her Correspondence from 1720–1761* 1:36, quoted in Porter and Porter, *In Sickness and in Health*, 243.

21. Cheyne, *Health and Long Life*, 4; Flynn, *Body in Swift and Defoe*, 52.

22. Cheyne, *Health and Long Life*, 171, 158; see Mullan, "Hypochondria and Hysteria"; on class, see Scull, *Most Solitary of Afflictions*, 53n.

23. Sydenham, "Epistolary Dissertation to Doctor Cole," in *Works of Sydenham* 2:85. See also Astruc, *Diseases Incident to Women*; Porter, *Mind-forg'd Manacles*, 48–50. See discussion in ch. 1 above.

24. Cheyne, *Health and Long Life*, 159.

25. David Hume to [?George Cheyne], ca. March 1734, in *Letters of David Hume* 1:15. This letter was never sent, and the identity of its intended recipient remains in dispute.

26. Cheyne to Richardson, 2 May 1742, *Letters to Richardson*, 94.

27. Cheyne to Richardson, 5 September 1742, ibid., 108; Cheyne to Richardson, 24 August 1741, ibid., 69; Cheyne to Countess of Huntingdon, 6 September 1735, *Letters to the Countess of Huntingdon*, 50; Bourignon, *Renovation of the Gospel-Spirit*, preface, xvi.

28. Cheyne, *Health and Long Life*, 144–53; the citation of Clarke is on 148–49. Cheyne used the proposition-axiom-scholium format of his earlier works in this chapter. On Clarke's views, see Shapin, "Of Gods and Kings."

29. Cheyne, *Health and Long Life*, 150–54; King, "George Cheyne," 525–26. On Stahl, see also Geyer-Kordesch, "Georg Ernst Stahl"; French, "Sickness and the Soul."

30. Cheyne, *Health and Long Life*, 156–59.

31. Ibid., 157–61. On religious melancholy, cf. Burton, *Anatomy of Melancholy.*

32. Cheyne, *Health and Long Life*, 157, 161–63.

33. "Platonick Love," British Library, Burney MS 390, ff. 8–9. This poem is ascribed in the MS to "Dr Cheyney."

34. On this aspect of Guyon, see especially Kristeva, *Tales of Love*, 297–317; Byrom, *Journal* 2, part 2 (May 1743): 363.

35. Bynum, *Holy Feast and Holy Fast*; Corrington, "Anorexia, Asceticism, and Autonomy." Also relevant is Bell, *Holy Anorexia*; Curran, *Grace before Meals.*

36. On knowledge of medieval mysticism in this period, see Rupp, *Religion in England*, 207–8; Tryon, *Miscellanea*, 35.

37. Bynum, *Holy Feast and Holy Fast*, 189–91 and passim. See my "A Diet for the Sensitive Soul."

38. On class, see Turner, "Government of the Body," and Turner, *Body and Society*, 76–80.

39. Barnard, *Lady Elizabeth Hastings*, 27.

40. William Stratford to Edward Harley, 4 August 1724, Historical Manuscripts Commission, *Manuscripts of His Grace the Duke of Portland* 7:381.

41. John Wesley to Susanna Wesley, 1 November 1724, *Letters of Wesley* 1:11; Byrom, *Journal* 1, part 1 (6 February 1726): 199.

42. Wynter, *Cyclus Metasyncriticus*, vii, xv–xvi, 4.

43. Wynter, *Of Bathing in the Hot Baths.*

44. Warner, *Original Letters*, 62–63.

45. Quinton, *De Thermis*, 19–20; Quinton, *Treatise of Warm Bath Water*, the first edition appeared as *Practical Observations in Physick* (1707; 2d ed., 1711).

46. *Remarks on Dr Cheyne's Essay of Health and Long Life*, xii–xvi, 14, and passim.

47. Broadside ballad from ?1725, quoted in Shuttleton, "My Own Crazy Carcase," 147.

48. *A Letter to George Cheyne, M.D., F.R.S.*, 2, 12, 51–53, 71–72.

49. *DNB*, s.v. "Strother, Edward"; Munk, *Roll*, 2. Strother, a Utrecht M.D., was admitted as a licentiate of the London College of Physicians in 1721.

50. Strother, *Essay on Sickness and Health*, 70–71, 138, 218.

51. *An Epistle to Ge——ge Ch——ne MD FRS*, i–ii, 3, 9, 15.

52. Cheyne, *Tractatus de infirmorum*. On Robertson see below. Rousseau, "Mysticism and Millenarianism," 103, n. 70, claims Clifton Winteringham (1689–1748) was the translator, but Winteringham only reissued Robertson's translation in 1742 with his own "nosological commentary."

53. Cheyne, *Tractatus de infirmorum*, preface, not paginated. Cheyne had been made a fellow in May 1724; in his preface he thanked his sponsor, John Drummond, president of the Edinburgh College from 1722 to 1727 and a friend of Pitcairne.

54. Sedgwick, *House of Commons, 1715–1754* 2:163–64; Linda Colley, *In Defiance of Oligarchy*, 98–99, 160–61. Hutcheson, a native of Ireland, acted as the duke of Ormonde's London agent and sat for Hastings from 1713 to 1727. His wife, Elizabeth, was later a follower of William Law; see below.

55. Cheyne, *De natura fibrae*. All translations that follow are mine except where indicated.

56. Ibid., 1–2.

57. Ibid., 9–10. This description is repeated in greater detail in Cheyne, *English Malady*, 10–13.

58. Cheyne, *De natura fibrae*, 9–11, 13–15.

59. Cheyne, *English Malady*, 14; this is translated from *De natura fibrae*, 12.

60. Cheyne, *De natura fibrae*, sections 16–18.

61. Cheyne, *Essay of Health and Long Life*, 213–20.

62. *DSB* 3:244.

63. On Boerhaave's theories, see King, *Medical World of the Eighteenth Century*, chs. 3–4; King, *Philosophy of Medicine*, 121–24. However, Cheyne told Richardson that he "despise[d] Boerhave for his wild Brags of some of his chemical Medicines," [May 1742], *Letters to Richardson*, 96.

64. Cheyne, *English Malady*, 61, 79. Cf. Clarke, "Doctrine of the Hollow Nerve," 137, who asserts that Cheyne "ignored" Leeuwenhoek's evidence.

65. Newton, *Opticks*, 354.

66. Mead, *Short Discourse Concerning Pestilential Contagion*, 11. Cheyne's essay "De morbis contagionis" was translated into English in 1753 and appended to the tenth edition of the *Essay on Gout*.

67. Cheyne, *De natura fibrae*, 84.

68. Newton, *Opticks*, 374, 375–76.

69. Cheyne, *English Malady*, 344–46, 356.

70. Ibid., 346–47.

71. Cheyne to Richardson, 23 December 1741, *Letters to Richardson*, 77.

72. Bordo, *Unbearable Weight*, 3–5.

73. Cheyne, *English Malady*, 347.

74. James Douglas (1675–1742) was a Scot, M.D. Rheims, who was chiefly known as an anatomist; see Thomas, *James Douglas*. Noel Broxholme (?1689–1748), a protégé of Mead, was elected a fellow of the London College in March 1725 and was later a physician to the prince of Wales; see *DNB*, s.v. "Broxholme, Noel"; Munk, *Roll*, 2. James Campbell was admitted a fellow of the Edinburgh College in 1727.

75. Cheyne, *English Malady*, 351. *OED*, s.v. "ichor"; cf. Pope, *Dunciad* 2:92. See also Flynn, "Running Out of Matter," 153–55.

76. Cheyne to Richardson, 30 June 1742, *Letters to Richardson*, 101; 14 March 1742, ibid., 88.

77. Cheyne, *English Malady*, 353–54. Rousseau, "Mysticism and Millenarianism," 85, claims that Cheyne's weight declined from 448 pounds to 130 but gives no citation for this claim, and I have found no evidence to support it. On the "cyclus metasyncriticus," *OED*, s.v. "metasyncrisis"; this was also the title of a 1725 book by Cheyne's Bath colleague John Wynter (see above).

78. Henderson, *Mystics of the North-east*, 166, n. 3, and passim.

79. Rousseau, "Mysticism and Millenarianism," Shuttleton, "My Own Crazy Carcase." See also T. L. Wetstein to John Walker, 26 February 1735, quoted in Byrom, *Journal* 2:472–73n. Wetstein, a scion of the Leiden publishing firm that published mystical works, mentioned "our friend and correspondent Dr. James Keith" and claimed that Thomas Carpenter was the only man in England who presently distributed the writings of Bourignon. He did not mention Cheyne.

80. Quoted in *DNB*, s.v. "Hooke, Nathaniel or Nathanael."

81. Nichols, *Literary Anecdotes*, 607–10; Nichols dates this to 1739, but the first translation of the *Travels of Cyrus* appeared in 1727, and the 1739 edition was merely a reprint of the revised edition of 1730. Cheyne subscribed to the 1730 edition. See Greenwood, *William King*, 96–98. On Ramsay and the *Travels of Cyrus*, see Walker, *Ancient Theology*, ch. 7, 231–63.

82. Walker, *Ancient Theology*, 236–37; I have no evidence that Ramsay and Cheyne met, but it seems likely.

83. Quoted in *DNB*, s.v. "Hooke, Nathaniel or Nathanael."

84. *Letters to the Countess of Huntingdon*, 25; *Letters to Richardson*, 98, 125, and passim; later Cheyne's married daughter, Frances Stewart, also served this function.

85. Cheyne to Richardson, 29 August 1739, *Letters to Richardson*, 55. Strahan was related to Cheyne's wife.

86. See *Letters to Richardson*, passim. Cheyne's relations with Leake seem to have been as stormy as those with Strahan; Cheyne complained to Richardson of Leake's "dark confused manner."

87. The widowed Richardson married Elizabeth Leake in 1733. Eaves and Kimpel, *Samuel Richardson*, 17–18, 20, 22–23, 30–31, 49, 62; Richardson later assumed the printing of Hutcheson's anti-Walpole pamphlets. Cheyne's correspondence with Richardson began in 1734; see ch. 7. On Leake's involvement with the Bath hospital, see Committee Minute Book, 1737–44, RNHRD. Leake actively sought subscriptions for the hospital in the 1730s. See also Neale, *Bath*, 23–24.

88. This included John Law of the Mississippi scheme. *Portland MSS*, VII, 279, 335.

89. Arbuthnot, *Nature of Aliments*, iii–iv.

90. Pope to Gay, 11 September 1722, Pope, *Correspondence* 2:133. On the Scriblerus Club, see Kerby-Miller, *Memoirs of Martinus Scriblerus*, introduction.

91. Pope, *Correspondence*, vol. 4, passim; his comments on Cheyne are discussed in ch. 7.

92. Barry, "Piety and the Patient"; Fissell, *Patients, Power, and the Poor*, 6–7 and passim; Schwartz, *French Prophets*, 157, 202–4. Schwartz speculates that James Cuninghame of Barns may have first encountered the prophets in Bristol while he was consulting Cheyne in Bath in 1709.

93. Barry, "Piety and the Patient," 167–68 and n.; Wesley, *Letters* 1:358–59, 3:104–10; Hill, *John Wesley*, 51–52; Wallis and Wallis, *Eighteenth-Century Medics*, 407, 506; they give Middleton's birthdate as 1710, which seems late but not impossible. Both Cheyne and Middleton subscribed to Patrick Cockburn's 1727 edition of Henry Scougal's *Life of God in the Soul of Man*. Robertson was admitted as an extra-licentiate of the Royal College of Physicians of London in 1732: Munk, *Roll* 2:119. See ch. 7 below.

94. Will of George Cheyne, 23 March 1738, PRO 727/193. For Heylyn, see *DNB*, s.v. "Heylyn, John"; Rupp, *Religion in England*, 218–19; Hobhouse, *Selected Writings of Law*, 388–89.

95. Orcibal, "Theological Originality of Wesley," 86.

96. Hobhouse, *Selected Writings of Law*, 388, states that Law was most likely curate when Heylyn was vicar of Haslingfield, Cambridgeshire, between 1714 and 1719. The facts of Law's life are much debated; apart from Hobhouse, the chief sources are Walton, *William Law* (I have used the copy Walton presented to Princeton University in 1861 with his own MS corrections); *DNB*, s.v. "Law, William" (by Leslie Stephen); Byrom, *Journal*; Rupp, *Religion in England*, 219–242 who is generally judicious and includes a short bibliography. He surmises Heylyn's influence (219).

97. Underhill, "William Law's Suspension at Cambridge," 42–44, refutes the generally believed notion that Law was suspended from his fellowship for the 1713 speech. He was stripped of his M.A., but this was restored two years later.

98. Law, *Treatise upon Christian Perfection*, 26.

99. Ibid., 45.

100. Ibid., 142–43.

101. Cheyne often recommended that Richardson distract himself with light though edifying reading, although he also continued to recommend reading theology: *Letters to Richardson*, passim. See ch. 7 below.

102. Perry, *Mary Astell*, 260–61; Lady Betty had subscribed five hundred pounds in 1726 (as did Walpole) toward "Dean Berkeley's design" for a college: *Portland MSS*, VII, 417. I

should add that any connection between Law and Lady Betty before 1730 is mere speculation on my part.

103. In January 1728/9 John Heylyn also emphasized Christian behavior in a sermon
delivered to the Societies for the Reformation of Manners: see Heylyn, *Sermon*.

104. Law, *Serious Call*, 38–39, 154, 67; on income levels, see Earle, *Making of the English
Middle Class*.

105. Law, Serious Call, 68–69. Like Cheyne, Law spent several pages on the virtues of
early rising.

106. Law, *Serious Call*, 75, 78.

107. Ibid., 68, 79.

108. Medhurst, *Lady Elizabeth Hastings*, 57, 227. On Wilson (1663–1755), see Keble, *Thomas
Wilson*; Rupp, Religion in England, 508.

109. Lady Elizabeth Hastings to Selina, Countess of Huntingdon, 9 August [no year],
Huntington Library, Hastings MSS, HA 4726. Although the Huntington cataloguer has
tentatively dated this letter 1728, a later date seems likely, since Lady Betty refers to the
countess's "sons." Selina Shirley married the earl of Huntingdon in June 1728, and the
first of their four sons was born the following year.

110. Cheyne to Lady Huntingdon, 12 August 1732, *Letters to Lady Huntingdon*, 9.

111. Cheyne to Lady Huntingdon, 28 August 1732, ibid., 10. Lady Huntingdon seemed
less concerned about her soul in 1732 than she would be later.

112. For Law's influence on Wesley, see Walsh, "Origins of the Evangelical Revival."
See also Orcibal, "Theological Originality of Wesley"; Barry, "Piety and the Patient,"
167–69.

113. Green, *Young Mr Wesley*, 307, 121, 145–47, 168, quoting the account of Richard
Morgan; John Wesley to Samuel Wesley, 10 December 1734, Wesley, *Letters* 1:169.

114. Byrom, *Journal* 1 (18 February 1729): 328–29.

115. Ibid. 1:327, 336–37; Green, *Young Mr Wesley*, 277–78, 311; Hobhouse, *Selected Writings of
Law*, 381–83; Hutin, *Disciples anglais*, 156.

116. Hutin, *Disciples anglais*, 297, n. 34.

117. Rupp, *Religion in England*, 267–71.

118. Green, *Young Mr Wesley*, 140, 231.

119. Quoted by Green, *Young Mr Wesley*, 170.

120. On the attribution to Law, see Green, *Young Mr Wesley*, 200–201.

121. Cheyne claimed that *English Malady* had "lain finish'd" for several years before its
publication and only appeared because of the "perhaps indiscreet *Zeal*" of his friends:

English Malady, ii. However, this was a claim Cheyne often made and may be taken as rhetorical, although some of the theoretical sections had already appeared (in Latin) in *De natura fibrae*.

122. These works included Henry Pemberton's introduction to Richard Mead's new edition of William Cowper, *Myotomia reformata* (London: R. Knaplock et al., 1724); Morgan, *Philosophical Principles of Medicine*; Nicholas Robinson, *New Theory of Physick and Diseases*; N. Robinson, *New System of the Spleen*; Bryan Robinson, *Treatise of the Animal Oeconomy*.

123. On Hutchinson, see Wilde, "Hutchinsonianism"; Wilde, "Matter and Spirit"; see also Barry, "Piety and the Patient," 167–70.

124. Sedgwick, *House of Commons* 1:444; Bateman lost his seat in 1734 and separated from his wife in 1738 for his alleged homosexuality. Cheyne later solicited his comments for his *Essay on Regimen*: Cheyne to Richardson, September 1737, Letters to Richardson, 35.

125. Cheyne to Lady Huntingdon, 25 February 1736/7, *Letters to Lady Huntingdon*, 58.

126. Cheyne, *English Malady*, preface and 254–55.

127. Burton, *Anatomy of Melancholy*; Sydenham, "Hysteria in Women; and Hypochondria in Men," in *Processus integri in morbis fere omnibus curandi*, trans. in *Works* 2:231–35; Stukeley, *Of the Spleen*; Blackmore, *Spleen and Vapours*; N. Robinson, *New System of the Spleen*; Mandeville, *Hypochondriack and Hysterick Diseases*.

128. Scull, *Most Solitary of Afflictions*, 179.

129. Cheyne, *English Malady*, i–ii.

130. Ibid., 49.

131. Ibid., i–ii, 54–56.

132. Ibid., 158–59.

133. Ibid., 2–4.

134. N. Robinson, *New System of the Spleen*, 29–31, 65–68, 78–88. For background and further discussion, see Guerrini, "Ether Madness."

135. B. Robinson, *Treatise of the Animal Oeconomy*, 82–85.

136. Cheyne, *English Malady*, 77–89. Pemberton, introduction, in Cowper, *Myotomia reformata*. Pemberton also identified Newton's ether as the animal spirits. For further discussion, see Guerrini, "Ether Madness."

137. Cheyne, *English Malady*, 69; Newton, *Opticks*, 404.

138. Cheyne, *English Malady*, 75.

139. Ibid., 85–89. See also Metzger, *Attraction universelle*, part 3; Westfall, *Science and Religion*, ch. 8.

140. Cheyne, *English Malady*, 99–105; Roy Porter, introduction to Cheyne, *English Malady*, xli.

141. Cheyne, *English Malady*, 220; Erickson, *Mother Midnight*, 95–96.

142. Robinson, *New System of the Spleen*, 211–12. See also Mandeville, *Hypochondriack and Hysterick Diseases*, 246–47; Mullan, "Hypochondria and Hysteria," 158–60.

143. Castle, "Female Thermometer," 13.

144. Cheyne, *English Malady*, 112–14.

145. Ibid., 128–35, 139–43, 144–46.

146. Ibid., dedication, not paginated.

147. Ibid., iv–v, 302. Barry, "Piety and the Patient," 170, claims that regimen books by Tory physicians in this period prescribed different regimens for different social classes as a means of restoring social stability. Barry does not cite any specific eighteenth-century texts, and his claim is not borne out by Cheyne, who wants everyone to eat like a yeoman.

148. Ibid., 49–51.

149. Ibid., 52–54.

150. Ibid., iii–vi, x–xii.

151. Ibid., 182.

152. Porter, *Mind-forg'd Manacles*, 80–81.

153. Cheyne, *English Malady*, 283.

154. Ibid., 260–62. Cf. Scull, *Most Solitary of Afflictions*, 178–79.

155. Laqueur, "Bodies, Details, and the Humanitarian Narrative," 176–78, 183–84. See also Wear, "Puritan Perceptions of Illness"; Porter and Porter, *In Sickness and in Health*, esp. ch. 13; Hunter, *Before Novels*, ch. 8.

156. Cheyne, *English Malady*, 264–65.

157. Ibid., 267–73, 269.

158. Ibid., 273, 275, 283.

159. Wright, "Metaphysics and Physiology," 270–71.

160. Cheyne, *English Malady*, 273, 279, 287, 293.

161. On moral treatment, see Scull, *Most Solitary of Afflictions*, 96–98; Porter, *Mind-forg'd Manacles*, 222–28. Both Scull and Porter minimize the role of religion in moral therapy.

Chapter 7. The Great Muse

1. *Letters to Richardson*, 38.

2. All of these are printed as an appendix to *Letters to Richardson*, 132–37. Richardson printed the *Weekly Miscellany* from its inception in 1732 through 1736: Eaves and Kimpel, *Samuel Richardson*, 58–59.

3. Chandler, *Description of Bath*; Green, "The Spleen," in *Oxford Anthology of English Poetry* 1:522. Thanks to Jeffrey Timmons for this reference.

4. B. Robinson, *Treatise of the Animal Oeconomy*, 2d ed., preface, iv.

5. Morgan, *Philosophical Principles of Medicine*, preface; Schofield, *Mechanism and Materialism*, 128–29. Morgan, ordained as a Presbyterian minister, entered a number of religious controversies, but religion does not seem to have been an issue in his debate with Robinson.

6. Morgan, *Mechanical Practice of Physick*.

7. Robinson, *A Letter to Dr Cheyne*; Morgan, *A Letter to Dr Cheyne*.

8 Duke of Chandos to Cheyne, 26 June 1728, Huntington Library, Stowe MSS 57 (Chandos Letterbooks), vol. 32, f. 18.

9. Cheyne to Richardson, 2 February 1742, *Letters to Richardson*, 83.

10. Cheyne to Richardson, 26 April 1742, ibid., 92.

11. Wallis and Wallis, *Eighteenth-Century Medics*, 111, list twelve subscriptions between 1710 and 1735.

12. Walcot Church Rate Records, Somerset Record Office, D/P/Wal, SW 4/1/1, copy in Bath City Archives. Cheyne's house appears in the church rate evaluations from 1734 onward, and his evaluation is consistently near the highest for the neighborhood. In 1742, Cheyne is listed at £1 12s, Frewin in Wood Street at £1 10s, and Oliver in Princes Street at £1 8s. On the streets of Bath and Monmouth Street in particular, see Wood, *Description of Bath*, 326–37, at 336. Cheyne's will, dated March 1738 (Public Record Office, 727/193) notes a mortgage of £7000, due in 1735.

13. Foster, *Alumni Oxonienses*, vol. 1, s.v. "Cheyne, John," and "Cheyne, William." Both matriculated at St. Mary Hall, John in April 1731 and William in March 1732.

14. Greenwood, *William King*, 96–98. See also *DNB*, s.v. "King, William (1685–1763)" (King had at least two ecclesiastical contemporaries of the same name, including the archbishop of Dublin and the author of the *Transactioneer*); Nichols, *Literary Anecdotes* 2:607–10, the source for much of the *DNB* article. King introduced Ramsay when he was granted an honorary degree at Oxford in 1730: Walker, *Ancient Theology*, 237.

15. Cheyne to Lady Huntingdon, 4 September 1733, *Letters to the Countess of Huntingdon*, 24. Richardson's Pamela remarked that Scots made good if unpolished tutors because of their poverty: cited in Eaves and Kimpel, *Richardson*, 150.

16. *DNB*, s.v. "Cheyne, George."

17. The date of Frances's marriage is given in Viets, "George Cheyne," 448. Viets does not list his source. William Stewart was named in 1738 as one of the executors of

Cheyne's will. On the office of remembrancer, see *OED*, s.v. "remembrancer"; this is the source of the Swift quotation.

18. On Peggy's health, see *Letters to Richardson*, 100, 103, 114. In a codicil to Cheyne's will dated April 1743, Margaret, being ill, is allotted an additional one thousand pounds besides the three thousand Cheyne bequeathed to each daughter. On her assistance to Richardson, see Richardson to Aaron Hill, 20 January 1746, cited in Eaves and Kimpel, *Richardson*, 187. Richardson's "favorite": *Letters to Richardson*, 103, 114, 118.

19. *Letters to Richardson*, 41, 44, 48, 78, 87, 112; *Letters to Lady Huntingdon*, 39.

20. Cheyne to [Grisell Baillie], 3 August 1738, Scottish Record Office, Hume of Marchmont papers, GD 158/2923.

21. Lyttelton to Pope, 4 December 1736, *Correspondence of Alexander Pope* 4:46.

22. Pope, *Correspondence*, vol. 4, passim. On Pope's health, see Nicolson and Rousseau, *This Long Disease, My Life.*

23. Pope to Samuel Gerrard, 17 May 1740, Pope, *Correspondence* 4:242. Several letters to and from Pope and Oliver are in this volume.

24. Pope to Allen, 17 June [1740], Pope, *Correspondence* 4:247; see also the same to the same, 19 April 1740, ibid., 4:235; Pope to Lyttelton, 12 December 1739, ibid., 4:208.

25. Cheyne to Richardson, 26 April 1742, *Letters to Richardson*, 93.

26. *DNB*, s.v. "Law, William." This was Archibald Hutcheson's deathbed wish.

27. Byrom, *Journal* 2, part 1: 330–32. Marsay wrote *Discourses on Subjects Related to the Spiritual Life.*

28. For Hartley see below. He is mentioned frequently in Byrom's journal and attended Cheyne on his deathbed.

29. On this circle, see Bechler, "Triall by What Is Contrary"; Schaffer, "Consuming Flame." Cheyne refers to "the Brethren" in *Letters to Richardson*, 112, 118. Letters from Cheyne to Byrom appear in Byrom, *Journal*; correspondence with Law is mentioned in Walton, *William Law*, 370n.

30. See *Letters to Richardson*, passim; "meer Rationalists": Cheyne to Richardson, 10 February 1738, 36; Cheyne to Byrom, 22 August 1742, Byrom, *Journal* 2, part 2: 32.

31. On Middleton, Robertson, and Bristol connections see Barry, "Piety and the Patient," esp. 166–69. See also Wallis and Wallis, *Eighteenth-Century Medics*, 407, 506; both Middleton and Robertson subscribed in 1753 to Richardson's *Sir Charles Grandison*; Fissell, *Patients, Power, and the Poor*, 63, 147; Hill, *John Wesley*, 51–52.

32. Wesley, *Journal* 4:82, 99; Wesley to Robertson, 24 September 1753, Wesley, *Letters* 3:104–10.

33. *Letters to Countess of Huntingdon*, 18, 61.

34. Ibid., 57, 49, 44; Welch, *Spiritual Pilgrim*, 29.

35 Chandos Letterbooks, vol. 28, f. 115; vol. 31, f. 334; vol. 41, f. 263.

36. Welch, *Spiritual Pilgrim* 20. The Huntingdons married in June 1728.

37. Ibid., 13–14, 19–20; Hastings MSS, Huntington Library, passim.

38. *Letters to Countess of Huntingdon*, 9; I have deduced Lady Huntingdon's pregnancies from an examination of the Hastings MSS, Huntington Library; see also Welch, *Spiritual Pilgrim*, 22. Only one child survived her.

39. Cheyne to Lady Huntingdon, date 1735, *Letters to Countess of Huntingdon*, 53; Welch, *Spiritual Pilgrim*, 24.

40. Cheyne to Dr. Harding, 3 March 1732/3, *Letters to Countess of Huntingdon*, 18.

41. Weiss-Amer, "Medieval Women's Guides," (thanks to the author for alerting me to this article and providing a copy); Lewis, *In the Family Way*, 131–32, 147–48.

42. Duke of Chandos to Cheyne, 15 June 1728, Huntington Library, Stowe MSS 57 (Chandos Letterbooks), vol. 31, f. 334.

43. Lady Elizabeth Hastings to Lady Huntingdon, 17 December [1731], Huntington Library, Hastings MS HA 4741.

44. Lady Huntingdon to Lord Huntingdon, n.d. [ca. 1735], Huntington Library, Hastings MS HA 5846.

45. Duke of Chandos to Cheyne, 24 May 1727, Huntington Library, Stowe MSS 57 (Chandos Letterbooks), vol. 30, f. 25.

46. Cheyne to Lady Huntingdon, 7 January 1733[/4], *Letters to Countess of Huntingdon*, 32–33.

47. "This place is as stupid as usual": Lady Huntingdon to Lord Huntingdon, 20 December, ca. 1743, Huntington Library, Hastings MSS HA 5856; Welch, *Spiritual Pilgrim*, 24.

48. Lady Elizabeth Hastings to Lady Huntingdon, 9 August, n.d. [ca. 1728–30], Huntington Library, Hastings MS HA 4726.

49. Lady Elizabeth Hastings to Lord Huntingdon, 21 June 1738, Huntington Library, Hastings MS HA 4758.

50. Lady Huntingdon to Lord Huntingdon, 28 February 1731/2, Historical Manuscripts Commission, *Report on the Manuscripts of the Late Reginald Rawdon Hastings, Esq.* 3:2. Hereafter HMC, *Hastings MSS.*

51. Welch, *Spiritual Pilgrim*, 64–67; Cheyne to Byrom, 17 December 1741, Byrom, *Journal* 2, part 1: 308.

52. Welch, *Spiritual Pilgrim*, 41. The account that follows is deeply indebted to Welch's excellent work.

53. Shuttleton, "Methodism," 328.

54. Welch, *Spiritual Pilgrim*, 40–49.

55. Wesley to Edmund Gibson, 11 June 1747, Wesley, *Letters* 2:285, referring to events of the 1730s; Wesley, *Journal* 5:373 (28 June 1770).

56. Montagu quoted in [Seymour], *Selina, Countess of Huntingdon* 1:35; Buckingham quoted in Mullett, *Letters to Countess of Huntingdon*, vi n.

57. Lady Huntingdon to Lord Huntingdon, 31 December 1741, HMC, *Hastings MSS*, 32.

58. Lady Huntingdon to Lord Huntingdon, 2 January 1741/2, HMC, *Hastings MSS*, 32.

59. Cheyne to Thomas Wilson [the younger], 13 August 1740, quoted in Keble, *Thomas Wilson*, 924.

60. Wesley, *Journal* 2:297, 3:17–18.

61. Welch, *Spiritual Pilgrim*, 66.

62. Cheyne to Richardson, 2 May 1742, *Letters to Richardson*, 96.

63. *Letters to Richardson*, introduction.

64. Cheyne to Richardson, 21 December 1734, *Letters to Richardson*, 31–32.

65. *Letters to Richardson*, 35, 93.

66. Cheyne to Richardson, 22 June 1738, *Letters to Richardson*, 38.

67. *Letters to Richardson*, 85; see also Eaves and Kimpel, *Samuel Richardson*, 63–64, 154–57.

68. *Letters to Richardson*, 71–72, 92.

69. Cheyne to Richardson, 20 April 1740, *Letters to Richardson*, 60.

70. Flynn, "Running Out of Matter," 147–48, 150.

71. *Letters to Richardson*, 38, 42.

72. 26 April 1742, *Letters to Richardson*, 93.

73. Ibid., 47, 104.

74. Flynn, "Running out of Matter," 148; see also De Porte, *Nightmares and Hobbyhorses*, 147.

75. *Letters to Richardson*, 93–94.

76. Cheyne to Richardson, 17 September 1742, *Letters to Richardson*, 111; Cheyne's prospectus for the catalog, titled "The Universal Cure of Lingering Disorders Either of the Mind or of the Body" is printed in ibid., 126; Hunter, *Before Novels*, 30.

77. Cheyne to Richardson, 5 September 1742, *Letters to Richardson*, 109–10.

78. Richardson, *Pamela*, preface.

79. Watt, *Rise of the Novel*, 173.

80. Richardson, *Pamela*, 112, 217–22.

81. Richardson, *Pamela*, 95–96, 231–33; Erickson, *Mother Midnight*, 94–97; Cheyne, *English Malady*, 220. Cf. Cattaneo, "Cheyne and Richardson," who argues that Cheyne afforded little specific influence on *Pamela*.

82. Cheyne to Richardson, 13 December 1740, *Letters to Richardson*, 63–64.

83. Cheyne to Richardson, 12 February 1741, ibid., 65. Pope had spent the winter at Bath at the home of his friend Ralph Allen: Pope, *Correspondence* 4:323.

84. Eaves and Kimpel, *Richardson*, 121.

85. Cheyne to Richardson, 24 August 1741, *Letters to Richardson*, 67–69.

86. Richardson to Cheyne, 31 August 1741, in *Selected Letters*, 46–51. This letter was apparently not sent.

87. Richardson to Stephen Duck, [1741], *Selected Letters*, 52–53.

88. Cheyne to Richardson, 30 December 1741, 3 September 1741, *Letters to Richardson*, 79, 69.

89. Cheyne to Richardson, February 1742, 9 March 1742, *Letters to Richardson*, 85, 88.

90. Cheyne to Wilson the younger, 13 August 1740, in Keble, *Life of Wilson*, 924. Cheyne coupled the "highest and greatest" with the "lowest and most abject."

91. Cheyne to Richardson, 23 August 1738, *Letters to Richardson*, 39.

92. Ibid., 39–41. For Baillie see *DNB*, s.v. "Baillie, Grizel," and "Baillie, Robert, d. 1684"; *House of Commons* 1:427–28.

93. Cheyne often commented on his advancing age to Richardson; see also Cheyne to Lady Huntingdon, 19 May 1739, *Letters to the Countess of Huntingdon*, 61.

94. Cheyne to Richardson, September 1737, *Letters to Richardson*, 35; 29 August 1739, ibid., 55.

95. Chesterfield to Lyttleton, 24 March 1739, quoted in ibid., 9–10.

96. Cheyne to Richardson, [1738], ibid., 41; 12 September 1739, ibid., 56.

97. Cheyne to Lady Huntingdon, 19 May 1739, *Letters to Countess of Huntingdon*, 61.

98. Cheyne, *Essay on Regimen*, dedication.

99. Ibid., 341.

100. Metzger, *Attraction universelle*, 142.

101. Cheyne, *Essay on Regimen*, preface, i–xvi.

102. Cheyne, *Essay on Regimen*, part 1 (separately paginated). See Flynn, "Running Out of Matter," 150.

103. Cheyne, *Essay on Regimen*, 6, 21–23, 26–30, 51.

104. Ibid., 54–58, 65.

105. Ibid., 66–67.

106. Cited in Schiebinger, *The Mind Has No Sex?*, 114.

107. Cheyne, *Essay on Regimen*, 78, 83–85.

108. On Boehme, see Hutin, *Disciples anglais*, chs. 1 and 7.

109. Cheyne, *Essay on Regimen*, 119–21, 182.

110. Metzger, *Attraction universelle*, 140–41; Walker, *Ancient Theology*, 242–43.

111. Cheyne, *Essay on Regimen*, 125, 186–87.

112. Ibid., 218–19.

113. Marsay, *Temoignage d'un enfant*. An English translation appeared in Edinburgh in 1749.

114. Cheyne to Byrom, 22 August 1742, Byrom, *Journal* 2, part 2: 330–31; Orcibal, "Theological Originality of John Wesley," 88.

115. Cheyne, *Essay on Regimen*, 333–34.

116. Cheyne to Richardson, 29 January 1739/40, 26 October [1739], *Letters to Richardson*, 58–59.

117. Cited in Rousseau, "Medicine and Millenarianism," n. 73.

118. [T. Johnson, pseud.] *Tryal of Colley Cibber*, 34. This passage was followed by a quote from Cheyne's first discourse.

119. Cheyne to Richardson, 26 October [1739], *Letters to Richardson*, 58.

120. *Letters to Richardson*, 63, 91.

121. Defoe, *Tour* (1742), 2:256–58.

122. Cheyne to Richardson, 31 October 1741, 15 November 1741, 2 December 1741, *Letters to Richardson*, 72–74.

123. Cheyne, *Natural Method*, dedication and preface, not paginated.

124. Ibid., preface (not paginated).

125. Ibid., 31–40.

126. Ibid., 57–58.

127. Ibid., 58–98.

128. Ibid., 138–52.

129. Ibid., 1-10; see above, ch. 3; and Gasking, *Concepts of Generation*; Roe, *Matter, Life, and Generation*.

130. On definitions of gender, see Laqueur, *Making Sex*.

131. Cheyne, *Natural Method*, 282; Cheyne to Richardson, February 1742, *Letters to Richardson*, 85.

132. *Letters to Richardson*, 85; *Letters to Countess of Huntingdon*, passim. Lady Huntingdon's second daughter, Selina, born 1735, was dead by 1736. For other examples see Lewis, *In the Family Way*, passim.

133. Cheyne, *Natural Method*, 276–83; Astruc, *Diseases Incident to Women*, 61; Mandeville, *Hypochondriack and Hysterick Diseases*, 2d ed., 271–82. See Crawford, "Attitudes to Menstruation"; Porter and Porter, *In Sickness and in Health*, 51, 83.

134. Cheyne to Richardson, 9 March 1742, *Letters to Richardson*, 88. A French translation appeared in 1749, and an Italian translation in 1765.

135. Cheyne to Richardson, 22 September 1741, 2 February 1742, *Letters to Richardson*, 70, 84.

136. Wesley, *Journal* 2:534 (12 April 1742). Wesley may have talked with Cheyne in Bath in December 1741: ibid., 517 and n.

137. Chesterfield to Cheyne, 20 April 1742, quoted in *Letters to Richardson*, 10.

138. Cheyne to Richardson, 10 January 1741/2, 27 January 1742[/3], *Letters to Richardson*, 82, 123. Mullett could not identify this work, and I have been no more successful.

139. Cheyne to Richardson, 9 March 1742, 29 August 1742, 27 January 1742[/3], *Letters to Richardson*, 88, 107, 123.

140. Cheyne to Richardson, 24 March 1743, *Letters to Richardson*, 125.

141. [Peggy Cheyne] to Richardson, 21 April 1743, *Letters to Richardson*, 130.

142. Wesley, *Journal* 3:161–62 (4 February 1745). On the ideal of death in the eighteenth century, see Porter and Porter, *In Sickness and in Health*, ch. 14, pp. 244–57.

143. *Letters to Richardson*, 126–29.

144. Byrom, *Journal* 2, part 2: 362–64.

145. Will of George Cheyne, Public Record Office 727/193, signed 23 March 1738, codicil 1 April 1743, proved 15 June 1743. If John was fourteen in 1731, he must have been twenty-five by the time his father died.

146. Walcot Church Rate Records, Somerset Record Office, D/P/Wal, SW 4/1/4, copy in Bath City Archives. "Mrs Cheney" is listed on Monmouth Street through the 1754 valuation; this may indicate that Peggy occupied the house for a time after her mother's death. Peggy's subsequent whereabouts are unknown. On Margaret Cheyne's death, see [Greenhill], *George Cheyne*, 125–26.

Conclusion: Cheyne in His Time and Ours

1. *Biographia Britannica*, 2d ed., 3:499.

2. Shuttleton, "My Own Crazy Carcase," passim.

3. Mullan, *Sentiment and Sociability*, 16.

4. Hunter, *Before Novels*, ch. 9.

5. Roy Porter, *Mind-forg'd Manacles*, 85.

6. See especially G. S. Rousseau, "Nerves, Spirits, and Fibers"; Mullan, "Hypochondria and Hysteria," Todd, *Sensibility*; Barker-Benfield, *Culture of Sensibility*.

7. Raymond Stephanson, "Richardson's 'Nerves'"; Mullan, "Hypochondria and Hysteria."

8. Stephanson, "Richardson's 'Nerves,'" especially 278–82.

9. Jina Politi, *The Novel and Its Presuppositions* (Amsterdam: Hakkert, 1976), 99, cited in Bechler, "Triall by What Is Contrary," 94.

10. Shuttleton, "My Own Crazy Carcase," 269–70; Troost, "Geography and Gender"; her death is recounted in Samuel Chandler, "Mary Chandler," in *Lives of the Poets* 5:351.

11. Walker, *Ancient Theology*, 231–63.

12. David Hartley, *Observations on Man*, vol. 1. See C. U. M. Smith, "Hartley's Newtonian Neuropsychology."

13. See Thom Verhave, introduction to Priestley, *Hartley's Theory of the Human Mind*; see also Webb, "David Hartley's *Observations on Man*."

14. Hartley, *Observations on Man* 2:196–97, 211–12, 218–20.

15. Lawrence, "Nervous System and Society," 19, 22, 25.

16. Wright, "Metaphysics and Physiology," 271; see above, ch. 6. Another example Porterfield used, that of the role of will in sustaining the concerted action of the eyes, had been mentioned in Newton's "De natura acidorum."

17. French, *Robert Whytt*, 82–83.

18. See ch. 6 above, and Lawrence, "Nervous System and Society," 24–27.

19. *Dr. Cheyne's Account of Himself and of His Writings*. On eighteenth-century handbooks after Cheyne, see Smith, "Prescribing the Rules of Health."

20. Armstrong, *Art of Preserving Health*. Armstrong (1709–79) wrote several medical works. His poem was reprinted a number of times over the next half-century; apart from Cheyne, it certainly also was inspired by the Bath physician Edward Baynard's *Health: A Poem*, which first appeared in 1716 and reached a ninth edition in 1764.

21. Turner, *Body and Society*, 77–78.

22. Wesley, *Primitive Physick*, preface, 9–10, 14–15. Wesley's own enthusiasm for "electrification" as a cure-all shows that he was not entirely untouched by modern science. See Schofield, "John Wesley and Science."

23. Wesley, *Primitive Physick*, 18, 19–22.

24. Rousseau, "John Wesley's *Primitive Physic* (1747)." Rousseau gives a checklist of editions on pp. 253–56. See also Hill, *John Wesley among the Physicians*.

25. Lawrence, "William Buchan: Medicine Laid Open"; Rosenberg, "Medical Text and Social Context."

26. Rosenberg, "Medical Text and Social Context," 54–55. On Tissot, see Emch-Dériaz, *Tissot*.

27. Bordo, *Unbearable Weight*, 3.

28. Ibid., 5, 116–17.

BIBLIOGRAPHY

1. Bibliography of Cheyne's works

(Note: I have endeavored to make this as comprehensive as possible, but gaps still remain.)

A New Theory of Continual Fevers: Wherein, Besides the Appearances of Such Fevers, and the Method of Their Cure, Occasionally, the Structure of the Glands, and the Manner and Laws of Secretion, the Operation of Purgative, Vomitive, and Mercurial Medicines, Are Mechanically Explain'd. London: George Strahan, 1701.

Another edition: Edinburgh: Printed for John Vallange, 1701.

A New Theory of Acute and Slow Continu'd Fevers: Wherein, Besides the Appearances of Such Fevers, and the Method of Their Cure, Occasionally, the Structure of the Glands, and the Manner and Laws of Secretion, the Operation of Purgative, Vomitive, and Mercurial Medicines, Are Mechanically Explain'd: Together with an Application of the Same Theory to Hectick Fevers, and an Essay Concerning the Improvements of the Theory of Medicine. 2d ed., "with many additions." London: George Strahan, 1702.

3d ed., "with many additions." London: H. Parker for George Strahan, 1722.

4th ed. London: George Strahan, 1724.

5th ed. London: George Strahan, 1740.

7th ed. London: Dan. Browne, 1753.

Latin translation: *Specimen de incrementis theoriae medicae: Novae theoriae febrium continuarum acutarum et lentarum praemissum.* Wittenberg, 1711.

Remarks on Two Late Pamphlets Written by Dr. Oliphant, against Dr. Pitcairn's Dissertations. Edinburgh: n.p., 1702.

Fluxionem methodus inversa: Sive quantitatum fluentium leges generaliores. ad celeberrimum virum, Archibaldum Pitcarnium. London: R.Smith, 1703

239

Rudimentorum methodi fluxionum inversae specimina: Quae responsionem continent ad animadversiones Ab. De Moivre in librum G. Cheynaei, M.D. S.R.S. London: G. Strahan, 1705.

Philosophical Principles of Natural Religion: Containing the Elements of Natural Philosophy, and the Proofs for Natural Religion, Arising from Them. London: George Strahan, 1705.

Philosophical Principles of Religion, Natural and Revealed. London: George Strahan, 1715. Reissued 1716.

2d ed. London: George Strahan, 1724.

3d ed., "corrected and enlarged." London: George Strahan, 1725.

4th ed. London: George Strahan, 1734.

5th ed. London: George Strahan, 1736.

Den Schepper in zyn Bestier te kennen in zyne Schepselen. Trans. Lambert ten Kate. 1716. Reprint. Amsterdam: A. van der Kroe, 1772.

Principi filosofici di religione naturale ovvero elementi della filosofia, e della religione da essi derivanti: Tradotta dall'idioma inglese dal cavaliere Tommaso Dereham. Naples: il Moscheni, 1729.

Observations Concerning the Nature and Due Method of Treating the Gout, for the Use of My Worthy Friend Richard Tennison, Esq. London: George Strahan, 1720.

An Essay of the Gout, with an Account of the Nature and Qualities of the Bath Waters: Intended for the Benefit of Richard Tennison, Esq.: The 2d edition. London: George Strahan, 1720.

An Essay on the Gout, with an Account of the Nature and Qualities of the Bath Waters. . . . 3d ed. London: G. Strahan, W. Mears, and H. Hammond, 1721.

An Essay of the True Nature and Due Method of Treating the Gout, Written for the Use of Richard Tennison, Esq.: Together with an Account of the Nature and Quality of the Bath Waters, the Manner of Using Them and the Diseases in Which They Are Proper: As Also of the Nature and Cure of Most Chronical Distempers, Not Publish'd Before. . . . The fourth ed., revis'd, corrected, and enlarg'd to more than double of the former. London: G. Strahan and H. Hammond, 1722.

5th ed. London: G. Strahan, W. Mears; Bath: J. Leak, 1723.

6th ed. London: G. Strahan et al., 1724.

7th ed. London: G. Strahan et al., 1725.

Unauthorized ed. Dublin: George Grierson, 1725.

8th ed. London: G. Strahan 1737.

9th ed. London: G. Strahan, 1738.

10th ed. London: D. Browne, 1753.

An Essay of Health and Long Life. London: George Strahan; Bath: J. Leake, 1724.

2d ed. London: G. Strahan; Bath: J. Leake, 1725.

3d ed. London: G. Strahan; Bath: J. Leake, 1725.

4th ed. London: G. Strahan; Bath: J. Leake, 1725.

5th ed. London: G. Strahan; Bath: J. Leake, 1725.

6th ed. London: G. Strahan; Bath: J. Leake, 1725.

7th ed. London: G. Strahan; Bath: J. Leake, 1725.

8th ed. London: George Strahan; Bath: J. Leake, 1734.

9th ed. London: George Strahan; Bath: J. Leake, 1745.

10th ed. London: George Strahan; Bath: J. Leake, 1745.

A Treatise on Health and Long Life: . . . To Which Is Added to This Edition (Not in Any Other One) the Life of the Author. 10th ed. [*sic*]. Mullingar: W. Kidd, 1787.

Rules and Observations for the Enjoyment of Health and Long Life: Extracted from the Celebrated Doctor Cheyne's Essay on Health and Long Life by a Lover of Mankind. Leeds: G. Wright and son, 1770.

An Essay on Health and Long Life. New York : Edward Gillespy, 1813.

Practical Rules for the Restoration and Preservation of Health London: James Smith, 1822.

2d ed. London: James Smith, 1823.

3d ed. London: James Smith, 1827 .

An Essay of Health and Long Life. Aging and Old Age. New York: Arno Press, 1979.

Tractatus de infirmorum sanitate tuenda, vitaque producenda: Libro ejusdem argumenti anglice edito lange auctior et limatior. London: G. Strahan; Bath: J. Leake, 1726.

Tractatus de infirmorum sanitate tuenda, vitaque producenda . . . cum ejusdem tractatu de natura fibrae . . . accessit huic editioni Clintoni Winteringham commentarium nosologicum. Paris: G. Cavelier, 1742.

Essai sur la santé et sur les moyens de prolonger la vie: Traduit de l'anglois. Paris: Chez Rollin, 1725.

Regles sur la santé, et sur les moyens de prolonger la vie. Paris: Rollin, 1726.

Regles sur la santé, et sur les moyens de prolonger la vie: Traduit de l'anglois. 2d ed. Brussels: Jean Léonard, 1727.

L'art de conserver le santé des personnes valétudinaires, et de leur prolonger la vie: Traduit de latin. . . . Paris: Laurent-Ch. D'Houry, fils, 1755.

Eene proeve om gezond en lang de leven. . . . Amsterdam: i. Tirion, 1734.

Hygiene; Das ist, Grundlicher Unterricht zur Gesundheit und zu einem langen Leben. Frankfurt am Main: Bey Stocks sel. Erben und Schilling, 1744.

De natura fibrae: Ejusque laxae sive resolutae morbis tractatus: Nunc primum editus. London: George Strahan; Bath: James Leake, 1725.
Reprint: Paris: G. Cavelier, 1741.

The English Malady; or, A Treatise of Nervous Diseases of All Kinds, as Spleen, Vapours, Lowness of Spirits, Hypochondriacal, and Hysterical Distempers, &c. London: George Strahan; Bath: James Leake, 1733.
Unauthorized ed. Dublin: George Risk, 1733.
2d ed. London: G. Strahan; Bath: J. Leake, 1734.
3d ed. London: G. Strahan; Bath: J. Leake, 1734.
5th ed. London: G. Strahan; Bath: J. Leake, 1735.
6th ed. London: G. Strahan; Bath: J. Leake, 1735.
The English Malady (1733): A Facsimile Reproduction. Introduction by Eric T. Carlson. Delmar, N.Y.: Scholars' Facsimiles & Reprints, 1976.
The English Malady (1733). Edited by Roy Porter. Tavistock Classics in the History of Psychiatry. London: Tavistock/Routledge, 1991.

An Essay on Regimen, Together with Five Discourses, Medical, Moral, and Philosophical: Serving to Illustrate the Principles and Theory of Philosophical Medicine, and Point Out Some of Its Moral Consequences. London: for C. Rivington; Bath: J. Leake, 1740.
2d ed. London: C. Rivington; Bath: J. Leake, 1740.
3d ed. London: Dan. Browne, 1753.

The Natural Method of Cureing the Diseases of the Body, and the Disorders of the Mind Depending on the Body. London: G. Strahan and John and Paul Knapton, 1742.
2d ed. London: G. Strahan et al., 1742.
3d ed. London: G. Strahan et al., 1742.
5th ed. London: Dan. Browne, 1753.
Méthode naturelle de guérir les maladies du corps et les déréglemens de l'esprit qui en dépendent: Traduite de l'anglois . . . par M. de La Chapelle. Paris: J. F. Quillau, fils, 1749.
Il metodo naturale di cura del Signor Giorgio Cheyne: Tradotto dall' inglese da Cosimo Mei. Padua: Nella Stamperia Volpi, 1765.

Dr Cheyne's Account of Himself & of His Writings, Faithfully Extracted from His Various Works.
      London: J. Wilford, 1743.
2d ed. London: J. Wilford, 1743.

The Letters of George Cheyne to the Countess of Huntingdon. Edited by Charles F. Mullett. San
      Marino, Calif.: Huntington Library, 1940.

The Letters of Doctor George Cheyne to Samuel Richardson (1733–1743). Edited by Charles F.
      Mullett. University of Missouri Studies, vol. 28, no. 1. Columbia: University of
      Missouri Press, 1943.

II. Manuscripts

Aberdeen. University Library.
      MS 2206/8 (David Gregory, Lectures 1692–96).
Bath. City Record Office.
      Walcot Church Rate Records, copy from Somerset Record Office.
Bath. Royal National Hospital for Rheumatic Diseases.
      Committee Minute Book.
Edinburgh. National Library of Scotland.
      Fettercairn MSS (accession 4796, box 104, folder B).
      MS 3440 (Pitcairne correspondence).
      Yester papers (MSS 7011, 7012, 7013, 7014, 7015, 7017, 7018, 7021, 7022).
Edinburgh. Scottish Record Office.
      GD 124 (Mar and Kellie MSS).
      GD 158 (Hume of Marchmont MSS).
      GD 205 (Ogilvy MSS).
      GD 248 (Cullen House MSS, Seafield papers).
      Jolly Kist (Episcopal Church of Scotland MSS).
Edinburgh. University Library.
      MS Dc.I.61 Gregory papers.
      MS Dc.I.62, "Praxeos Pitcarnianae specimina."
      MS Dc.4.35 Gregory's *Notae in Isaaci Newtoni Principia Philosophiae.*
      MS La.II.36 MS copy of Pitcairne's *Epistola Archimedis ad regem Gelonem.*
      MS La.II.303 Letter of Cheyne to Jekyll.
      MS La.III.535 Thomas Bower.
      MS Gen. (Dyer) 130 letter concerning Cheyne.

London. British Library.

    Sloane MSS 3216, 4034, 4039, 4042, 4045, 4046, 4059, 4078.

    Add. MSS 4291 (correspondence).

    Add. MSS 15,911 (correspondence of James Keith).

    Add. MSS 23,204 (correspondence of James Keith).

    Add. MSS 29,243 (Gregory's medical notebook).

    Burney MS 390 (Cheyne's "Platonick Love").

    Lansdowne MSS 841 (correspondence of James Keith).

London. Public Record Office (Chancery Lane).

    Probate records.

London. Royal Society.

    MS 82 (Brook Taylor's commentary on Cheyne's *Philosophical Principles*).

    MS 346 (Gregory papers).

London. Wellcome Institute for the History of Medicine.

    MS 2451 (lecture notes of John Fullerton, 1713–14).

    MS 3915 (lecture notes of George Hepburn, 1693).

Oxford. Bodleian Library.

    Ballard MSS.

    Lister MSS.

Oxford. Christ Church.

    Gregory MSS 131, 346, 350.

    (Also books from David Gregory's library).

San Marino, California. Huntington Library.

    Stowe MSS (ST 57, Chandos letterbooks).

    Loudoun MSS.

    Hastings MSS.

III. Primary sources

Anstey, Christopher. *The Poetical Works of Christopher Anstey, Esq.* London: T. Cadell and W. Davies, 1808.

An Answer to the Pretended Refutation of Dr. Olyphant's Defence. Edinburgh: J.W. for Thomas Carruthers, 1699.

Arbuthnot, John. *An Essay Concerning the Nature of Aliments, and the Choice of Them, According to the Different Constitutions of Human Bodies.* 1731. 4th ed. London: J. and R. Tonson, 1756.

Armstrong, John. *The Art of Preserving Health: A Poem.* London: A. Millar, 1744.

Astruc, Jean. *A Treatise on All the Diseases Incident to Women.* trans. J.R., M.D. London: T. Cooper, 1743.

Barnard, Thomas. *An Historical Character Relating to the Holy and Exemplary Life of the Right Honourable the Lady Elizabeth Hastings.* Leeds: J. Lister for John Swale, 1742.

Bentley, Richard. *Eight Boyle Lectures on Atheism.* 1693. Reprint. New York: Garland, 1976.

Blackmore, Richard. *A Treatise of the Spleen and Vapours.* London: Pemberton, 1725.

Borelli, G. A. *De motu animalium.* 2 vols. Rome: A. Bernabò, 1680–81.

Bourignon, Antoinette. *The Light of the World . . . Faithfully Translated into English: To Which Is Added a Preface to the English Reader.* [Translated and preface by George Garden]. London, 1696.

———. *The Renovation of the Gospel-Spirit: In Three Parts . . . To Which Is Prefix'd a Preface to the English Reader.* [Translated and preface by George Garden]. London: R. Burrough and J. Baker, 1707.

———. *A Warning against the Quakers . . . To Which Is Prefix'd a Preface to the English Reader.* [Translated by George Garden]. London: R. Burrough and J. Baker, 1708.

Bourignon, Antoinette, and Pierre Poiret. *La Vie de Damlle. Antoinette Bourignon: Écrite partie par elle-meme, partie par une personne de sa connoissance.* Amsterdam: Jean Riewerts and Pierre Arents, 1683.

Burton, Robert. *The Anatomy of Melancholy.* Edited by Floyd Dell and Paul Jordan-Smith. New York: George H. Doran, 1927.

Byrom, John. *The Private Journal and Literary Remains of John Byrom.* Edited by Richard Parkinson. 2 vols. in 4 parts. Manchester: Chetham Society, 1854–57.

Chamberlen, Hugh. *Remarks on Giving Vomits in Fevers: In a Letter to a Friend.* [London], 1700.

Chandler, Mary. *A Description of Bath: A Poem: Humbly Inscribed to Her Royal Highness the Princess Amelia.* 2d ed. London: J. Leake and J. Gray, 1734.

Clarke, Samuel. *A Demonstration of the Being and Attributes of God.* London: J. Knapton, 1705.

Cockburn, John. *Bourignianism Detected; or, The Delusions and Errors of Antonia Bourignon and Her Growing Sect, Which May Also Serve for a Discovery of All Other Enthusiastical Impostures. Narrative I.* London: C. Browne, W. Keblewhite, H. Hindmarsh, 1698.

Cockburn, William. *Profluvia Ventris; or, The Nature and Causes of Loosenesses Plainly Discovered.* London: B.Barker and G. Strahan, 1701.

———. *Sea Diseases.* 2d ed. London: George Strahan, 1706.

Cowper, William. *Myotomia Reformata.* London: R. Knaplock et al., 1724.

Craig. John. "Specimen methodi generalis determinandi figurarum quadraturas . . . ad D. Georgium Cheynaeum, M.D." *Philosophical Transactions* 23 (1703): 1346.

—————. *Mathematical Principles of Christian Theology.* Edited by Richard Nash. Carbondale/ Edwardsville: Southern Illinois University Press, 1991.

Defoe, Daniel. *A Tour thro' the Whole Island of Great Britain.* 3d ed. 4 vols. London: J. Osborn et al., 1742.

—————. *A Tour through the Whole Island of Great Britain.* 1727. Edited and abridged by Pat Rogers. Harmondsworth: Penguin, 1971.

De Moivre, Abraham. *Animadversiones in D. Georgii Cheynaei tractatum de fluxionum methodo inversa.* London: E. Midwinter, D. Midwinter, and T. Leigh, 1704.

Descartes, René. *Oeuvres.* Edited by Charles Adam and Paul Tannery. 13 vols. Paris: Vrin, 1964–75.

Dryden, John. *Works.* Edited by Walter Scott. London: W. Miller, 1808.

Fiennes, Celia. *The Illustrated Journeys of Celia Fiennes.* Edited by Christopher Morris. London: Macdonald, 1982.

Floyer, John and Edward Baynard. *[Psychroloysia]; or, The History of Cold-Bathing, Both Ancient and Modern: In Two Parts: The First Written by Sir John Floyer, of Litchfield, kt.: The Second, Treating of the Genuine Use of Hot and Cold Baths . . . by Dr. Edward Baynard.* 1707. 5th ed. London: William and John Innys, 1722.

Forbes, John. *The First Book of the Irenicum of John Forbes of Corse.* Edited by E. G. Selwyn. Cambridge: Cambridge University Press, 1923.

Freind, John. *Emmenologia.* 1703. Translated by Thomas Dale. London: T. Cox, 1729.

Garden, George. "A Discourse concerning the Modern Theory of Generation, by Dr. George Garden of Aberdeen." *Philosophical Transactions* 16, no. 192 (1690/1).

—————. *An Apology for M. Antonia Bourignon.* London: D. Brown et al., 1699.

Garden, James. *Comparative Theology; or, The True and Solid Grounds for Pure and Peaceable Theology.* London, 1700. First published in Latin, 1699.

Green, Matthew. "The Spleen." In *The Oxford Anthology of English Poetry,* vol. 1, edited by John Wain. New York: Oxford University Press, 1990.

Gregory, David. *Astronomiae physicae et geometricae elementa.* Oxford, 1702.

—————. *David Gregory, Isaac Newton, and Their Circle.* Edited by W. S. Hiscock. Oxford: Oxford University Press, 1937.

Halley, Edmond. *Correspondence and Papers of Edmond Halley.* Edited by E. F. MacPike. Oxford: Clarendon Press, 1932.

Hamilton, David. *The Diary of David Hamilton, 1709–1714*. Edited by Philip Roberts. Oxford: Clarendon Press, 1975.

Harris, Walter. *An Exact Enquiry into, and Cure of the Acute Diseases of Infants: Englished by W.C., M.S.: With a Preface in Vindication of the Work*. London: for Sam. Clement, 1693.

Hartley, David. *Observations on Man, His Frame, His Duty, and His Expectations*. In 2 parts. London: S. Richardson for James Leake and Wm. Frederick, Bath, and Charles Hitch and Stephen Austin, London, 1749.

Harvey, William. *Exercitatio anatomica de motu cordis et sanguinis in animalibus*. English translation by Chauncey D. Leake. Springfield, Ill., and Baltimore, Md.: C. C. Thomas, 1931.

Heylyn, John. *A Sermon Preached to the Societies for Reformation of Manners, at St. Mary-le-Bow, on Wednesday, January the 8th, 1728*. London: Downing, 1729.

Historical Manuscripts Commission. *Downshire MSS*. London: HMSO, 1924.

———. *Manuscripts of J. B. Fortescue, Esq., Preserved at Dropmore*. vol. 1. London: HMSO, 1892.

———. *Portland MSS*. London: HMSO, 1897.

———. *Report on the Manuscripts of His Grace the Duke of Portland, K.G., Preserved at Welbeck Abbey*. vol. 7. London: HMSO, 1901.

———. *Report on the Manuscripts of the Late Reginald Hastings, Esq*. vol. 3. London: HMSO, 1934.

Hume, David. *The Letters of David Hume*. Vol. 1. Edited by J. Y. T. Greig. Oxford: Clarendon Press, 1932.

[Johnson, T., pseud.]. *The Tryal of Colley Cibber, Comedian &c for Writing a Book Intitled An Apology for His Life, &c. Being a Thorough Examination Thereof: Wherein He Is Proved Guilty of High Crimes and Misdemeanors against the English Language . . . And the Arraignment of George Cheyne, Physician at Bath, for the Philosophical, Physical, and Theological Heresies, Uttered in His Last Book on Regimen*. London: for the Author, by W. Lewis, E. Curll, et al., 1740.

Kerby-Miller, Charles, ed. *The Memoirs of Martinus Scriblerus*. 1950. Reprint. New York: Oxford University Press, 1988.

Law, William. *A Practical Treatise upon Christian Perfection*. 1726. 4th ed. London: William Innys, 1741.

———. *A Serious Call to Devout and Holy Life*. 1728. Reprint. London: Dent, Everyman, 1967.

———. *An Appeal to all That Doubt, or Disbelieve the Truths of the Gospel, Whether They Be Deists, Arians, Socinians, or Nominal Christians. . . .* London: W. Innys, 1742.

————. *Selected Mystical Writings of William Law.* Edited by Stephen Hobhouse. London: Salisbury Press, 1948.

LeClerc, Jean. *Bibliothèque ancienne et moderne.* Vol. 3. Amsterdam: David Mortier, 1715.

Leibniz, G. W. *Der Briefwechsel des Gottfried Wilhelm Leibniz in der Koniglichen offentlichen Bibliothek zu Hannover.* Edited by Eduard Bodemann. 1889. Reprint. Hildesheim: Olms, 1966.

Leighton, Robert. *The Works of Robert Leighton, D.D.* London: T. Nelson, 1860.

A Letter to George Cheyne, M.D., F.R.S., Shewing, the Danger of Laying Down General Rules to Those Who Are Not Acquainted with the Animal Oeconomy, &c. . . . London: J. Graves, J. Hooke, and T. Jeffries, [1724].

Lister, Martin. "A Letter from Dr Martin Lister, F.R.S., to Dr Tancred Robinson, F.R.S., Concerning Pouder'd Blues Passing the Lacteal Veins, &c." *Philosophical Transactions* 22 (1701): 819–20.

Mandeville, Bernard. *A Treatise of the Hypochondriack and Hysterick Diseases: In Three Dialogues.* 1711. 2d ed. London: J. Tonson, 1730.

————. *The Fable of the Bees.* Edited by Phillip Harth. Harmondsworth: Penguin, 1970.

Marsay, Charles Hector de St. Georges de. *Témoignage d'un enfant de la verité & droiture de voyes de l'esprit; ou, Explication des trois premiers chapitres de la Genèse; ou, L'on traite de plusieurs merveilles & mystères de la Création.* Berlebourg: Christoffle Michel Regelein, 1731.

————. *Discourses on Subjects Related to the Spiritual Life.* Edinburgh: J. and W. Ruddimans, 1749.

Mead, Richard. *A Mechanical Account of Poisons in Several Essays.* London: J. R. for Ralph South, 1702.

————. *Of the Influence of the Sun and Moon on Humane Bodies.* London: R. Wellington, 1712.

————. *A Short Discourse Concerning Pestilential Contagion, and the Methods to Be Used to Prevent It.* 6th ed. London: for Sam. Buckley and Ralph Smith, 1720.

Morgan, Thomas. *Philosophical Principles of Medicine.* London: J. Osborne et al., 1725.

————. *The Mechanical Practice of Physick: In Which the Specific Method Is Examine'd and Exploded, and the Beleineian Hypothesis of Animal Secretion and Muscular Motion Consider'd and Refuted.* London: T. Woodward, 1735.

————. *A Letter to Dr Cheyne, Occasioned by Dr Robinson's Letter to Him: In Defence of His Treatise of the Animal Oeconomy, against Dr Morgan's Objections in His Mechanical Practice.* London: Thos. Cox, 1738.

Morland, Samuel. "An Abstract of Dr. Mead's Mechanical Account of Poisons." *Philosophical Transactions* 23 (1703): 1320–28.

Newton, Isaac. *Philosophiae naturalis principia mathematica*. Edited by I. B. Cohen and Alexandre
    Koyré. 2 vols. Cambridge, Mass.: Harvard University Press, 1972.

————. *Opticks*. 4th ed. 1730. Reprint. New York: Dover, 1952.

————. *The Correspondence of Isaac Newton*. Edited by H. W. Turnbull, J. F. Scott, A. R. Hall,
    and Laura Tilling. 7 vols. Cambridge: Cambridge University Press, 1959–77.

Nichols, John. *Literary Anecdotes of the Eighteenth Century*. 2 vols. London: Nichols, 1812.

Oliphant, Charles. *A Short Discourse to Prove the Usefulness of Vomiting in Fevers, by Plain Reasoning
    and the Authority of the Best Physicians, Ancient and Modern*. Edinburgh: Thomas
    Carruthers, 1699.

————. *A Refutation of the Short Answer to the Examination of Dr. Pitcairn's Dissertations*.
    Edinburgh: 1702.

————. *A Short Answer to Two Lybels Lately Published against D.O. by Drs. Cheyne and Pitcairn*.
    [Edinburgh], 1702.

Oliver, William. *A Practical Dissertation on Bath Waters . . . To Which Is Added, a Relation of a Very
    Extraordinary Sleeper near Bath*. London: A. Bell, 1707.

*The Oxford Methodists: Being Some Account of a Society of Young Gentlemen in That City, So Denomi-
    nated: Setting Forth Their Rise, Views, and Designs: With Some Occasional Remarks on a Letter
    Inserted in Fog's Journal of December 9th, Relating to Them: In a Letter from a Gentleman near
    Oxford, to His Friend in London*. London: J. Roberts, 1733.

Peirce, Robert. *Bath Memoirs; or, Observation in Three and Forty Years Practice, at the Bath*. Bristol:
    printed for H. Hammond, 1697.

[Pillo-Tisanus, pseud.] *An Epistle to Ge———ge Ch———ne MD FRS upon His Essay of Health
    and Long Life with Notes Physical and Metaphysical: By Pillo-Tisanus, a Lover of the Mathe-
    maticks, and Practitioner of the Occult Sciences*. London: J. Roberts, 1725.

Pitcairne, Archibald. *The Assembly*. 1692. Edited by Terence Tobin. Lafayette, In.: Purdue
    University Studies, 1972.

————. *Apollo Staticus; or, The Art of Curing Fevers by the Staticks. . . .* Edinburgh: J. W. for James
    Wardlow, 1695.

————. *Dissertation de curatione febrium, quae per evacuationes instituitur*. [Edinburgh]: G.
    Mosman, 1695.

————. *The Philosophical and Mathematical Elements of Physick*. Translated by John Quincy.
    London: Andrew Bell and John Osborn, 1718.

————. *The Whole Works of Dr Archibald Pitcairn*. Translated by George Sewell and J. T.
    Desaguliers. 1715. 2d ed. London: E. Curll, J. Pemberton, and W. and J. Innys,
    1727.

———. *Elementa medicinae physico-mathematica . . . item ejusdem opuscula medica.* Venice: A. Bortoli, 1740.

———. *The Best of Our Owne: Letters of Archibald Pitcairne, 1652–1713.* Edited by W. T. Johnston. Edinburgh: Saorsa Books, 1979.

Pope, Alexander. *The Correspondence of Alexander Pope.* Edited by George Sherburn. 6 vols. Oxford: Clarendon Press, 1956.

Priestley, Joseph. *Hartley's Theory of the Human Mind.* 1775. Reprint. New York: AMS Press, 1973.

Purcell, John. *A Treatise of Vapours, or Hysterick Fits.* London: E. Place, 1707.

Quinton, John. *Practical Observations in Physick, but Especially of the Nature of Mineral Waters and Metallick Medicines.* 2d ed. London: J. Morphew, 1711.

———. *De Thermis; or, Of Natural and Artificial Baths.* London: J. Roberts, 1726.

———. *A Treatise of Warm Bath Water, and of Cures Made Lately at Bath in Somersetshire. . . .* 2 vols. Oxford: n.p., 1733–34.

Remarks on Dr Cheyne's Essay of Health and Long Life: Wherein Some of the Doctor's Notorious Contradictions, and False Reasonings are laid open . . . By a Fellow of the Royal Society. London: Aaron Ward and T. Cos, [1724].

Richardson, Samuel. *Pamela; or, Virtue Rewarded.* 1740. Reprint. New York: New American Library, 1980.

———. *Selected Letters of Samuel Richardson.* Edited by John Carroll. Oxford: Clarendon Press, 1964.

Robinson, Bryan. *A Treatise of the Animal Oeconomy.* Dublin: George Grierson, 1732.

———. *A Treatise of the Animal Oeconomy.* 2d ed. Dublin: S. Powell for George Ewing and William Smith, 1734.

———. *A Letter to Dr Cheyne, Containing an Account of the Motion of Water through Orifices and Pipes: And an Answer to Dr. Morgan's Remarks on Dr Robinson's Treatise of the Animal Oeconomy.* Dublin: G. Ewing and W. Smith, 1735.

Robinson, Nicholas. *A New Theory of Physick and Diseases, Founded on the Principles of the Newtonian Philosophy.* London: C. Rivington, J. Lacy, and J. Clarke, 1725.

———. *A New System of the Spleen, Vapours, and Hypochondriack Melancholy.* London: A Bettesworth, W. Innys, and C. Rivington, 1729.

Sacheverell, Henry. *The Perils of False Brethren, Both in Church and State.* London: Henry Clements, 1709.

Scott-Moncrief, Robert, ed. *The Household Book of Lady Grisell Baillie, 1692–1733.* Edinburgh: University of Edinburgh Press for the Scottish History Society, 1911.

Scougal, Henry. *The Life of God in the Soul of Man.* London: for Charles Smith and William Jacob, 1677.

Sibbald, Robert. *Memoirs.* Edited by Francis Paget Hett. London: Oxford University Press, 1932.

Smollett, Tobias. *The Expedition of Humphry Clinker.* 1771. Reprint. Harmondsworth: Penguin, 1967.

The Spectator. Edited by Donald F. Bond. 5 vols. Oxford: Clarendon Press, 1965.

Strother, Edward. *An Essay on Sickness and Health: Wherein Are Contain'd, All Necessary Cautions and Directions, for the Regulation of Diseas'd and Healthy Persons: In Which Dr. Cheyne's Mistaken Opinions in His Late Essay, Are Occasionally Taken Notice Of.* London: H. P. for Charles Rivington, 1725.

Stukeley, William. *Of the Spleen.* London: for the author, 1723.

———. *Of the Gout.* London: J. Roberts, 1734.

Sydenham, Thomas. *The Works of Thomas Sydenham, M.D.* Translated by R. G. Latham. Vol. 2. London: Sydenham Society, 1850.

Tryon, Thomas [Phylotheus Physiologus]. *Monthly Observations for the Preserving of Health, with a Long and Comfortable Life, in This Our Pilgrimage on Earth: But More Particularly for the Spring and Summer Seasons.* London, A. Sowle, 1688.

———. *Miscellanea.* London: T. Sowle, 1696.

Ward, Ned. *The London Spy.* 1703. Edited by Arthur L. Hayward. London: Cassell, 1927.

Warner, Rebecca, ed. *Original Letters.* London: Longman, Hurst, Rees, Orme, and Brown, 1817.

Wesley, John. *Primitive Physick.* Reprint of Chicago, 1880, edition retitled *Primitive Remedies.* Santa Barbara, Calif.: Woodbridge, 1975.

———. *The Journal of John Wesley.* Edited by N. Curnock. 5 vols. London: Charles Kelly, 1909.

———. *Letters of the Rev. John Wesley.* Edited by John Telford. 6 vols. London: Epworth Press, 1931.

Whiston, William. *Historical Memoirs of the Life of Dr. Samuel Clarke.* 2d ed. London: Fletcher Gyles and J. Roberts, 1730.

Wodrow, Robert. *Analecta.* 3 vols. Edinburgh, 1842.

Wood, John. *A Description of Bath.* 2d ed. 2 vols. in 1. London: W. Bathoe and T. Lownds, 1765.

Wordsworth, Christopher. *Scholae academicae.* 1877. Reprint. London: Frank Cass, 1968.

Woodward, John. *The State of Physick: And of Diseases, with an Inquiry into the Causes of the Late Increase of Them: But More Particularly of the Small-pox: With Some Considerations upon the New Practice of Purgeing in That Disease.* London, T. Horne, 1718.

————. *The Art of Getting into Practice in Physick, Here at Present in London: In a Letter to That Very Ingenious and Most Learned Physician, (Lately Come to Town) Dr. Timothy Vanbustle, M.D., A.B.C., &c.* London: J. Peele, 1722.

Wynter, John. *Cyclus Metasyncriticus; or, An Essay on Chronical Diseases.* London: W. and J. Innys, and J. Leake at Bath, 1725.

————. *Of Bathing in the Hot Baths, at Bathe: Chiefly with Regard to the Palsie, and Some Diseases in Women: In a Letter Addressed to Doctor Freind.* London: W. Innys; Bath: James Leake, 1728.

IV. Reference Works

Anderson, P. J., ed. *Officers and Graduates of University and King's College, 1495–1860.* Aberdeen: New Spalding Club, 1893.

————. *Fasti academiae mariscallanae, 1593–1860.* 3 vols. Aberdeen: New Spalding Club, 1889–98.

Biographia Britannica. Edited by Andrew Kippis. 1st ed. 5 vols. London: W. Innys et al., 1747–66. 2d ed. 5 vols. London: C. Bathurst, W. Strahan, et al., 1778–93.

Fasti Aberdonenses: Selections from the Records of the University and King's College in Aberdeen, 1494–1854. Aberdeen: Spalding Club, 1854.

Foster, Joseph. *Alumni Oxonienses, 1715–1886.* Oxford: Parker, 1888.

————. *Members of Parliament, Scotland.* 2d ed. London: Hazell, Watson, and Viney, 1882.

List of Pollable Persons in the Shire of Aberdeen, 1696. Vol. 2. Aberdeen: William Bennett, 1844.

The Lives of the Poets of Great Britain and Ireland. Edited by Robert Shiels, revised by Theophilus Cibber. 5 vols. London: R. Griffiths, 1753.

Munk, W. *Roll of the Royal College of Physicians of London.* Vols. 1, 2. London, 1878.

Nieuw Nederlandsch biografisch woordenboek. Edited by P. C. Molhuysen and P. J. Blok. 10 vols. Leiden: A. W. Sijthoff's uitgevers-matschappij, 1911–37.

Paul, J. B., ed. *Scots Peerage.* Edinburgh: David Douglas, 1910.

Plomer, Henry. *A Dictionary of the Printers and Booksellers Who Were at Work in England, Scotland, and Ireland from 1688 to 1725.* London: for the Bibliographical Society by Oxford University Press, 1922.

Register of Marriages for the Parish of Edinburgh, 1595–1700. Edited by Henry Paton. Edinburgh: James Skinner for the Scottish Historical Society, 1905.

Register of the Privy Council of Scotland. 3d ser., vol. 16 (1691). Edinburgh: HMSO, 1970.

Register of the Society of Writers to Her Majesty's Signet. Edinburgh: Clark Constable, 1983.

Roll of Edinburgh Burgesses, 1406–1700. Edited by C. B. Boog Watson. Edinburgh: James Skinner for the Scottish Historical Society, 1929.

Sedgwick, Romney. ed. *The House of Commons, 1715–1754.* 2 vols. *History of Parliament.* New York: Oxford University Press, 1970.

Smith, R. W. Innes. *English-Speaking Students of Medicine at the University of Leiden.* Edinburgh: Oliver and Boyd, 1932.

Wallis, P. J., and R. V. Wallis. *Eighteenth-Century Medics.* 2d ed. Newcastle upon Tyne: Project for Historical Biobibliography, 1988.

V. Secondary Sources

Aitken, George. *The Life and Works of John Arbuthnot.* Oxford: Clarendon Press, 1892.

Andrew, Donna. *Philanthropy and Police.* Princeton, N.J.: Princeton University Press, 1989.

Andrews, Jonathan. "A Respectable Mad Doctor? Dr Richard Hale, F.R.S. (1670–1728)." *Notes and Records of the Royal Society* 44 (1990): 169–203.

Appleby, Joyce. "One Good Turn Deserves Another." *American Historical Review* 94 (1989): 1326–32.

Arber, Agnes. "Analogy in the History of Science." In *Studies and Essays in the History of Science and Learning Offered in Homage to George Sarton*, edited by M. F. Ashley Montagu, 221–33. New York: Henry Schuman, 1946.

Balsama, George. "Madame Guyon, Heterodox." *Church History* 42 (1973): 350–65.

Barbeau, A. *Life and Letters at Bath in the XVIII Century.* London: William Heinemann, 1902.

Barfoot, Michael. "Hume and the Culture of Science in the Early Eighteenth Century." In *Studies in the Philosophy of the Scottish Enlightenment*, edited by M. A. Stewart, 151–90. Oxford: Clarendon Press, 1990.

Barker-Benfield, G. J. *The Culture of Sensibility.* Chicago: University of Chicago Press, 1992.

Barry, Jonathan. "Piety and the Patient." In *Patients and Practitioners*, edited by Roy Porter, 145–75. Cambridge: Cambridge University Press, 1985.

Bates, Donald G. "Thomas Sydenham and the Medical Meaning of 'Method.'" *Bulletin of the History of Medicine* 51 (1977): 324–38.

Beattie, Lester. *John Arbuthnot.* Cambridge, Mass.: Harvard University Press, 1935.

Bechler, Rosemary. "'Trial by What Is Contrary': Samuel Richardson and Christian Dialectic." In *Samuel Richardson: Passion and Prudence*, edited by Valerie Grosvenor Myer, 93–113. London: Vision; Totowa, N.J.: Barnes and Noble, 1986.

Bechler, Zev. "Introduction: Some Issues of Newtonian Historiography." In *Contemporary Newtonian Research*, edited by Zev Bechler, 1–20. Dordrecht: Reidel, 1982.

Beier, Lucinda McCray. *Sufferers and Healers*. London: Routledge, 1987.

Bell, Rudolph. *Holy Anorexia*. Chicago: University of Chicago Press, 1985.

Bennett, G. V. "King William III and the Episcopate." In *Essays in Modern Church History in Memory of Norman Sykes*, edited by G. V. Bennett and J. D. Walsh, 104–31. New York: Oxford University Press, 1966.

Biagioli, Mario. *Galileo Courtier*. Chicago: University of Chicago Press, 1993.

Bono, James. "Science, Discourse, and Literature: The Role/Rule of Metaphor in Science." In *Literature and Science*, edited by Stuart Peterfreund, 59–89. Boston: Northeastern University Press, 1990.

Bordo, Susan. *Unbearable Weight: Feminism, Western Culture, and the Body*. Berkeley and Los Angeles: University of California Press, 1993.

———. *Twilight Zones*. Berkeley and Los Angeles: University of California Press, 1997.

Borsay, Anne. "Cash and Conscience: Financing the General Hospital at Bath c. 1738–1750." *Social History of Medicine* 6 (1991): 207–29.

Borsay, Peter. *The English Urban Renaissance*. Oxford: Clarendon Press, 1989.

Bower, Alexander. *The History of the University of Edinburgh*. 2 vols. Edinburgh: Oliphant, Waugh, and Innes, 1817.

Bowles, Geoffrey. "Physical, Human, and Divine Attraction in the Life and Thought of George Cheyne." *Annals of Science* 31 (1974): 473–88.

———. "The Place of Newtonian Explanation in English Popular Thought, 1687–1727." D.Phil. thesis, Oxford, 1977.

Brewer, John. "Commercialization and Politics." In *The Birth of a Consumer Society: The Commercialization of Eighteenth-Century England*, edited by Neil McKendrick, John Brewer, and J. H. Plumb, 197–262. Bloomington: Indiana University Press, 1982.

Brooke, John Hedley. *Science and Religion: Some Historical Perspectives*. Cambridge: Cambridge University Press, 1991.

Brown, T. M. "The College of Physicians and the Acceptance of Iatromechanism in England, 1665–1695." *Bulletin of the History of Medicine* 44 (1970): 12–30.

———. "The Mechanical Philosophy and the 'Animal Oeconomy.'" Ph.D. diss. Princeton University, 1968. New York: Arno, 1981.

Brumberg, Joan Jacobs. *Fasting Girls*. 1988. Reprint. New York: Plume, 1989.

Buckroyd, Julia. *Church and State in Scotland, 1660–1681*. Edinburgh: John Donald, 1980.

Bulloch, J. M. "An Aberdeen Falstaff: Dr. George Cheyne, Our Double M.D." *Aberdeen University Library Bulletin* 7 (1930): 393–411.

Burnett, George. *The Family of Burnett of Leys, with Collateral Branches.* Edited by James Allardyce. Aberdeen: New Spalding Club, 1901.

Bynum, Caroline Walker. *Jesus as Mother.* Berkeley and Los Angeles: University of California Press, 1982.

———. *Holy Feast and Holy Fast.* Berkeley and Los Angeles: University of California Press, 1987.

Cantor, G. N. "The Eighteenth-Century Problem." *History of Science* 20 (1982): 44–63.

Castelli, Elizabeth. "'I Will Make Mary Male': Pieties of the Body and Gender Transformation of Christian Women in Late Antiquity." In *Body Guards: The Cultural Politics of Gender Ambiguity*, edited by Julia Epstein and Kristina Straub, 29–49. New York: Routledge, 1991.

Castle, Terry. "The Female Thermometer." *Representations* 17 (1987): 1–27.

Cattaneo, Arturo. "Dr Cheyne and Richardson: Epistolary Friendship and Scientific Advice." In *Science and Imagination in XVIIIth-Century British Culture*, edited by Sergio Rossi, 113–32. Milan: Edizioni Unicopli, 1987.

Chalklin, C. W. *The Provincial Towns of Georgian England.* London: Edward Arnold, 1974.

Child, Paul W. "Discourse and Practice in Eighteenth-Century Medical Literature: The Case of George Cheyne." Ph.D. diss. University of Notre Dame, 1992.

Christie, J. R. R. "The Origins and Development of the Scottish Scientific Community, 1680–1760." *History of Science* 12 (1974): 122–41.

Clark, G. N. *The Later Stuarts, 1660–1714.* 2d ed. Oxford: Clarendon Press, 1955.

Clark, J. C. D. *English Society, 1688–1832.* Cambridge: Cambridge University Press, 1985.

Clarke, Edwin. "The Doctrine of the Hollow Nerve in the Seventeenth and Eighteenth Centuries." In *Medicine, Science, and Culture*, edited by Lloyd G. Stevenson and Robert Multhauf, 123–41. Baltimore: Johns Hopkins University Press, 1968.

Clive, John. "The Social Background of the Scottish Renaissance." In *Scotland in the Age of Improvement*, edited by N. T. Phillipson and Rosalind Mitchison, 225–44. Edinburgh: Edinburgh University Press, 1970.

Cohen, Paula Marantz. *The Daughter's Dilemma: Family Process and the Nineteenth-Century Domestic Novel.* Ann Arbor: University of Michigan Press, 1991.

Coleman, William. "Health and Hygiene in the *Encyclopédie*: A Medical Doctrine for the Bourgeoisie." *Journal of the History of Medicine* 29 (1974): 399–421.

———. "Mechanical Philosophy and Hypothetical Physiology." In *The Annus Mirabilis of Isaac Newton*, edited by Robert Palter, 322–32. Cambridge, Mass.: MIT Press, 1970.

Coley, Noel. "Physicians, Chemists, and the Analysis of Mineral Waters: 'The Most Difficult Part of Chemistry.'" In *The Medical History of Waters and Spas*, edited by Roy Porter, Medical History, supplement 10 (1990): 55–66.

Colie, Rosalie. *Light and Enlightenment*. Cambridge: Cambridge University Press, 1957.

Colley, Linda. *In Defiance of Oligarchy: The Tory Party, 1714–1760*. Cambridge: Cambridge University Press, 1982.

Cook, Harold J. *The Decline of the Old Medical Regime in Stuart London*. Ithaca, N.Y.: Cornell University Press, 1986.

———. "Practical Medicine and the British Armed Forces after the 'Glorious Revolution.'" *Medical History* 34 (1990): 1–26.

———. "The Rose Case Reconsidered: Physic and the Law in Augustan England." *Journal of the History of Medicine* 45 (1990): 527–55.

———. "Sir John Colbatch and Augustan Medicine: Experimentalism, Character, and Entrepreneurialism." *Annals of Science* 47 (1990): 475–505.

Corfield, Penelope. *The Impact of English Towns, 1700–1800*. Oxford: Oxford University Press, 1982.

Corrington, Gail Paterson. "Anorexia, Asceticism, and Autonomy: Self-Control as Liberation and Transcendence." *Journal of Feminist Studies in Religion* 2 (1986): 51–63.

Coudert, Allison. "Forgotten Ways of Knowing." In *The Shapes of Knowledge from the Renaissance to the Enlightenment*, edited by D. R. Kelley and R. H. Popkin, 83–99. Dordrecht: Kluwer, 1991.

Craig, W. R. *History of the Royal College of Physicians of Edinburgh*. Oxford: Blackwell, 1976.

Crawford, Patricia. "Attitudes to Menstruation in Seventeenth-Century England." *Past and Present* 91 (May 1981): 47–73.

Cressy, David. "Kinship and Kin Interaction in Early Modern England." *Past and Present* 113 (November 1986): 38–69.

Cunningham, Andrew. "Sydenham versus Newton: The Edinburgh Fever Dispute of the 1690s between Andrew Brown and Archibald Pitcairn." *Medical History* supp. 1 (1981): 71–98.

———. "How the Principia Got Its Name; or, Taking Natural Philosophy Seriously." *History of Science* 29 (1991): 377–92.

Curran, Patricia. *Grace before Meals: Food Rituals and Body Discipline in Convent Culture*. Urbana: University of Illinois Press, 1989.

Curtis, T. C., and W. A. Speck. "The Societies for the Reformation of Manners." *Literature and History* 3 (1976): 45–64.

Davis, Natalie Zemon. "City Women and Religious Change." In *Society and Culture in Early Modern France*, 65–95. Stanford, Calif.: Stanford University Press, 1975.

Dear, Peter. "Totius in verba: Rhetoric and Authority in the Early Royal Society." *Isis* 76 (1985): 145–61.

De Baar, Mirjam. "Prophecy, Femininity, and Spiritual Leadership in the Seventeenth Century: The Case of Antoinette Bourignon." Unpub. ms. 1990.

De Maria, Robert. *Samuel Johnson and the Life of Reading*. Baltimore: Johns Hopkins University Press, 1997.

De Porte, Michael. *Nightmares and Hobbyhorses*. San Marino, Calif.: Huntington Library, 1974.

Dewhurst, Kenneth. *Dr. Thomas Sydenham, 1624–1689: His Life and Original Writings*. Berkeley and Los Angeles: University of California Press, 1966.

Dickson, P. G. M. *The Financial Revolution in England*. London: Macmillan, 1967.

Dobbs, B. J. T. *The Foundations of Newton's Alchemy*. Cambridge: Cambridge University Press, 1975.

———. *The Janus Faces of Genius*. Cambridge: Cambridge University Press, 1992.

Donnison, Jean. *Midwives and Medical Men*. London: Heinemann, 1977.

Duden, Barbara. *The Woman beneath the Skin*. Translated by Thomas Dunlap. Cambridge, Mass.: Harvard University Press, 1991.

Eagles, Christina M. "The Mathematical Work of David Gregory, 1659–1708." Ph.D. diss. University of Edinburgh, 1977.

Earle, Peter. *The Making of the English Middle Class*. London: Methuen, 1989.

Eaves, T. C. Duncan, and Ben D. Kimpel. *Samuel Richardson: A Biography*. Oxford: Clarendon Press, 1971.

Elias, Norbert. *The Court Society*. Translated by Edmund Jephcott. New York: Pantheon, 1983.

———. "Scientific Hierarchies." In *Scientific Establishments and Hierarchies*, edited by Norbert Elias, Herminio Martins, and Richard Whitley, 3–69. Sociology of the Sciences 6. Dordrecht: Reidel, 1982.

Emch-Dériaz, Antoinette. *Tissot: Physician of the Enlightenment*. New York: P. Lang, 1992.

Emerson, Roger L. "Latitudinarianism and the English Deists." In *Deism, Masonry, and the Enlightenment*, edited by J. A. Leo Lemay, 19–48. Newark: University of Delaware Press, 1987.

———. "Sir Robert Sibbald, Kt, the Royal Society of Scotland, and the Origins of the Scottish Enlightenment." *Annals of Science* 45 (1988): 41–72.

———. "Science and Moral Philosophy in the Scottish Enlightenment." In *Studies in the Philosophy of the Scottish Enlightenment*, edited by M. A. Stewart, 11–36. Oxford: Clarendon Press, 1990.

Erickson, Robert. *Mother Midnight*. New York: AMS Press, 1986.

'Espinasse, Margaret. "The Decline and Fall of Restoration Science." *Past and Present* 14 (July 1958): 71–89.

Falconer, R. W. *History of the Royal Mineral Water Hospital, Bath*. 3d issue. Bath: for the Royal Mineral Water Hospital, 1888.

Ferguson, William. *Scotland's Relations with England*. Edinburgh: John Donald, 1977.

Figlio, Karl. "Chlorosis and Chronic Disease in Nineteenth-Century Britain." *Social History* 3 (1978): 167–97.

Fischer-Homberger, Esther. "Hypochondriasis of the Eighteenth Century: Neurosis of the Present Century." *Bulletin of the History of Medicine* 46 (1972): 391–401.

Fisher, F. J. "The Development of London as a Centre of Conspicuous Consumption in the Sixteenth and Seventeenth Centuries." *Transactions of the Royal Historical Society*, 4th ser., 30 (1948): 37–50.

Fissell, Mary. *Patients, Power, and the Poor in Eighteenth-Century Bristol*. Cambridge: Cambridge University Press, 1991.

Flinn, M. W. *The European Demographic System, 1500–1820*. Baltimore: Johns Hopkins University Press, 1981.

Flynn, Carol Houlihan. *The Body in Swift and Defoe*. Cambridge: Cambridge University Press, 1990.

———. "Running out of Matter: The Body Exercised in Eighteenth-Century Fiction." In *The Languages of Psyche*, edited by G. S. Rousseau, 147–85. Berkeley and Los Angeles: University of California Press, 1990.

Force, J. E. *William Whiston, Honest Newtonian*. Cambridge: Cambridge University Press, 1985.

Force, James E., and Richard F. Popkin. *Essays on the Context, Nature, and Influence of Isaac Newton's Theology*. Dordrecht: Kluwer, 1990.

Foucault, Michel. *The Order of Things*. Trans. 1970. Reprint. New York: Vintage, 1973.

———. *The Birth of the Clinic*. Translated by A. M. Sheridan Smith. 1973. Reprint. New York: Vintage, 1975.

Frank, Robert G., Jr. "The Physician as Virtuoso in Seventeenth-Century England." In *English Scientific Virtuosi in the Sixteenth and Seventeenth Centuries*. Los Angeles: William Andrews Clark Library, 1979.

——. *Harvey and the Oxford Physiologists*. Berkeley and Los Angeles: University of California Press, 1980.

Fraser, Kevin J. "William Stukeley and the Gout." *Medical History* 36 (1992): 160–86.

Freidson, Eliot. *Profession of Medicine*. 1970. Reprint. Chicago: University of Chicago Press, 1988.

——. *Professional Powers*. Chicago: University of Chicago Press, 1986.

French, Roger. *Robert Whytt, the Soul, and Medicine*. London: Wellcome Institute for the History of Medicine, 1969.

——. "Sickness and the Soul: Stahl, Hoffmann, and Sauvages on Pathology." In *The Medical Enlightenment of the Eighteenth Century*, edited by Andrew Cunningham and Roger French, 88–110. Cambridge: Cambridge University Press, 1990.

Funkenstein, Amos. *Theology and the Scientific Imagination*. Princeton, N.J.: Princeton University Press, 1986.

Gadd, David. *Georgian Summer: The Rise and Development of Bath*. 2d ed. Newbury, Berkshire: Countryside Books, 1987.

Garrison, Fielding. "Medicine in the *Tatler, Spectator*, and *Guardian*." *Bulletin of the Institute of the History of Medicine, Johns Hopkins University* 2 (1934): 477–503.

Gasking, Elizabeth. *Investigations into Generation, 1650–1800*. Baltimore: Johns Hopkins University Press, 1967.

Geertz, Clifford. *The Interpretation of Cultures*. New York: Basic Books, 1973.

George, M. Dorothy. *London Life in the Eighteenth Century*. 1925. Reprint. New York: Capricorn Books, 1965.

Geyer-Kordesch, Johanna. "Georg Ernst Stahl's Radical Pietist Medicine and Its Influence on the German Enlightenment." In *The Medical Enlightenment of the Eighteenth Century*, edited by Andrew Cunningham and Roger French, 67–87. Cambridge: Cambridge University Press, 1990.

Golinski, Jan. *Science as Public Culture*. Cambridge: Cambridge University Press, 1992.

Gondal, Marie-Louise. *Madame Guyon, 1648–1717: Un Nouveau visage*. Paris: Beauchesne, 1989.

Granshaw, Lindsay, and Roy Porter, eds. *The Hospital in History*. London: Routledge, 1989.

Grant, Alexander. *The Story of the University of Edinburgh.* 2 vols. London: Longmans, Green, 1884.

Green, V. H. H. *The Young Mr Wesley: A Study of John Wesley and Oxford.* New York: St Martin's Press, 1961.

Greenblatt, Stephen. *Renaissance Self-Fashioning from More to Shakespeare.* Chicago: University of Chicago Press, 1980.

[Greenhill, W. A.]. *Life of George Cheyne, M.D.* Oxford: J. H. Parker; London: John Churchill, 1846.

Greenwood, David. *William King: Tory and Jacobite.* Oxford: Clarendon Press, 1969.

Gregg, Edward. *Queen Anne.* 1980. Reprint. London: Ark, 1984.

Guerrini, Anita. "Newtonian Matter Theory, Chemistry, and Medicine, 1690–1713." Ph.D. diss. Indiana University, 1983.

———. "James Keill, George Cheyne, and Newtonian Physiology, 1690–1740." *Journal of the History of Biology* 18 (1985): 247–66.

———. "The Tory Newtonians: Gregory, Pitcairne and Their Circle." *Journal of British Studies* 25 (1986): 288–311.

———. "Archibald Pitcairne and Newtonian Medicine." *Medical History* 31 (1987): 70–83.

———. "The Ethics of Animal Experimentation in Seventeenth-Century England." *Journal of the History of Ideas* 50 (1989): 391–407.

———. "Isaac Newton, George Cheyne, and the 'Principia Medicinae.'" In *The Medical Revolution of the Seventeenth Century.* edited by Andrew Wear and Roger French, 222–45. Cambridge: Cambridge University Press, 1989.

———. "'A Club of Little Villains': Rhetoric, Professional Identity, and Medical Pamphlet Wars." In *Literature and Medicine during the Eighteenth Century,* edited by Roy Porter and Marie Roberts, 226–44. London: Routledge, 1993.

———. "Ether Madness: Newtonianism, Religion, and Insanity." In *Action and Reaction,* edited by Adele Seeff and Paul Theerman, 232–54. Newark: University of Delaware Press, 1993.

———. "Chemistry Teaching at Oxford and Cambridge, circa 1700." In *Alchemy and Chemistry in the XVI and XVII Centuries,* edited by Antonio Clericuzio and P. M. Rattansi, 183–99. Dordrecht: Kluwer, 1994.

———. "Case History as Spiritual Autobiography: George Cheyne's 'Case of Author.'" *Eighteenth-Century Life* 19 (May 1995): 18–27.

———. "Newtonian Medicine and Religion." In *Religio medici,* edited by Andrew Cunningham and O. P. Grell, 293–312. Aldershot: Scolar, 1996.

————. "The Varieties of Mechanical Medicine: Borelli, Malpighi, Bellini, Pitcairne." In *Marcello Malpighi, Anatomist and Physician*, edited by D. Bertoloni Meli, *Nuncius* 27, 111–28. Florence: Leo Olschki, 1997.

————. "A Diet for the Sensitive Soul: Vegetarianism in the Eighteenth Century." *Eighteenth-Century Life*, forthcoming.

————. "The Hungry Soul: George Cheyne and the Construction of Femininity in the Eighteenth Century." *Eighteenth-Century Studies* 32 (1999): 279–99.

Guerrini, Anita, and Jole R. Shackelford. "John Keill's *De operationum chymicarum ratione mechanica*." *Ambix* 36 (1989): 138–52.

Hall, A. R. *Philosophers at War*. Cambridge: Cambridge University Press, 1980.

Hall, M. B. *Promoting Experimental Learning*. Cambridge: Cambridge University Press, 1991.

Hamlin, Christopher. "Chemistry, Medicine, and the Legitimization of English Spas, 1740–1840." In *The Medical History of Waters and Spas*, edited by Roy Porter, *Medical History* supplement 10 (1990): 67–81.

Harlan, David. "Intellectual History and the Return of Literature." *American Historical Review* 94 (1989): 581–609.

Heilbron, John. *Physics at the Royal Society during Newton's Presidency*. Los Angeles: William Andrews Clark Library, 1983.

Heimann, P. M., and J. E. McGuire. "Newtonian Forces and Lockean Powers: Concepts of Matter in Eighteenth-Century Thought." *Historical Studies in the Physical Sciences* 3 (1971): 233–306.

Hembry, Phyllis. *The English Spa, 1560–1815: A Social History*. London: Athlone Press, 1990.

Henderson, G. D. *Mystics of the North-east*. Aberdeen: New Spalding Club, 1934.

————. *Chevalier Ramsay*. London: Nelson, 1952.

————. *The Burning Bush: Studies in Scottish Church History*. Edinburgh: Saint Andrew Press, 1957.

Hesse, M. B. *Forces and Fields*. 1961. Reprint. Totowa, N.J.: Littlefield, Adams, 1965.

Hill, A. W. *John Wesley among the Physicans*. London: Epworth Press, 1958.

Hill, Christopher. "John Mason and the End of the World." In *Puritanism and Revolution*, 323–36. New York: Schocken Books, 1958.

————. "William Harvey and the Idea of Monarchy." *Past and Present* 27 (1964): 55–72.

————. "Sir Isaac Newton and His Society." In *Change and Continuity in Seventeenth-Century England*, 251–77. Cambridge, Mass.: Harvard University Press, 1975.

Holmes, Geoffrey. *British Politics in the Age of Anne*. London: Macmillan, 1967.

————. "The Sacheverell Riots." *Past and Present* 72 (August 1972): 55–85.

———. *The Trial of Doctor Sacheverell.* London: Eyre Methuen, 1973.

———. "Science, Reason, and Religion in the Age of Newton." *British Journal for the History of Science* 11 (1978): 164–71.

———. *Augustan England: Professions, State, and Society. 1680–1730.* London: Allen and Unwin, 1982.

———. "Religion and Party in Late Stuart England." In *Politics, Religion, and Society in England, 1672–1742,* 181–215. London: Hambledon Press, 1986.

Holmes, Geoffrey, and W. A. Speck, eds. *The Divided Society.* New York: St. Martin's Press, 1968.

Howie, W. D. "Sir Archibald Stevenson, His Ancestry, and the Riot in the College of Physicians in Edinburgh." *Medical History* 11 (1967): 269–84.

Hunt, Lynn, ed. *The New Cultural History.* Berkeley and Los Angeles: University of California Press, 1989.

Hunter, J. Paul. *Before Novels: The Cultural Contexts of Eighteenth-Century English Fiction.* New York: Norton, 1990.

Hunter, Michael. *Science and Society in Restoration England.* Cambridge: Cambridge University Press, 1981.

———. "Reconstructing Restoration Science: Problems and Pitfalls in Institutional History." *Social Studies of Science* 12 (1982): 451–66.

———. *The Royal Society and Its Fellows, 1660–1700.* Chalfont St Giles: British Society for the History of Science, 1982.

———. *Establishing the New Science.* Woodbridge: Boydell, 1989.

Hunter, Michael, and Paul B. Wood. "Towards Solomon's House." *History of Science* 24 (1986): 49–108.

Hutin, Serge. *Les Disciples anglais de Jacob Boehme au xvii et xviii siècles.* Paris: Denoel, 1960.

Irwin, Joyce. "Anna Maria von Schurman and Antoinette Bourignon: Contrasting Examples of Seventeenth-Century Pietism." *Church History* 60 (1991): 301–15.

Jackson, Stanley W. "Melancholia in the Eighteenth Century." *Journal of the History of Medicine* 38 (1983): 298–319.

———. *Melancholia and Depression from Hippocratic Times to Modern Times.* New Haven, Conn.: Yale University Press, 1986.

Jacob, Margaret C. *The Newtonians and the English Revolution, 1689–1720.* Ithaca, N.Y.: Cornell University Press, 1976.

———. *The Radical Enlightenment: Pantheists, Freemasons, and Republicans.* London: Allen and Unwin, 1981.

———. *The Cultural Meaning of the Scientific Revolution.* New York: Knopf, 1988.

Jewson, N. D. "Medical Knowledge and the Patronage System in Eighteenth-Century England." *Sociology* 8 (1974): 369–85.

Keble, John. *The Life of the Right Reverend Father in God, Thomas Wilson, D.D.* 2 vols. Oxford: Parker, 1863.

Keevil, J. J. *Medicine and the Navy, 1200–1900.* Vol. 2, *1649–1714.* Edinburgh: E. & S. Livingstone, 1958.

King, Lester S. *The Medical World of the Eighteenth Century.* Chicago: University of Chicago Press, 1958.

———. "George Cheyne, Mirror of Eighteenth-Century Medicine." *Bulletin of the History of Medicine* 48 (1974): 517–39.

———. *The Philosophy of Medicine: The Eighteenth Century.* Cambridge, Mass.: Harvard University Press, 1978.

Klein, Lawrence. "Liberty, Manners, and Politeness in Early Eighteenth-Century England." *Historical Journal* 32 (1989): 583–605.

———. "Politeness for Plebes: Some Social Identities in Early Eighteenth-Century England." Paper presented at a Clark Library seminar, January 1991.

Kleinman, Arthur. *Patients and Healers in the Context of Culture.* Berkeley and Los Angeles: University of California Press, 1980.

———. *The Social Origins of Distress and Disease.* New Haven, Conn.: Yale University Press, 1986.

———. *The Illness Narratives.* New York: Basic Books, 1988.

Kramer, John C. "Opium Rampant: Medical Use, Misuse, and Abuse in Britain and the West in the Seventeenth and Eighteenth Centuries." *British Journal of Addiction* 74 (1979): 377–89.

Kramnick, Jonathan Brody. "Dr. George Cheyne and the Eighteenth-Century Body: A Study in Representation." Senior honors thesis. Cornell University, 1989.

Kristeva, Julia. *Tales of Love.* Translated by Leon S. Roudiez. New York: Columbia University Press, 1987.

Kubrin, David. "Newton and the Cyclical Cosmos." *Journal of the History of Ideas* 28 (1967): 325–46.

Kuhn, Thomas. "Mathematical versus Experimental Traditions in the Development of Physical Science." In *The Essential Tension,* 31–65. Chicago: University of Chicago Press, 1977.

LaCapra, Dominick. "Rethinking Intellectual History and Reading Texts." In *Modern European Intellectual History,* edited by Dominick LaCapra and Steven L. Kaplan, 47–85. Ithaca, N.Y.: Cornell University Press, 1982.

Laqueur, Thomas. "Bodies, Details, and the Humanitarian Narrative." In *The New Cultural History*, edited by Lynn Hunt, 176–204. Berkeley and Los Angeles: University of California Press, 1989.

———. *Making Sex*. Cambridge, Mass.: Harvard Univeristy Press, 1990.

Lane, Joan. "'The Doctor Scolds Me': The Diaries and Correspondence of Patients in Eighteenth-Century England." In *Patients and Practitioners*, edited by Roy Porter, 205–48. Cambridge: Cambridge University Press, 1985.

Lawrence, Christopher. "The Nervous System and Society in the Scottish Enlightenment." In *Natural Order: Historical Studies of Scientific Culture*, edited by Barry Barnes and Steven Shapin, 19–40. Beverly Hills, Calif.: Sage, 1979.

———. "William Buchan: Medicine Laid Open." *Medical History* 19 (1975): 20–35.

Lawrence, P. D., and A. G. Molland. "David Gregory's Inaugural Lecture at Oxford." *Notes and Records of the Royal Society* 25 (1970): 143–44.

Lenman, Bruce. "The Scottish Episcopal Clergy and the Ideology of Jacobitism." In *Ideology and Conspiracy: Aspects of Jacobitism, 1689–1759*, edited by E. Cruikshanks. Manchester: Manchester University Press, 1979.

———. "Physicians and Politics in the Jacobite Era." In *The Jacobite Challenge*, edited by Eveline Cruickshanks and Jeremy Black, 74–91. Edinburgh: John Donald, 1988.

Lewis, Judith Schneid. *In the Family Way: Childbearing in the British Aristocracy, 1760–1860*. New Brunswick, N.J.: Rutgers University Press, 1986.

Lindeboom, G. A. "Pitcairn's Leyden Interlude Described from the Documents." *Annals of Science* 19 (1963): 273–84.

Lonie, I. M. "Hippocrates the Iatromechanist." *Medical History* 25 (1981): 113–50.

McClellan, James, III. *Science Reorganized*. New York: Columbia University Press, 1985.

McCrae, Thomas. "George Cheyne, An Old London and Bath Physician, 1671–1743." *Johns Hopkins Hospital Bulletin* 15, no. 156 (March 1904): 84–94.

MacDonald, Michael. *Mystical Bedlam*. Cambridge: Cambridge University Press, 1981.

———. "*The Fearefull Estate of Francis Spira*: Narrative, Identity, and Emotion in Early Modern England." *Journal of British Studies* 31 (1992): 32–61.

Macewen, Alec R. *Antoinette Bourignon, Quietest*. London: Hodder and Stoughton, 1910.

McGee, J. S. "Conversion and the Imitation of Christ in Anglican and Puritan Writing." *Journal of British Studies* 15 (1976): 21–39.

McGuire, J. E. "Transmutation and Immutability: Newton's Doctrine of Physical Qualities." *Ambix* 14 (1967): 69–95.

———. "Force, Active Principles, and Newton's Invisible Realm." *Ambix* 15 (1968): 154–208.

————. "Atoms and the 'Analogy of Nature': Newton's Third Rule of Philosophizing."
    Studies in the History and Philosophy of Science 1 (1970): 3–58.

————. "Neoplatonism and Active Principles: Newton and the *Corpus Hermeticum*." In
    Hermeticism and the Scientific Revolution, R. S. Westman and J. E. McGuire, 95–142.
    Los Angeles: William Andrews Clark Library, 1977.

McGuire, J. E., and P. M. Rattansi. "Newton and the 'Pipes of Pan.'" *Notes and Records of
    the Royal Society* 21 (1966): 108–43.

MacInnes, Angus. "The Emergence of a Leisure Town: Shrewsbury, 1660–1760." *Past and
    Present* 120 (August 1988): 53–87.

McIntyre, Sylvia. "Bath: The Rise of a Resort Town, 1660–1800." In *Country Towns in Pre-
    Industrial England*, edited by Peter Clark, 197–249. Leicester: Leicester University
    Press, 1981.

Mack, Phyllis. *Visionary Women: Ecstatic Prophecy in Seventeenth-Century England*. Berkeley and
    Los Angeles: University of California Press, 1992.

McKendrick, Neil. "The Consumer Revolution in Eighteenth-Century England." In *The
    Birth of a Consumer Society: The Commercializaiton of Eighteenth-Century England*, edited
    by Neil McKendrick, John Brewer, and J.H. Plumb, 9–33. Bloomington: Indiana
    University Press, 1982.

[Macmichael, William]. *The Gold-Headed Cane.* 1827. Reprint. Springfield, Ill.: Charles C.
    Thomas, 1953.

Mallet-Joris, Françoise. *Jeanne Guyon.* Paris: Flammarion, 1978.

Manuel, Frank. *Isaac Newton, Historian.* Cambridge, Mass.: Harvard University Press,
    1963.

————. *The Religion of Isaac Newton.* Oxford: Clarendon Press, 1974.

Markley, Robert. "Representing Order: Mathematics, Natural Philosophy, and Theology
    in the Newtonian Revolution." In *Chaos and Order*, edited by N. Katherine
    Hayles, 125–48. Chicago: University of Chicago Press, 1991.

————. *Fallen Languages.* Ithaca, N.Y.: Cornell University Press, 1994.

Martin, R. J. J. "Explaining John Freind's *History of Physick*." *Studies in the History and
    Philosophy of Science* 19 (1988): 399–418.

Medhurst, Charles Edward. *Life and Work of Lady Elizabeth Hastings.* Leeds: Richard Jackson,
    1914.

Melville, Lewis. *Bath under Beau Nash.* London: Eveleigh Nash, 1907.

Metzger, Hélène. *Attraction universelle et religion naturelle chez quelques commentateurs anglais de
    Newton.* Paris: Hermann, 1938.

Micale, Mark. "Hysteria and Its Historiography: A Review of Past and Present Writings."
    History of Science 27 (1989): 223–62, 319–51.

Miller, D. P. "'Into the Valley of Darkness': Reflections on the Royal Society in the
    Eighteenth Century." *History of Science* 27 (1989): 154–66.

Moore, James, and Michael Silverthorne. "Gershom Carmichael and the Natural Juris-
    prudence Tradition in Eighteenth-Century Scotland." In *Wealth and Virtue*, edited
    by Istvan Hont and Michael Ignatieff, 73–87. Cambridge: Cambridge Univer-
    sity Press, 1983.

Moscucci, Ornella. *The Science of Woman.* Cambridge: Cambridge University Press, 1990.

Mousnier, Roland. *Social Hierarchies, 1450 to the Present.* Translated by Peter Evans, edited by
    Margaret Clarke. New York: Schocken Books, 1973.

Mullan, D. G. *Episcopacy in Scotland: The History of an Idea, 1560–1638.* Edinburgh: John
    Donald, 1986.

Mullan, John. "Hypochondria and Hysteria: Sensibility and the Physicians." *The Eighteenth
    Century: Theory and Interpretation* 25 (1984): 141–74.

———. *Sentiment and Sociability.* Oxford: Clarendon Press, 1988.

Mullet, Charles F. *Public Baths and Health in England, 16th–17th Century. Bulletin of the History of
    Medicine,* supplement 5, Baltimore: Johns Hopkins University Press, 1946.

Mulligan, Lotte, and Glenn Mulligan. "Reconstructing Restoration Science: Styles of
    Leadership and Social Composition of the Early Royal Society." *Social Studies of
    Science* 11 (1981): 327–64.

Neale, R. S. *Bath, 1680–1750: A Social History.* London: Routledge and Kegan Paul, 1981.

———. "Bath: Ideology and Utopia, 1700–1760." In *The Eighteenth-Century Town,* edited by
    Peter Borsay, 223–42. London: Longman, 1990.

Nicholson, M., and G. S. Rousseau. *"This Long Disease, My Life": Alexander Pope and the Sciences.*
    Princeton, N.J.: Princeton University Press, 1966.

Nicolson, Malcolm. "The Metastatic Theory of Pathogenesis and the Professional Interests
    of the Eighteenth-Century Physician." *Medical History* 32 (1988): 277–300.

Nussbaum, Felicity. *The Autobiographical Subject.* Baltimore: Johns Hopkins University Press,
    1989.

Orcibal, Jean. "The Theological Originality of John Wesley and Continental Spirituality."
    In *A History of the Methodist Church in Great Britain,* vol. 1, edited by Rupert Davies
    and Gordon Rupp, 83–111. London: Epworth Press, 1965.

Ouston, Hugh. "York in Edinburgh: James VII and the Patronage of Learning in Scotland,
    1679–1688." In *New Perspectives on the Politics and Culture of Early Modern Scotland,*

edited by John Dwyer, Roger A. Mason, and Alexander Murdoch. Edinburgh: John Donald, 1982.

Paster, Gail Kern. *The Body Embarrassed: Drama and the Disciplines of Shame in Early Modern England.* Ithaca, N.Y.: Cornell University Press, 1993.

Perry, Ruth. *The Celebrated Mary Astell.* Chicago: University of Chicago Press, 1986.

Plumb. J. H. *Sir Robert Walpole: The Making of a Statesman.* Boston: Houghton Mifflin, 1956.

Politi, Jina. *The Novel and Its Presuppositions.* Amsterdam: Hakkert, 1976.

Porter, Dorothy, and Roy Porter. *Patient's Progress.* Stanford, Calif.: Stanford University Press, 1989.

Porter, Roy. "The Drinking Man's Disease: The Prehistory of Alcoholism in Georgian Britain." *British Journal of Addiction* 80 (1985): 384–96.

———. "Lay Medical Knowledge in the Eighteenth Century: The Evidence of the *Gentleman's Magazine.*" *Medical History* 29 (1985): 138–68.

———. "Laymen, Doctors, and Medical Knowledge in the Eighteenth Century: The Evidence of the *Gentleman's Magazine.*" In *Patients and Practitioners,* edited by Roy Porter, 283–314. Cambridge: Cambridge University Press, 1985.

———. "Medicine and Religion in Eighteenth-Century England: A Case of Conflict?" *Ideas and Production* 7 (1987): 4–17.

———. *Mind-forg'd Manacles: A History of Madness in England from the Restoration to the Regency.* Cambridge, Mass.: Harvard University Press, 1987.

———. "The Gift Relation." In *The Hospital in History,* edited by Lindsay Granshaw and Roy Porter, 149–78. London: Routledge, 1989.

———. *Health for Sale.* Manchester: Manchester University Press, 1989.

———. *English Society in the Eighteenth Century.* 2d ed. Harmondsworth: Penguin, 1990.

———, ed. *Patients and Practitioners.* Cambridge: Cambridge University Press, 1985.

Porter, Roy, and Dorothy Porter. *In Sickness and in Health.* New York: Blackwell, 1989.

Redwood, John. *Reason, Ridicule, and Religion.* Cambridge, Mass.: Harvard University Press, 1976.

Reinach, Salomen. *Cultes, mythes et religions.* vol. 1. Paris: Ernest Leroux, 1922.

Riddell, W. R. "George Cheyne and the 'English Malady.'" *Annals of Medical History* 4 (1922): 304–10.

Riley, James. *The Eighteenth-Century Campaign to Avoid Disease.* New York: St. Martin's Press, 1987.

Riley, P. W. J. *The Union of England and Scotland.* Manchester: Manchester University Press, 1978.

———. *King William and the Scottish Politicians.* Edinburgh: John Donald, 1979.

Risse, Guenter B. *Hospital Life in Enlightenment Scotland.* Cambridge: Cambridge University Press, 1986.

Ritchie, R. Peel. *The Early Days of the Royall Colledge of Physitians, Edinburgh.* Edinburgh: G. P. Johnston, 1899.

Ritterbush, Philip. *Overtures to Biology.* New Haven, Conn.: Yale University Press, 1964.

Roe, Shirley. *Matter, Life, and Generation: Eighteenth-Century Embryology and the Haller-Wolff Debate.* Cambridge: Cambridge University Press, 1981.

Rogers, Pat. "'This Calamitous Year': *A Journal of the Plague Year* and the South Sea Bubble." In *Eighteenth-Century Encounters*, 151–67. Brighton: Harvester Press; Totowa, N.J.: Barnes and Noble, 1985.

Rolls, Roger. *The Hospital of the Nation.* Bath: Bird, 1988.

Rosen, George. "Enthusiasm: The 'Dark Lanthorn of the Spirit.'" *Bulletin of the History of Medicine* 42 (1968): 393–421.

Rosenberg, Charles. "Medical Text and Social Context: Explaining William Buchan's *Domestic Medicine.*" 1983. Reprint in Charles Rosenberg, *Explaining Epidemics*, 32–56. Cambridge: Cambridge University Press, 1992.

Rosner, Lisa. *Medical Education in the Age of Improvement.* Edinburgh: Edinburgh University Press, 1991.

Rossi, Paolo. *The Dark Abyss of Time.* Translated by Lydia Cochrane. Chicago: University of Chicago Press, 1984.

Rousseau, G. S. "John Wesley's *Primitive Physic* (1747)." *Harvard Library Bulletin* 16 (1968): 242–56.

———. "Nerves, Spirits, and Fibres: Towards Defining the Origins of Sensibility." In *Studies in the Eighteenth Century*, vol. 3, edited by R. F. Brissenden and J. C. Earle, 137–57. Toronto: University of Toronto Press, 1976.

———. "Mysticism and Millenarianism: 'Immortal Dr Cheyne.'" In *Millenarianism and Messianism in English Literature and Thought, 1650–1800*, edited by Richard Popkin, 81–126. Leiden: Brill, 1988.

———. "'A Strange Pathology': Hysteria in the Early Modern World, 1500–1800." In *Hysteria beyond Freud*, edited by Sander L. Gilman et al., 91–221. Berkeley and Los Angeles: University of California Press, 1993.

Rudwick, Martin J. S. *The Meaning of Fossils.* 2d ed. 1976. Reprint. Chicago: University of Chicago Press, 1985.

Rupp, Gordon. *Religion in England, 1688–1791.* Oxford History of the Christian Church. Oxford: Clarendon Press, 1986.

Schaffer, Simon. "Halley's Atheism and the End of the World." *Notes and Records of the Royal Society* 32 (1977): 17–40.

———. "Natural Philosophy." In *The Ferment of Knowledge,* edited by Roy Porter and G. S. Rousseau, 55–91.Cambridge: Cambridge University Press, 1980.

———. "Newtonian Cosmology and the Steady State." Ph.D. diss. Cambridge University, 1980.

———. "The Glorious Revolution and Medicine in Britain and the Netherlands." *Notes and Records of the Royal Society* 43 (1989): 167–90.

———. "The Consuming Flame: Electric Showmen and Tory Mystics in the World of Goods." In *Consumption and the World of Goods,* edited by Roy Porter and John Brewer. London: Routledge, 1993.

Schiebinger, Londa. *The Mind Has No Sex?* Cambridge, Mass.: Harvard University Press, 1989.

Schofield, Robert E. "John Wesley and Science in Eighteenth-Century England." *Isis* 44 (1953): 331–40.

———. *Mechanism and Materialism: British Natural Philosophy in an Age of Reason.* Princeton, N.J.: Princeton University Press, 1970.

———. "An Evolutionary Taxonomy of Eighteenth-Century Newtonianisms." *Studies in Eighteenth-Century Culture* 7 (1978): 175–92.

Schwartz, Hillel. *The French Prophets.* Berkeley and Los Angeles: University of California Press, 1980.

Scull, Andrew. *The Most Solitary of Afflictions: Madness and Society, 1700–1900.* New Haven, Conn.: Yale University Press, 1993.

Sedgwick, Adam. *Jansenism in Seventeenth-Century France.* Charlottesville: University of Virginia Press, 1977.

Sekora, John. *Luxury: The Concept in Western Thought, Eden to Smollett.* Baltimore: Johns Hopkins University Press, 1977.

[Seymour, Aaron Crossley]. *The Life and Times of Selina, Countess of Huntingdon.* 2 vols. London, 1839–40.

Shapin, Steven. "Of Gods and Kings: Natural Philosophy and Politics in the Leibniz-Clarke Disputes." *Isis* 72 (1981): 187–215.

———. "The House of Experiment in Seventeenth-Century England." *Isis* 79 (1988): 373–404.

———. "'A Scholar and a Gentleman': The Problematic Identity of the Scientific Practitioner in Early Modern England." *History of Science* 29 (1991): 279–327.

Shapin, Steven, and Simon Schaffer. *Leviathan and the Air-Pump*. Princeton, N.J.: Princeton University Press, 1985.

Shapiro, Barbara. "History and Natural History in Sixteenth- and Seventeenth-Century England: An Essay on the Relationship between Humanism and Science." In B. J. Shapiro and R. G. Frank, Jr. *English Scientific Virtuosi in the Sixteenth and Seventeenth Centuries*, 1–55. Los Angeles: William Andrews Clark Library, 1979.

———. *Probability and Certainty in Seventeenth-Century England*. Princeton, N.J.: Princeton University Press, 1983.

Shepherd, Christine King. "Philosophy and Science in the Arts Curriculum of the Scottish Universities in the Seventeenth Century." Ph.D. diss. University of Edinburgh, 1975.

———. "The Arts Curriculum at Aberdeen at the Beginning of the Eighteenth Century." In *Aberdeen and the Enlightenment*, edited by Jennifer Carter and Joan Pittock, 146–54. Aberdeen: University of Aberdeen Press, 1987.

Shirlaw, Leslie. "Dr. Archibald Pitcairn and Sir Isaac Newton's 'Black Years' (1692–1694)." *Chronicle of the Royal College of Physicians of Edinburgh* (January 1975): 23–26.

Shuttleton, David E. "'My Own Crazy Carcase': The Life and Works of Dr George Cheyne, 1672–1743." Ph.D. diss., University of Edinburgh, 1992.

———. "Methodism and Dr George Cheyne's 'More Enlightening Principles.'" In *Medicine and the Enlightenment*, edited by Roy Porter, 323–42. Wellcome Institute Series. Amsterdam: Rodopi, 1995.

Siddall, R. S. "George Cheyne, M.D." *Annals of Medical History* n.s. 4 (1942): 95–109.

Smith, Ginnie. "Prescribing the Rules of Health: Self-help and Advice in the Late Eighteenth Century." In *Patients and Practitioners*, edited by Roy Porter, 249–62. Cambridge: Cambridge University Press, 1985.

Smout, T. C. *A History of the Scottish People, 1560–1830*. 1969. Reprint. London: Fontana, 1972.

Snow, W. G. Sinclair. *The Times, Life, and Thought of Patrick Forbes, Bishop of Aberdeen, 1618–1635*. London: SPCK, 1952.

Speck, W. A. *Stability and Strife: England, 1714–1760*. Cambridge, Mass.: Harvard University Press, 1977.

Spiegel, Gabrielle. "History and Post-Modernism, IV." *Past and Present* 135 (May 1992): 194–208.

Steensma, Robert. *Dr. John Arbuthnot*. New York: Twayne, 1979.

Stephenson, Raymond. "Richardson's 'Nerves': The Physiology of Sensibility in Clarissa." *Journal of the History of Ideas* 49 (1988): 267–85.

Stevenson, Lloyd G. "'New Diseases' in the Seventeenth Century." *Bulletin of the History of Medicine* 39 (1965): 1–21.

Stewart, A. G. *The Academic Gregories*. Edinburgh: Oliphant, Anderson, and Ferrier, 1901.

Stewart, Dugald. *The Life and Letters of Robert Leighton*. London: Hodder and Stoughton, 1903.

Stewart, Larry. "Samuel Clarke, Newtonianism, and the Factions of Post-Revolutionary England." *Journal of the History of Ideas* 42 (1981): 53–72.

———. "Public Lectures and Private Patronage in Newtonian England." *Isis* 77 (1986): 47–58.

———. "The Selling of Newton: Science and Technology in Early Eighteenth-Century England." *Journal of British Studies* 25 (1986): 178–92.

———. *The Rise of Public Science*. Cambridge: Cambridge University Press, 1992.

Stigler, Stephen M. "Apollo Mathematicus: A Story of Resistance to Quantification in the Seventeenth Century." *Proceedings of the American Philosophical Society* 136 (1992): 93–126.

Stone, Lawrence. "Social Mobility." *Past and Present* 33 (April 1966): 16–55.

———. "The Revival of Narrative." *Past and Present* 85 (November 1979): 1–24.

———. *The Family, Sex, and Marriage in England, 1500–1800*. New York: Harper and Row, 1977.

———. "The Residential Development of the West End of London in the Seventeenth Century." In *After the Reformation*, edited by B. C. Malament, 177–212. Manchester: Manchester University Press, 1980.

Stott, Rosalie. "The Incorporation of Surgeons and Medical Education and Practice in Edinburgh, 1696–1755." Ph.D. diss. University of Edinburgh, 1984.

Straka, Gerald. "The Final Phase of Divine Right Theory in England, 1688–1702." *English Historical Review* 77 (1962): 638–58.

Sykes, Norman. *Church and State in England in the XVIIIth Century*. Cambridge: Cambridge University Press, 1934.

Talbott, J. H. *Gout*. 3d ed. New York: Grune and Stratton, 1967.

Tayler, Alistair, and Henrietta Tayler. *Jacobites of Aberdeenshire and Banffshire in the Rising of 1715*. Edinburgh: Oliver and Boyd, 1934.

Thackray, Arnold. "'Matter in a Nutshell': Newton's Opticks and Eighteenth-Century Chemistry." *Ambix* 15 (1968): 29–53.

————. "'The Business of Experimental Philosophy': The Early Newtonian Group at the Royal Society." *Actes XIIe Cong. Int. Hist. Sci.* (1970): 155–59.

Thomas, K. Bryn. *James Douglas of the Pouch and His Pupil William Hunter.* London: Pitman, 1964.

Thomas, Keith. *Religion and the Decline of Magic.* 1971. Reprint. Harmondsworth: Penguin, 1973.

Todd, Janet. *Sensibility: An Introduction.* London: Methuen, 1986.

Tomaselli, Sylvana. "Reflections on the History of the Science of Woman." *History of Science* 29 (1991): 185–205.

Trail, R. R. "Sydenham's Impact on English Medicine." *Medical History* 9 (1965): 356–64.

Troost, Linda Veronika. "Geography and Gender: Mary Chandler and Alexander Pope." In *Pope, Swift, and Women Writers,* edited by Donald Mell, 67–85. Newark: University of Delaware Press, 1996.

Tuana, Nancy. *The Less Noble Sex: Scientific, Religious, and Philosophical Conceptions of Woman's Nature.* Bloomington: Indiana University Press, 1993.

Turner, Bryan. "The Government of the Body: Medical Regimens and the Rationalizations of Diet." *British Journal of Sociology* 33 (1982): 254–69.

————. *The Body in Society.* Oxford: Blackwell, 1984.

Tuveson, E. L. *Millennium and Utopia.* Berkeley and Los Angeles: University of California Press, 1949.

Underhill, Timothy. "William Law's Suspension at Cambridge." *Notes and Queries* n.s. 39, no. 237 (March 1992): 42–44.

Valadez, F. M., and C. D. O'Malley. "James Keill of Northampton." *Medical History* 15 (1971): 317–35.

Van der Does, Marthe. *Antoinette Bourignon.* Amsterdam: Holland University Press, 1974.

Varey, Simon. *Space and the Eighteenth-Century English Novel.* Cambridge: Cambridge University Press, 1990.

Veith, Ilza. *Hysteria: The History of a Disease.* Chicago: University of Chicago Press, 1965.

Vermij, Rienk. *Secularisering en naturwetenschap in de zeventiende en achttiende eeuw: Bernard Nieuwentijt.* Amsterdam: Rodopi, 1991.

Viets, Henry R. "George Cheyne, 1673–1743." *Bulletin of the History of Medicine* 23 (1949): 435–52.

Walker, D. P. *The Ancient Theology.* Ithaca, N.Y.: Cornell University Press, 1972.

Walsh, John. "Origins of the Evangelical Revival." In *Essays in Modern Church History in Memory of Norman Sykes,* edited by G. V. Bennett and J. D. Walsh, 132–62. New York: Oxford University Press, 1966.

Walton, Christopher. *Notes and Materials for an Adequate Biography of the Celebrated Divine and Theosopher William Law*. London: Printed for Private Circulation, 1854.

Watt, Ian. *The Rise of the Novel*. Berkeley and Los Angeles: University of California Press, 1957.

Wear, Andrew. "Puritan Perceptions of Illness in Seventeenth-Century England." In *Patients and Practitioners*, edited by Roy Porter, 55–99. Cambridge: Cambridge University Press, 1985.

————. "Medical Practice in Late Seventeenth- and Early Eighteenth-Century England: Continuity and Union." In *The Medical Revolution of the Seventeenth Century*, edited by Roger French and Andrew Wear. Cambridge: Cambridge University Press, 1989.

Weatherill, Lorna. *Consumer Behaviour and Material Culture in Britain, 1660–1760*. London: Routledge, 1988.

Webb, Martha Ellen. "A Reexamination of the Inception, Development, and 'Newtonianism' of David Hartley's *Observations on Man* (1749)." Ph.D. diss. University of Oklahoma, 1981.

Webster, Charles. *An Account of the Life and Writings of the Celebrated Dr Archibald Pitcairn*. Edinburgh: Gordon and Murray; London: Richardson and Urquhart, 1781.

Webster, Charles. *The Great Instauration*. London: Duckworth, 1975.

Weiss-Amer, Melitta. "Medieval Women's Guides to Food during Pregnancy: Origins, Texts, and Traditions." *Canadian Bulletin of Medical History* 10 (1993): 5–23.

Welch, Edwin. *Spiritual Pilgrim: A Reassessment of the Life of the Countess of Huntingdon*. Cardiff: University of Wales Press, 1995.

Westfall, R. S. *Science and Religion in Seventeenth-Century England*. New Haven, Conn.: Yale University Press, 1958.

————. *Never at Rest: A Biography of Isaac Newton*. Cambridge: Cambridge University Press, 1980.

————. "Isaac Newton's *Theologiae Gentilis Origines Philosophicae*." In *The Secular Mind*, edited by W. Warren Wagar, 15–34. New York: Holmes and Meier, 1982.

————. "Newton's Theological Manuscripts." In *Contemporary Newtonian Research*, edited by Z. Bechler, 129–43. Dordrecht: Reidel, 1982.

White, John S. "William Harvey and the Primacy of the Blood." *Annals of Science* 43 (1986): 239–55.

Wightman, W. P. D. "David Gregory's Commentary on Newton's *Principia*." *Nature* 179 (1957): 393–94.

Wilde, C. B. "Hutchinsonianism, Natural Philosophy. and Religious Controversy in Eighteenth-Century Britain." *History of Science* 18 (1980): 1–24.

————. "Matter and Spirit as Natural Symbols in Eighteenth-Century Britain." *British Journal for the History of Science* 15 (1982): 99–131.

Wilson, Adrian. "The Politics of Medical Improvement in Early Hanoverian London." In *The Medical Enlightenment of the Eighteenth Century*, edited by Andrew Cunningham and Roger French, 4–39. Cambridge: Cambridge University Press, 1990.

Wilson, Charles. *England's Apprenticeship, 1603–1763*. 2d ed. London: Longman, 1884.

Wood, Paul. "Science and the Pursuit of Virtue in the Aberdeen Enlightenment." In *Studies in the Philosophy of the Scottish Enlightenment*, edited by M. A. Stewart, 127–49. Oxford: Clarendon Press, 1990.

Wright, John P. "Metaphysics and Physiology: Mind, Body, and the Animal Economy in Eighteenth-Century Scotland." In *Studies in the Philosophy of the Scottish Enlightenment*, edited by M. A. Stewart, 251–301. Oxford: Clarendon Press, 1990.

Wrigley, E. A. "A Simple Model of London's Importance in Changing English Society and Economy. 1650–1750." *Past and Present* 37 (July 1967): 44–45.

Zuckerman, Arnold. "Dr. Richard Mead, 1673–1754: A Biographical Study." Ph.D. diss. University of Illinois, 1965.

INDEX

Aberdeen, Scotland, 9–10, 46, 145
Adair, James Mackittrick, 183
Aldrich, Henry, 52, 204n.29
Allen, Ralph, 156, 234n.83
Angela da Foligno, 17
Anne, Queen, 50–52, 61, 85, 92, 96, 103, 105, 109, 114
Anorexia, 108–109, 113
Anstey, Christopher, 97, 100
Applebee's Journal, 106
Arbuthnot, John, 35, 48, 50–52, 59, 69, 71, 73, 91, 135, 138, 149, 158, 170, 177
Arbuthnot, Robert, 51
Argyll, Duke of, 48
Aristotle, 76–77
Armstrong, John, 184, 237n.20
Astell, Mary, 115
Astruc, Jean, 7, 176

Bacon, Francis, 25, 31, 44, 49–50
Baillie, George, 91, 95, 100, 155, 167, 214n.17
Baillie, Grisell, 91, 95, 100
Barfoot, Michael, 89
Barker-Benfield, G. J., 99
Bateman, William, Lord Bateman, 144, 155, 168, 228n.124

Bath, England, 21, 80, 90–117, 121, 127, 129, 135, 138, 141, 144–45, 148–49, 154, 158–59, 173–74, 177; hospital, 114–17, 137
Bave, Charles, 100, 116
Baynard, Edward, 96, 121, 237n.20
Beier, Lucinda, 97, 99, 100
Bellini, Lorenzo, 36–37, 58, 64, 67, 73, 154
Bennet of Grubet, William, 60
Bentley, Richard, 43, 55, 72–74, 77, 79
Bernard of Clairvaux, 14
Bernoulli, Johann, 69–70
Bibliothèque ancienne et moderne, 90
Biographia Britannica, 180
Blackmore, Sir Richard, 144
Blount, Charles, 84
Boehme, Jacob, 3, 80, 142, 161, 171, 177
Boerhaave, Herman, 133
Bordo, Susan, 135, 185–86
Borelli, Giovanni Alfonso, 36–37, 41, 64, 73
Borsay, Peter, 93
Bossuet, Jacques Benigne, 82
Bourignon, Antoinette, 13, 15–18, 81–82, 85, 88, 105, 108, 121–22, 124, 126, 139, 169
Bower, Thomas, 24, 70
Bowles, Geoffrey, 77
Boyle, Robert, 3, 24, 39